UROLOGY
SECRETS

MARTIN I. RESNICK, M.D.
Lester Persky Professor of Urology
Chairman, Department of Urology
Case Western Reserve University
  School of Medicine
Department of Urology
University Hospitals of Cleveland
Cleveland, Ohio

ANDREW C. NOVICK, M.D.
Chairman, Department of Urology
The Cleveland Clinic Foundation
Cleveland, Ohio

HANLEY & BELFUS, INC./ Philadelphia
MOSBY/ St. Louis • Baltimore • Boston • Chicago
London • Philadelphia •Sydney • Toronto

113510381

Publisher: HANLEY & BELFUS, INC.
              210 S. 13th Street
              Philadelphia, PA 19107
              (215) 546-7293

North American and worldwide sales and distribution:

              MOSBY
              11830 Westline Industrial Drive
              St. Louis, MO 63146

In Canada: Times Mirror Professional Publishing, Ltd.
              130 Flaska Drive
              Markham, Ontario L6G 1B8
              Canada

UROLOGY SECRETS   ISBN 1-56053-108-8

Last digit is the print number: 9 8 7 6 5 4 3 2 1

CONTENTS

I. PATIENT EVALUATION

v

Contents

III. CONGENITAL AND ACQUIRED DISEASE

IV. INFLAMMATION AND INFECTION

CONTRIBUTORS

Kenneth W. Angermeier, M.D.
Staff Physician, Department of Urology, The Cleveland Clinic Foundation, Cleveland, Ohio

Rodney A. Appell, M.D., FACS
Head, Section of Female Urology and Urodynamics, Department of Urology, The Cleveland Clinic Foundation, Cleveland, Ohio

Donald R. Bodner, M.D.
Associate Professor of Urology, Department of Urology, Case Western Reserve University School of Medicine, Cleveland, Ohio

Kurt H. Dinchman, M.D.
MetroHealth Medical Center, Cleveland, Ohio

Jack S. Elder, M.D.
Professor of Urology and Pediatrics, Case Western Reserve University School of Medicine; Director of Pediatric Urology, Rainbow Babies & Children's Hospital, Cleveland, Ohio

Stuart M. Flechner, M.D.
Section of Renal Transplantation, Department of Urology, The Cleveland Clinic Foundation, Cleveland, Ohio

David A. Goldfarb, M.D.
Department of Urology, The Cleveland Clinic Foundation, Cleveland, Ohio

Nehemia Hampel, M.D.
Associate Professor, Department of Urology, Case Western Reserve University School of Medicine, Cleveland, Ohio

Ernest E. Hodge, M.D.
Head, Section of Renal Transplantation, Department of Urology, The Cleveland Clinic Foundation, Cleveland, Ohio

Robert Kay, M.D.
Head, Section of Pediatric Urology, Department of Urology, The Cleveland Clinic Foundation, Cleveland, Ohio

Eric A. Klein, M.D.
Head, Section of Urologic Oncology, Department of Urology, The Cleveland Clinic Foundation, Cleveland, Ohio

Elroy D. Kursh, M.D.
Professor of Urology, Department of Urology, Case Western Reserve University School of Medicine, Cleveland, Ohio

Milton M. Lakin, M.D.
Head, Section of Male Sexual Medicine, Department of Urology, The Cleveland Clinic Foundation, Cleveland, Ohio

David A. Levy, M.D.
Chief Resident, Department of Urology, Case Western Reserve University School of Medicine, Cleveland, Ohio

Drogo K. Montague, M.D.
Director, Center for Sexual Function, Department of Urology, The Cleveland Clinic Foundation, Cleveland, Ohio

Andrew C. Novick, M.D.
Chairman, Department of Urology, The Cleveland Clinic Foundation, Cleveland, Ohio

Martin I. Resnick, M.D.
Lester Persky Professor of Urology, and Chairman, Department of Urology, Case Western Reserve University School of Medicine, Cleveland, Ohio

Jonathan H. Ross, M.D.
Section of Pediatric Urology, Department of Urology, The Cleveland Clinic Foundation, Cleveland, Ohio

David S. Sandock, M.D.
Resident in Urology, Department of Urology, Case Western Reserve University School of Medicine, Cleveland, Ohio

Bashir R. Sankari, M.D.
Staff Physician, Department of Urology, The Cleveland Clinic Foundation, Cleveland, Ohio

Allen D. Seftel, M.D.
Assistant Professor of Urology, Department of Urology, Case Western Reserve University School of Medicine, Cleveland, Ohio

J. Patrick Spirnak, M.D.
Associate Professor of Urology, Department of Urology, Case Western Reserve University School of Medicine; Director of Urology, MetroHealth Medical Center, Cleveland, Ohio

Stevan B. Streem, M.D.
Head, Section of Stone Disease and Endourology, Department of Urology, The Cleveland Clinic Foundation, Cleveland, Ohio

Anthony J. Thomas, Jr., M.D.
Head, Section of Male Infertility, Department of Urology, The Cleveland Clinic Foundation, Cleveland, Ohio

Sandip Vasavada, M.D.
Resident, Department of Urology, The Cleveland Clinic Foundation, Cleveland, Ohio

Mark A. Wainstein, M.D.
Resident, Department of Urology, Case Western Reserve University School of Medicine, Cleveland, Ohio

Lawrence M. Wyner, M.D.
Associate Staff, Department of Urology, The Cleveland Clinic Foundation, Cleveland, Ohio

PREFACE

Over the past two decades the specialty of urology has witnessed many changes in both the assessment and management of patients with various diseases of the genitourinary system. Stone disease best exemplifies these changes with the development of percutaneous procedures and extracorporeal shock wave lithotripsy. However, concepts have also changed in the management of patients with various malignancies, urinary incontinence, and impotence. Urologists are interacting more with other specialists, and the care of many patients has become a collaborative effort.

Urology Secrets provides information that should be of value to house officers and medical students learning this specialty. A broad selection of topics is reviewed, and information is provided that should be useful in both the operating room and office. This book is not intended to be a comprehensive textbook on the subject. The questions and short answers as well as the informal tone are employed to make the text enjoyable as well as useful.

New concepts regarding disease processes continue to evolve, operative techniques continue to be developed, technologic advances are ongoing, and the office practice of urology is continuing to expand. These changes will enhance the care provided to patients with urologic problems. It is hoped that the material presented here will provide a strong foundation for providing the highest quality of care.

Martin I. Resnick, M.D.
Andrew C. Novick, M.D.
Cleveland, Ohio

I. Patient Evaluation

1. PHYSICAL EXAMINATION

Kenneth W. Angermeier, M.D.

1. Are the kidneys palpable in a normal patient?
The right kidney may be palpable in children and thin adults. The left kidney is difficult to palpate, as it lies higher within the retroperitoneum than the right kidney. Examination is best performed bimanually, with one hand behind the patient in the costovertebral angle and the other anteriorly just below the costal margin. With inspiration, the kidney may be felt as it moves downward. In neonates, examination is performed by palpating the flank between the thumb anteriorly and the remaining fingers posteriorly in the costovertebral angle. Both kidneys can be outlined reliably in this fashion.

2. What is the significance of an abdominal bruit?
Although not a specific finding, auscultation of a bruit in the epigastrium or upper abdomen may suggest the presence of renal artery stenosis in the appropriate clinical setting. This finding is particularly indicative when the bruit is continuous (systolic-diastolic). A bruit may vary in intensity with fluctuation of the systemic blood pressure, or disappear if renal artery stenosis progresses to near or total occlusion. An abdominal bruit may also occur in association with a renal artery aneurysm or arteriovenous malformation.

3. Where is renal pain usually localized on examination?
Renal pain due to inflammation or obstruction may result in vague, diffuse back discomfort. A renal source often can be identified by the finding of localized tenderness in the costovertebral angle, just lateral to the sacrospinalis muscle and inferior to the twelfth rib. This is usually best elicited by percussion of the area with the fist.

4. At what filling volume can the adult bladder be detected on physical examination?
In the adult, a normal bladder cannot be palpated or percussed until there is a urine volume of at least 150 ml. For the most part, percussion is superior to palpation when evaluating a patient for bladder distention. Patients with frank urinary retention may have visible bladder distention that may extend to the level of the umbilicus.

5. When is examination of the bladder under anesthesia important?
Bimanual examination under anesthesia is useful in assessing the local extent of carcinoma of the bladder and its mobility. In the female, this is done by compressing the bladder between one hand on the abdomen and the other in the vagina. Male patients are examined with a hand on the abdomen and a finger in the rectum.

6. What is paraphimosis?
Paraphimosis is a condition that may arise when the foreskin of the penis has been retracted beyond the corona of the glans, and is not subsequently reduced. This can lead to constriction of the glans penis, resulting in pain, edema, and possible vascular compromise. Failure to reduce the foreskin after insertion of a urethral catheter is one situation in which paraphimosis may occur.

Paraphimosis is a urologic emergency that requires immediate dorsal slit or circumcision if the foreskin cannot be manually reduced.

7. What disease process is characterized by a palpable scar or "plaque" along the shaft of the penis?
Peyronie's disease is a condition in which a fibrotic scar develops within the tunica albuginea of the corpora cavernosa, and may result in curvature of the erect penis. The scar most commonly involves the dorsal aspect of the penis, although it can extend laterally or occur on the ventrum in some cases. Calcification is present in approximately 30% of patients, and indicates that the scar is mature.

8. Describe the physical findings in hypospadias.
Hypospadias occurs as a result of incomplete fusion of the urethral plate during embryogenesis. The urethral meatus is abnormally located and may be present along the ventral shaft of the penis, scrotum, or perineum. The foreskin is usually incomplete ventrally, being described as "hooded." Dysgenetic tissue along the urethral plate may result in ventral penile curvature (chordee).

9. What is the appearance of genital herpes?
Genital herpes is characterized by superficial vesicles grouped on an erythematous base. The lesions are often painful and may coalesce. The incubation period is 2–7 days. The majority of patients with genital herpes have herpes simplex virus type II.

10. What is priapism?
Priapism is a prolonged, painful erection, often of several hours' duration. Physical examination reveals rigid corpora cavernosa that may be somewhat tender. The glans penis is usually flaccid. This condition is often seen in patients with sickle cell anemia, but may also be idiopathic. Priapism may occur in patients on a pharmacologic erection program. Emergent treatment is indicated, as prolonged priapism may result in intracorporal fibrosis and impotence.

11. When should a rectal examination be performed in the male?
Digital rectal examination should be performed annually beginning at age 40, or in any male presenting for urologic evaluation. It should include an estimation of anal sphincter tone, palpation of the prostate and rectum, and testing of the stool for occult blood.

12. Compare the findings on rectal examination in benign prostatic hyperplasia (BPH) and prostatic carcinoma.
In BPH, the prostate is variably enlarged and has a rubbery consistency. The enlargement is usually symmetric and may be associated with deepening of the lateral sulci and obliteration of the median furrow. Prostatic carcinoma may be palpable as a discrete, firm, or hard nodule within one prostatic lobe. This can progress to firm induration of an entire lobe or diffuse involvement of the prostate. The presence of extracapsular extension or seminal vesicle involvement should be noted. Prostatic carcinoma can also be present in a patient with a benign rectal examination, with the diagnosis usually being made because of an elevated prostate-specific antigen level or following transurethral resection of the prostate.

13. What condition is suggested by the presence of a soft, cystic mass palpable in the midline near the base of the prostate?
This finding may indicate the presence of a mullerian duct cyst or an enlarged utricle. These entities arise from remnants of the fetal mullerian system, which regresses in the male during normal development. An enlarged utricle is occasionally seen in patients with proximal hypospadias.

14. What is the significance of a palpable testicular mass?
The majority of solid testicular masses represent malignant germ cell tumors. It is important to ascertain on physical examination whether the mass is located within the testicle or is arising from

the spermatic cord or epididymis. Extratesticular masses are more often benign, although malignancies may occur in these locations as well.

15. Describe the characteristics of a hydrocele and a spermatocele.

A **hydrocele** is a collection of fluid within the scrotum that is contained by the parietal and visceral components of the tunica vaginalis. It is palpable as a relatively smooth fluid collection filling the hemiscrotum and surrounding the testicle. The hydrocele may be tense or somewhat fluctuant. The testicle may be difficult to palpate in the presence of a hydrocele. A **spermatocele** is a cystic fluid collection primarily involving the epididymis, and may be tense or firm on palpation. The diagnosis of both of these entities is confirmed by transillumination using a bright light in a dark room. A hydrocele or spermatocele should completely transilluminate, whereas a solid mass will not.

16. What is a varicocele?

A varicocele occurs as a result of enlargement of the spermatic vein (pampiniform plexus) above the testicle, more commonly on the left side. The enlarged, tortuous veins are palpable as a "bag of worms" within the superior aspect of the involved hemiscrotum. Typically, the veins fill and enlarge with the patient in the upright position or with the Valsalva maneuver, and decompress with recumbency. The ipsilateral testicle may be smaller in size than the opposite one, and in some patients a varicocele is associated with infertility.

17. What is the significance of a varicocele that does not decompress with the patient in the supine position?

Patients with a varicocele that does not decompress with recumbency should be suspected of having obstruction of the spermatic vein where it enters the renal vein on the left, or the inferior vena cava on the right. This may be caused by a retroperitoneal neoplasm, such as renal cell carcinoma with tumor thrombus in the renal vein or inferior vena cava. Acute onset of a varicocele or a right-sided varicocele should raise similar suspicions.

BIBLIOGRAPHY

1. Lowe FC, Brendler, CB: Evaluation of the urologic patient: History, physical examination, and urinalysis. In Walsh PC, Retik AB, Stamey TA, Vaughan ED Jr (eds): Campbell's Urology, 6th ed. Philadelphia, W. B. Saunders, 1992, pp 311–316.
2. Tanagho EA: Physical examination of the genitourinary tract. In Tanagho EA, McAninch JW (eds): Smith's General Urology. Norwalk, CT, Appleton & Lange, 1992, pp 40–47.

2. INSTRUMENTATION AND ENDOSCOPY

Stevan B. Streem, M.D.

1. Name the usual indications for urethral catheterization.
The most frequent procedure, "straight catheterization," may be indicated for diagnosis of possible urinary infection in women, especially when a voided urine shows significant vaginal contamination. Catheterization for this purpose alone is rarely indicated in men.

Urethral catheterization may be indicated to assess the amount of residual urine after voiding or as part of a urodynamic evaluation of bladder and urethral function. It may also be used for retrograde instillation of radiographic contrast medium to obtain a cystogram or voiding cystourethrogram for radiographic evaluation is some patients.

2. What types of catheters are best to use for these studies?
To obtain urine for microbiologic study or to check for residual urine, straight catheters of 14–16 French size are generally used. When the catheter is to be left in place, such as for patients with urinary retention, a self-retaining balloon catheter, or Foley catheter, is used.

3. What do those French sizes mean?
The French scale is a measure of circumference. One French equals approximately 0.33 mm in diameter, so that an 18-French catheter is about 6 mm wide.

4. What do I do if I can't pass a catheter easily in a man?
Call a urology resident or urologist. He or she will show you how to use the specialized catheters, such as coudé catheters with curved tips for patients who have had prostate surgery, or filiform and follower catheters for men with urethral strictures.

5. What are "sounds"?
Sounds are specialized metal catheters most commonly used to treat urethral strictures. Only urologists or urology residents should use sounds in the urethra.

6. How do you treat a man who is in pain from a distended bladder, but in whom the catheter cannot be passed?
Sometimes the best approach is placement of a small-caliber suprapubic tube via a percutaneous approach. This requires only local anesthetic and provides immediate relief of urinary retention.

7. List the three most frequent indications for cystoscopy.
Evaluation of hematuria, infection, or voiding dysfunction.

8. What instruments are used for cystoscopy?
Usually, rigid instruments ranging from 16–22 French are used for diagnostic purposes. Two lenses with different angles of vision are used to visualize the entire urethra and bladder.

9. Compare the advantages of flexible and rigid cystoscopes.
Flexible instrumentation is more comfortable for the patient if the procedure is not done under anesthesia. Rigid instrumentation offers a greater field of vision and allows more therapeutic options.

10. When should you perform diagnostic retrograde pyelography at the time of cystoscopy?
Retrograde x-rays of the upper urinary tracts are done when intravenous urography does not adequately visualize the pyelocalyceal system and ureters, or when intravenous urography is

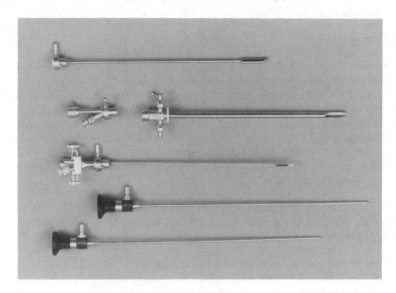

Standard rigid instrumentation for cystourethroscopy.

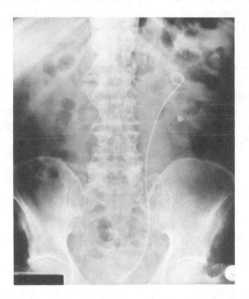

Plain x-ray showing an indwelling, self-retaining ureteral stent.

contraindicated, such as in patients with significant renal insufficiency or a history of a significant adverse reaction to intravenous contrast.

11. What instruments are used to evaluate the upper tracts?

Like the bladder, the ureter and pyelocalyceal system can be intubated with catheters or with rigid or flexible endoscopes.

12. Name some frequent indications for ureteral catheterization.
   1. Obtaining retrograde x-rays
   2. Temporarily bypassing an obstruction, such as from ureteral calculi or strictures
   3. Obtaining differential urine from each collection system to assess problems such as abnormal cytologic findings or to localize bacteriuria.

13. Explain the difference between a ureteral catheter and a ureteral stent.
Ureteral catheters are placed cystoscopically to the renal pelvis and exit via the urethra. They frequently migrate distally and are a source of infection. Therefore, they are used only for temporary upper tract access. In contrast, ureteral stents, which are also usually placed cystoscopically, are self-retaining and completely indwelling. They can be left for days or weeks with little risk of infection or migration.

14. Can the upper tracts be visualized directly with telescopes?
Yes. Upper tract endoscopy can be done for diagnostic or therapeutic purposes with both rigid and flexible ureteropyeloscopes.

15. What are the indications for upper tract endoscopy?
The most frequent indications include evaluation of "filling defects," evaluation of intrinsic obstructing lesions, and management of ureteral calculi.

16. When should direct percutaneous instrumentation of the upper collecting system be used?
Usually, a percutaneous nephrostomy is placed to relieve ureteral obstruction in the face of infection or obstructive uropathy when retrograde catheterization is unsuccessful or otherwise contraindicated.

17. Can endoscopy be performed via a percutaneous approach?
Yes. Percutaneous nephroscopy (actually, pyeloscopy is a better term) can be performed with rigid or flexible instruments analogous to those used for cystoscopy and ureteroscopy. Percutaneous nephroscopy can be diagnostic or therapeutic. It is particularly valuable for managing large renal calculi, though occasionally it can be used to manage upper tract transitional cell carcinoma in select patients.

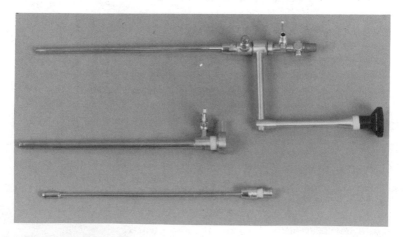

A rigid nephroscope is similar to a cystoscope except that it is shorter and of wider caliber. The optical system is offset to allow passage of the rigid working instrumentation. The part across from the eyepiece can accommodate an ultrasound wand to be used for percutaneous ultrasonic stone fragmentation and extraction.

BIBLIOGRAPHY

1. Bagley DH, Huffman JL, Lyons ES: Flexible ureteropyeloscopy: Diagnosis and treatment in the upper urinary tract. J Urol 138:280–285, 1987.
2. Blute ML, Segura JW, Patterson DE, et al: Impact of endourology on diagnosis and management of upper urinary tract urothelial cancer. J Urol 141:1298–1301, 1989.
3. Carter HB: Instrumentation and endoscopy. In Walsh PC, Retik AB, Stamey TA, Vaughan ED Jr (eds): Campbell's Urology, 6th ed. Philadelphia, W. B. Saunders, 1992, pp 331–341.
4. Guz B, Streem SB, Novick AC, et al: Role of percutaneous nephrostomy in patients with upper tract transition cell carcinoma. Urology 37:331, 1991.
5. Huffman JL, Bagley DH, Lyon ES: Extending cystoscopic techniques into the ureter and renal pelvis. JAMA 250:2002–2205, 1983.
6. Smith AD, Reinke DB, Miller RP, Lange PH: Percutaneous nephrostomy in the management of ureteral and renal calculi. Radiology 133:49, 1979.
7. Streem SB, Pontes JE, Novick AC, et al: Ureteropyeloscopy in the evaluation of upper tract filling defects. J Urol 136:383–385, 1986.

3. URINALYSIS AND URINE FUNCTION STUDIES

Kurt H. Dinchman, M.D.

1. What types of information can be obtained from a urinalysis? What is their importance?
Urinalysis is the most commonly performed laboratory test in a general medical practice. It is routinely performed in two parts: (1) use of a dipstick and (2) microscopic examination of spun urine. The most common dipsticks give results such as pH, specific gravity, presence or absence of blood, protein, and leukocytes, and various other tests, including assessment of glucose, ketones, bilirubin, and urobilinogen.

2. What is the normal pH of urine?
The normal pH of urine is between 5 and 8, depending on diet and other factors. Urine pH is important in determination of renal tubular acidosis, which may cause a pH below 5.5. Uric acid stones may be suspected with acidic urine. Alkaline urine may be observed in the presence of urea-splitting organisms, such as *Proteus* sp.

3. What is the significance of abnormal findings on a urine dipstick examination?
The presence of glucose in urine may indicate glycosuria secondary to undiagnosed diabetes mellitus. Leukocytes may indicate an inflammatory or infectious process within the urinary tract; interpretation, however, must be verified by microscopic examination. Protein in the urine may indicate a reabsorption problem in the kidneys, whereas ketones may indicate ketoacidosis, as seen with diabetes or a state of starvation or malnutrition. Bilirubin may be seen in the urine of patients with early stages of liver abnormalities. Erythrocytes or free hemoglobin from lysed erythrocytes should alert the investigator to examine the urine microscopically for red blood cells.

4. How is a clean specimen obtained for microscopic examination of urine?
It is important for the investigator to obtain a "clean-catch urine." Women should clean themselves with a sanitary wipe and spread the labia to get a clean, clear stream into the specimen bottle. Uncircumcized men should retract the foreskin before giving the specimen.

5. How is a proper microscopic examination of urine performed?
The clean-catch specimen is centrifuged for approximately 3–5 minutes at 2–3,000 rpm. The sediment (button) at the bottom of the centrifuge tube is suspended in approximately 0.2 ml of urine. The resuspended button then is poured onto a glass slide and covered with a coverslip. First a low-power scanning of the specimen is performed to detect red blood cell casts, crystals and pathogens such as trichomonads. High-power analysis identifies bacteria, yeast, red blood cells, and white blood cells.

6. What is the significance of findings in a microscopic urine examination?
High-power examination may reveal urine casts that contain erythrocytes encased in a noncellular matrix. This finding may indicate glomerular hemorrhage, as seen in glomerulonephritis. Other casts with renal tubular cells may indicate renal tubular damage. The examiner also may observe urinary crystals of phosphate, oxalate, and cystine in stone-forming patients; however, crystals also may be seen in non–stone-forming patients. Leukocytes in the urine sediment may indicate an inflammatory process secondary to infection, calculi, or interstitial renal disease. Microscopic examination also may reveal erythrocytes. The differential diagnosis for erythrocytes in urine is quite extensive. Patients with microhematuria should be evaluated for infection, calculus disease, carcinoma, inflammatory process, trauma, sickle-cell enemia, bleeding disorder, and glomerulonephritis. Epithelial cells are seen frequently in urinalysis, especially squamous

epithelial cells in postpubertal and nonmenopausal women. Abnormal transitional cells in the urine indicate malignant transitional cell carcinoma.

7. What are the most commonly used renal function tests?
The most commonly used renal function tests are urine specific gravity, serum creatinine, blood urea nitrogen, serum electrolytes, and complete blood count.

8. How is urine specific gravity used to test renal function?
Urine specific gravity is a simple test of the ability of the kidneys to concentrate urine. Decreasing ability to concentrate urine parallels a decrease in overall renal function. Urine specific gravity remains the simplest method of determining the ability to concentrate and dilute urine.

9. How is serum creatinine helpful in determining renal function?
Creatinine, an end product of metabolism in skeletal muscle, is excreted by the kidneys and is not influenced by hydration status. Because of the constancy of daily creatinine production in a normal, active patient, levels of serum creatinine remain within a fairly reliable range and therefore can be used to determine renal function.

10. How is creatinine clearance calculated? What does it mean?
Calculation of creatinine clearance requires determination of the concentration of creatinine in urine and in plasma and the volume of urine excreted per minute. Creatinine clearance is calculated by the formula: clearance = UV/P, where U is urine creatinine concentration, V is urine volume, and P is plasma creatinine concentration. Creatinine clearance of 90–110 ml/min is normal. Because creatinine production is stable and filtered through the glomeruli, creatinine clearance is close to the glomerular filtration rate. Therefore decreased creatinine clearance indicates a decrease in the glomerular filtration rate.

11. How is blood urea nitrogen (BUN) related to glomerular filtration rate?
Urea, an end product of protein catabolism, also is excreted by the kidneys, but it is not as accurate as creatinine clearance in determining glomerular filtration rate. The BUN-to-creatinine ratio, however, may be used to obtain certain clinical information. A classic example is seen in dehydrated patients with prerenal azotemia, in which the BUN:creatinine ratio may be 10:1. Patients with obstruction or postrenal azotemia may have a ratio of 20–30:1.

12. How are blood count and electrolyte studies helpful in assessing renal function?
Anemia may be seen in patients with renal insufficiency due to decreased production of erythopoietin. Serum sodium and potassium abnormalities are often seen in patients with renal insufficiency. The degree of hyperkalemia is paramount in determining the initiation of renal dialysis.

BIBLIOGRAPHY

1. Schrier RW, Gottschalk CW (eds): Diseases of the Kidney, vol. 1, 5th ed. Boston, Little, Brown, 1993.
2. Tanagho EA, McAninch JW (eds): Smith's General Urology, 8th ed. Norwalk, CT, Appleton & Lange, 1992.
3. Walsh PC, Retik AB, Stamey TA, Vaughan ED Jr (eds): Campbell's Urology, 6th ed. Philadelphia, W. B. Saunders, 1992.

4. INTRAVENOUS UROGRAPHY AND ANGIOGRAPY

David A. Goldfarb, M.D.

1. In what urologic conditions is intravenous urography useful?

Hematuria	Suspected renal obstruction
Pain arising from the urinary tract	Evaluation of postsurgical complications
Recurrent urinary infection	Evaluation of congenital anomalies
Suspected renal calculus disease	Trauma

2. What types of contrast material are available?
Ionic and nonionic.

3. What are the risks of intravenous contrast material?
Allergic reaction and renal toxicity.

4. Who is at risk for an allergic contrast reaction?
Those with a prior history of contrast reaction or of other severe allergies and asthma.

5. Which diseases place patients at high risk for renal toxicity from intravenous contrast material?
Diabetic nephropathy, multiple myeloma, hyperuricosuria, amyloidosis, preexisting chronic renal failure.

6. What is the usual film sequence for urography?
   1. **Plain film**—the kidneys, ureters, and bladder (KUB) must be visualized to evaluate calcifications and bony structures.
   2. **1 minute**—the nephrogram visualizes the renal parenchyma.
   3. **5 minutes**—early visualization of the upper collecting system (calices, pelvis, upper ureter).
   4. **Tomograms**—performed to assess renal outlines and fine calcifications. Routine on patients >40 years old and used selectively below age 40.
   5. **15/20 minutes**—late visualization should include the lower ureters and bladder.

7. What tricks are useful to improve the diagnostic yield?
   1. **Delayed films**—to assess the level of obstruction in hydronephrotic kidneys.
   2. **Plain tomograms**—before contrast, these are used to assess renal calcifications.
   3. **Ureteral compression**—a compression band surrounding the lower abdomen helps to fill the upper ureters better.
   4. **Prone films**—demonstrate better visualization of the pelvic portion of the ureters.
   5. **Oblique films**—help to visualize abnormalities in three dimensions.
   6. **Postvoid film**—provides a better assessment of bladder pathology and residual urine.

8. What features of the IV urogram are useful diagnostically?
   1. **Plain film**—to assess bony structures and any calcifications
   2. **Nephrogram**—to assess function (normal, delayed, or not visualized)
   3. **Tomograms**—to assess renal outlines for the presence of a mass and to assess smaller calcifications within the kidney
   4. **Early films**—to assess upper collecting system for hydronephrosis, filling defect, distorted calices, malposition, mass

5. **Late films**—to assess ureter for filling defects, dilation, constriction. The bladder should be assessed for size, filling defects, mucosal pattern (thickened, trabeculated), and shape (teardrop: pelvic lipomatosis; Christmas tree: neurogenic bladder).

9. How can calcifications observed on plain films be localized?
Oblique views and plain tomography.

10. What is the differential diagnosis of renal calcifications?
- Collecting system stone
- Tumor (speckled)
- Cyst (rim)
- Renal artery aneurysm
- Caliceal diverticulum

11. Name the causes of extrarenal calcification seen on plain films.
Vascular, mesenteric nodes, gallstones, adrenal, and splenic.

12. What important diagnoses can be made by plain films?
- Cancer metastases (sclerotic/lytic)
- Paget's disease (thickened cortex with course trabeculation)
- Myelodysplasia (increased interpedicular distance)
- Sacral agenesis (absence of sacrum)
- Exstrophy of the bladder (widening of the pubis)

13. What is the differential diagnosis of a filling defect in the kidney?
Stone, tumor, blood clot, sloughed papilla, fungus ball, vascular impression.

14. What is the differential diagnosis of a filling defect in the ureter?
Stone, tumor, blood clot, inflammation, fibroepithelial polyp.

15. What is the differential diagnosis of a filling defect in the bladder?
Stone, tumor, blood clot, middle lobe prostate, foreign body, ureterocele, fungus ball.

16. What is the differential diagnosis in nonvisualization of a kidney? What further studies are required?

Condition	Next step in diagnosis
Renal agenesis	Ultrasound or CT
High-grade obstruction	Ultrasound/retrograde pyelography/CT
Mass	CT or U/S
Vascular compromise	Renal scan
Prior nephrectomy	Confirm by history

17. Name the indications for renal angiography.
- Hematuria—when noninvasive studies suggest a vascular abnormality
- Surgical planning for:
    Large renal, adrenal, retroperitoneal or pelvic masses
    Nephron-sparing renal surgery
- To evaluate renal vascular disease
- Trauma—to evaluate vascular integrity of the kidney when this is questioned by studies such as IVP or CT
- To evaluate postsurgical vascular complications (thrombosis)
- Renal mass—to evaluate vascular pattern

18. Name the indications for renal venography and/or venacavography.
- Evaluation of a tumor thrombus (renal cell carcinoma)
- Definitive evaluation for renal vein thrombosis
- Renal vein renin determination in renovascular hypertension

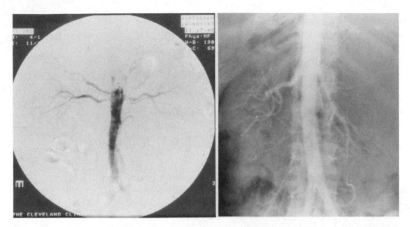

Left, Digital subtraction angiogram demonstrating high-grade bilateral renal artery stenosis. *Right,* Standard catheter angiogram showing downward displacement of the left renal artery from a large hypovascular left adrenal mass.

19. List three angiographic techniques.
1. Cut-film arteriography (standard arteriogram)
2. Intraarterial digital subtraction angiography (IADSA)
3. Intravenous digital subtraction angiography (IVDSA)

20. Describe the advantages and disadvantages of each angiographic technique.

	CONTRAST DOSE	INVASIVENESS	IMAGE QUALITY
Standard arteriogram	+++	+++	+++
IADSA	+	++	+++
IVDSA	+++	+	+

21. What are the complications of angiography?

Hematoma   Allergic reaction to contrast material
Pseudoaneurysm   Nephrotoxicity from contrast material
Atheroembolism   Vessel dissection

22. Describe the indications for angiographic renal embolization.
- Renal cell carcinoma—to facilitate operative management of large tumors with vena caval thrombi
- Control hemorrhage from:
    Percutaneous biopsy
    Arteriovenous malformation

BIBLIOGRAPHY

1. Dunbar JS: Excretory urography in infants and children. In Walsh PC, Retik AB, Stamey TA, Vaughan ED Jr, (eds): Campbell's Urology, 6th ed. Philadelphia, W. B. Saunders, 1992, p 434.
2. Friedenberg RM: Excretory urography in the adult. In Walsh PC, Retik AB, Stamey TA, Vaughan ED Jr (eds): Campbell's Urology, 6th ed. Philadelphia, W. B. Saunders, 1992, p 412–433.
3. Hartman GW, Hattery RR, Witten DW, Williamson B: Mortality during excretory urography: Mayo Clinic experience. AJR 139:919–922, 1982.
4. Kinnison ML, Powe NR, Steinberg ED: Results of randomized controlled trials of low vs. high-osmolality contrast media. Radiology 170:381, 1989.
5. Pollack HM: Clinical Urography: An Atlas and Textbook of Urologic Imaging. Philadelphia, W. B. Saunders, 1990.

5. ULTRASONOGRAPHY

Martin I. Resnick, M.D.

1. What is the sound frequency of diagnostic ultrasound?
3–15 MHz.

2. How is the frequency related to depth of tissue penetration and resolution?
The higher the frequency of the ultrasound wave, the less tissue penetration but greater resolution of near objects. Similarly, the lower frequencies result in greater penetration but at the expense of resolution. Typically, abdominal ultrasound imaging for viewing the kidneys uses 3.5-MHz transducers, whereas transrectal techniques use 7.5-MHz transducers for imaging the prostate.

3. How do tissue interfaces affect ultrasound waves?
Ultrasound waves pass through tissue but are reflected or scattered at interfaces between tissues. It is this reflection of the ultrasound waves that allows for the delineation of different structures. If no interfaces exist, ultrasound waves tend to pass unimpeded through the structure, which typically occurs with fluid-filled masses (e.g., simple renal cyst).

4. How are ultrasound waves generated?
An electrical current applied to a piezoelectric ceramic crystal results in vibration of the crystal with the development of ultrasound waves. Reflected ultrasound waves impinge on the crystal and generate an electrical potential that can be processed to provide an image on a cathode tube.

5. What is A-mode? B-mode?
In **A-mode** imaging (amplitude mode), the magnitude or intensity of the signal is displayed as a spike of varying height along a time or distance axis. This one-dimensional display is rarely used clinically. In **B-mode** (brightness mode), the presence of an echo is indicated by the appearance of a bright spot, while the intensity of the echo is indicated by the brightness of the spot.

6. What is gray scale?
Current ultrasound instruments usually display brightness of echoes in 64 or 128 shades of gray (gray scale). A two-dimensional, clinically useful image is obtained.

7. What is real time imaging?
In real-time scanning, the transducer constantly changes location, providing in essence a rapid B-mode scan that gives the examiner the sense of "live" imaging analogous to x-ray fluoroscopy.

8. Explain the purpose of Doppler studies. What is color-flow Doppler?
Doppler imaging allows for simultaneous viewing in real time and evaluating blood flow. The Doppler effect or Doppler shift refers to the alteration in frequency that occurs after a sound wave is reflected off a moving target. The red blood cell is an individual moving target and each scatters a single sound wave. The combined effect of multiple sound waves is received by the transducer, and different colors (typically blue and red) are superimposed on the gray scale image depending on whether the reflected waves are of higher or lower frequency, i.e., the red blood cells are moving away from or toward the transducer.

9. Describe the ultrasound characteristics of a renal cyst.
Typically, a renal cyst is a mass associated with the kidney. There are no internal echoes present, the walls of the cyst are thin and can be noted circumferentially, and there is an enhancement of transmitted waves on the back wall of the cyst.

10. Describe the ultrasound characteristics of renal tumors.
Renal tumors are masses associated with the kidney which often distort the collecting system. They usually have a heterogeneous internal architecture with poorly defined margins that are, at times, difficult to separate from the renal parenchyma.

11. Is ultrasound helpful in detecting hydronephrosis?
The normal central echo pattern within the mid-portion or hilum of the kidney is hyperechoic due to the fat and vascular structures. In the hydronephrotic kidney, the collecting system becomes distended with urine (fluid), which can easily be detected by ultrasound. Ultrasound imaging is very useful in detecting the presence of distention of the intrarenal collecting system to help establish a diagnosis of hydronephrosis.

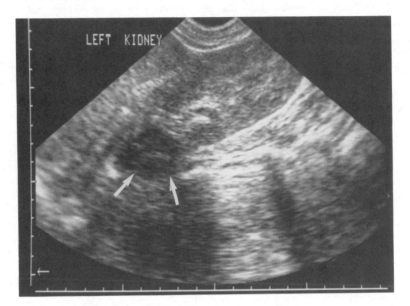

12. What are the ultrasound characteristics of a stone?
Typically, the calcification in the urinary tract appears as a hyperechoic interface with shadowing behind it due to the nontransmittal of ultrasound waves. These typical characteristics are present in calcifications throughout the urinary tract, including the kidney, bladder, and prostate.

13. How is ultrasound useful in evaluating bladder outlet obstruction?
Ultrasound of the urinary bladder can detect and measure the volume of residual urine. Volume measurement can be calculated by obtaining anterior-posterior, transverse, and longitudinal (cephalad-caudad) diameters of the bladder.

14. Describe the ultrasound characteristics of a ureterocele.
Ureteroceles are often associated with duplicated collecting systems and are not infrequently detected in children, particularly girls presenting with urinary tract infections. Ureterocele appears as a fluid mass within the bladder with a thin but clearly defined membrane. Many patients with ureteroceles will have associated hydroureteronephrosis of that segment draining the ureterocele. Ultrasound is useful making this determination.

15. Can ultrasound detect a testicular tumor?
Typically, the testicle is echogenic, and tumors within the testicle, though small, are well delineated. The tumors usually are uniform and of low echogenicity, but can be heterogeneous. If the tumor is large, it can replace the entire testicle so that no normal testicular tissue is evident.

16. How is the Doppler useful in evaluating varicoceles?
Doppler studies are able to detect blood flow. By checking for flow within the spermatic cord during a Valsalva maneuver, one is able to detect retrograde flow to the testicle and establish the presence of a varicocele. The clinical significance of subclinical varicoceles (i.e., those that are detected by ultrasound but are not palpable) remains controversial.

17. How is ultrasound used to assess testicular torsion?
Testicular torsion is associated with the interruption of blood flow to the testicle and, if untreated, results in infarction. Doppler studies are useful in detecting the presence or absence of blood flow when torsion is suspected. Flow studies are very useful in making this determination. Radionuclide studies have also been used to establish this diagnosis.

18. Are there typical ultrasound characteristics of carcinoma of the prostate?
On transrectal ultrasonography, carcinoma of the prostate presents as a hypoechoic area within the peripheral zone of the prostate. However, not all prostatic malignancies are associated with changes on ultrasonography. Many are isoechoic and cannot be distinguished from normal surrounding prostatic tissue.

19. Describe the typical appearance of benign prostatic hyperplasia on ultrasound.
Benign prostatic hyperplasia has its origin in the transition zone of the prostate. With benign prostatic hyperplasia, there is an increase in the anterior-posterior diameter of the prostate, and the gland has a more rounded appearance. The large increase in size of the transition zone results in compression of the peripheral zone, and the distinction between these zones is usually most evident.

20. How is ultrasound used to measure prostate size?
Ultrasound measurements of prostate size use the formula for calculating the volume of a prolate ellipse. The three largest diameters of the prostate (anterior-posterior, transverse, and longitudinal) are multiplied by each other and by pi (3.14159). Three measurements are usually obtained with transrectal ultrasound.

21. What is prostate-specific antigen density (PSAD)?
PSAD has been used to test for the presence of carcinoma of the prostate. The PSAD is derived by dividing the serum PSA level by the volume of the prostate (measured by ultrasound). A value >0.15 suggests carcinoma of the prostate, and these patients require evaluation.

22. Is ultrasound used in the evaluation of impotence?
Yes. Doppler flow studies are useful in measuring penile blood flow changes following injection of vasoactive substances. Patients with vasculogenic impotence will not demonstrate changes in arterial diameter or an increase in blood flow. These studies have also been used to assess for impotence secondary to venous insufficiency.

BIBLIOGRAPHY

1. Coleman BG: Genitourinary Ultrasound: A Text/Atlas. New York, Igaku-Shoin, 1988.
2. Pollack HM: Clinical Urography: An Atlas and Textbook of Urological Imaging. Philadelphia, W. B. Saunders, 1990.
3. Resnick MI: Prostatic Ultrasonography. Philadelphia, B. C. Decker, 1990.
4. Resnick MI, Rifkin MD: Ultrasonography of the Urinary Tract, 3rd ed. Baltimore, Williams & Wilkins, 1991.

6. COMPUTED TOMOGRAPHY

Nehemia Hampel, M.D.

1. What is computed tomography (CT)?

In regular radiography a broad beam passes through the subject to produce an image on the x-ray film (detector). In CT scanning a thin, collimated beam of x-ray is directed through the subject and is sensed on a series of x-ray detectors. During scanning, thin slices through the body are recorded. The process is repeated in consecutive slices and later reconstructed by digital computers to assemble and integrate the data and to reconstruct a cross-sectional image. The image can be displayed on screen or photographed. The reconstructed two-dimensional image uses measurements of linear attenuation coefficients collected from the multiple projections around the body.

2. When was CT scan developed?

Sir Godfrey N. Hounsfield at EMI Limited in England developed the first CT scanner in 1973.

3. What are Hounsfield units (HU)?

HUs are a relative density scale that assigns a value of −1000 to air, 0 to water, and +1000 to dense bone. The density of a structure is proportionate to the amount of x-ray attenuation. The higher the density, the higher the CT number. Approximate typical values: fat, −90 HU; soft tissue, +40 HU; and clotted blood, +70 HU.

4. How wide is a CT scan slice?

CT scanning commonly uses contiguous 1-cm slices. Thinner slices of 0.5 cm are used to obtain a more accurate delineation of small or unclear lesions.

5. What patient positions and techniques are used in performing abdominal or pelvic CT scanning?

After a 12-hour fast, patients are usually placed in the supine position and given a limited bowel preparation. An oral contrast medium is used to avoid mistaking non-opacified loops of bowel for peritoneal or retroperitoneal masses. The need for a preliminary noncontrast scan is somewhat controversial. For the evaluation of renal masses, renal or retroperitoneal calcification, suspected urine extravasation, or trauma, CT scans should be performed both before and after intravenous contrast enhancement.

6. When is CT used in urology?

CT is used for the evaluation of renal, perirenal, or retroperitoneal processes. It is effective in defining complications associated with renal transplants, assessing adrenal lesions, and detecting retroperitoneal lymph nodes and lung lesions in patients with testicular cancer. It also has a role in staging bladder and prostate cancer as well as in evaluating pelvic masses.

7. When is CT used in renal and perirenal evaluation?

CT is used most commonly in detection or delineation of a renal mass. It is one of the best modalities for detecting masses and separating solid from cystic masses. It also is used in the detection and staging as well as in the follow-up of malignant renal tumors. In inflammatory renal, perirenal, and retroperitoneal masses, CT detects the process and defines its extent. It is the imaging modality of choice in staging renal trauma. CT is extremely sensitive in detecting calculus disease. Usually uric acid stones are undetected on plain radiographs, but they are intensely radiopaque on CT scans.

8. Can CT be used as a guide for interventional procedures?

CT may be used as guide for biopsy, aspiration, and drainage techniques, particularly for renal lesions. Usually ultrasonography is faster, less expensive, and readily available, but in some cases the approach or lesions are better demonstrated with CT. Although undetected on plain radiographs, hydronephrosis may be detected by CT scan; ultrasonography, however, is an accurate and less expensive method. CT is somewhat less sensitive than ultrasonography in distinguishing solid from cystic masses.

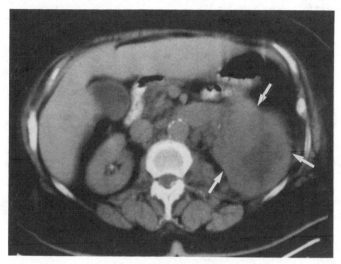

CT scan of left renal tumor.

9. Is CT effective in staging carcinoma of the prostate?

CT has only a limited value for staging carcinoma of the prostate. Lymphatic metastases in the pelvis are difficult to visualize. Differentiation of cancer from the normal gland is seldom possible in localized disease. Cancer is detected only in advanced extraprostatic extension into the bladder base or seminal vesicles. CT should not be used in the routine staging of prostate carcinoma.

10. What is the most important contribution of CT in urology?

CT is most important in the evaluation and assessment of renal masses. It is the modality of choice in detecting and staging solid renal lesions.

BIBLIOGRAPHY

1. Bosniack MA: Problems in the radiologic diagnosis of renal parenchymal tumors. Urol Clin North Am 20:217–230, 1993.
2. Gillenwater JY, Grayhack JT, Howards SS, Duckett JW (eds): Adult and Pediatric Urology, 2nd ed. Chicago, Year Book, 1991.
3. Hounsfield GN: Computed medical imaging. Med Phys 7:283–290, 1980.
4. Miraldi F: Imaging principles in computed tomography. In Haaga JR, Alfide RJ (eds): Computed Tomography of the Whole Body. St. Louis, Mosby, 1983.
5. Walsh PC, Retik AB, Stamey TA, Vaughan ED Jr (eds): Campbell's Urology, 6th ed. Philadelphia, W. B. Saunders, 1992.

7. MAGNETIC RESONANCE IMAGING

David A. Goldfarb, M.D.

1. What element forms the basis for MRI?
Hydrogen.

2. How does MRI work?
A large magnet aligns the hydrogen nuclei within the tissue under examination. A radio frequency pulse is applied and deflects the net magnetization of the hydrogen nuclei in the tissue. The excited nuclei precess about the axis of the magnetic field and produce an electric signal detected in a receiver coil. The decay of the signal as the nuclei return to equilibrium is monitored. The return to equilibrium is called magnetic relaxation and is a unique property of each tissue, described by T1 and T2 relaxation times. These are important determinants of image contrast and signal intensity in MRI.

3. What pulse sequence is used for MRI?
Spin-echo.

4. What pulse sequence highlights flow in large blood vessels?
Gradient-echo.

5. Compare the advantages and disadvantages of MRI and CT.

MRI Versus CT

MRI	CT
No ionizing radiation	Ionizing radiation
No iodinated contrast	Iodinated contrast
High cost	Low cost
Less widely available	Widely available
Three-dimensional imaging	Two-dimensional imaging
Improved imaging of vascular structures	—
Better soft-tissue characterization	—

6. What are contraindications to MRI?
Claustrophobia, ferromagnetic prosthetic device, pacemaker, and certain intracerebral clips.

7. Outline the T1- and T2-weighted appearances of urologic tissues on MRI.

MRI Appearance of Urologic Tissues

TISSUE	T1-WEIGHTED	T2-WEIGHTED
Calcium	Dark	Dark
Fat	Very bright*	Bright
Urine (water)	Very bright	Very bright
Renal cortex	Intermediate	Bright
Renal medulla	Dark	Intermediate
Adrenal	Intermediate	Intermediate
Bladder wall	Intermediate	Intermediate*
Prostate	Intermediate	Intermediate*
Seminal vesicles	Intermediate	Bright
Blood vessels	Dark	Dark

The asterisks indicate the best sequence to visualize structures. No signal is obtained from flowing blood.

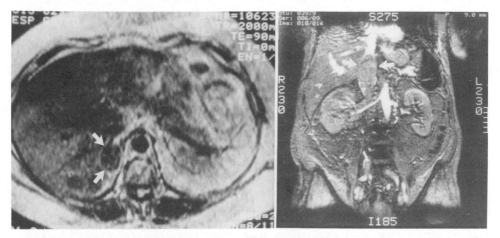

Left, T2-weighted MRI with a right adrenal mass that is iso-intense to the liver, which is an adenoma. *Right,* Gradient echo image of the abdomen. This demonstrates the full extent of a vena caval thrombus from a right renal cell carcinoma.

8. How is MRI useful in the evaluation of renal disorders?

1. **Staging of renal cell carcinoma.** MRI is comparable to CT for evaluating local tumor extension and adenopathy. Because of its ability to evaluate blood vessels, MRI can be used noninvasively to assess the precise limits of vena caval involvement.

2. **Renal masses.** Ultrasound and CT are generally better and less expensive than MRI. MRI has been used to assess renal masses in azotemic patients who cannot receive iodinated contrast.

3. **Obstruction.** Other methods, such as ultrasound and urography, are better and less expensive than MRI.

9. Can adrenal masses be differentiated by MRI?

Signal Intensity Compared to Liver

CONDITION	T1-WEIGHTED	T2-WEIGHTED
Adenoma	Isointense	Isointense
Carcinoma/metastasis	Isointense	Heterogeneous, intermediate increase
Pheochromocytoma	Isointense	Hyperintense

10. What is the role of MRI in staging of prostate cancer?

Prostate cancer is best viewed on T2-weighted images as an area of low signal intensity in the peripheral zone. Staging of localized disease using a whole body coil is only 60% accurate, but staging is improved when an endorectal surface coil is used, approaching 80% accuracy. Most staging errors are due to the inability to detect microscopic capsular invasion.

BIBLIOGRAPHY

1. Goldfarb DA, Novick AC, Bretan PN, et al: Magnetic resonance imaging for assessment of vena caval tumor thrombi: A comparative study with vena cavography and CT scanning. J Urol 144:1100, 1990.
2. Kressel HX: Magnetic resonance imaging. In Walsh PC, Retik AB, Stamey TA, Vaughn ED Jr (eds): Campbell's Urology, 6th ed. Philadelphia, W. B. Saunders, 1992, pp 485–495.
3. Rackley R, Lorig R, Goldfarb DA, Kay R: Magnetic resonance imaging of pelvic tumors in pediatric patients. J Urol 1994.
4. Reinig JW, Doppman JL, Dwyer AJ, Frank J: MRI of indeterminate adrenal masses. AJR 147:493–496, 1986.
5. Rifkin MD, Zerhouni EA, Gatsonis CA, et al: Comparison of magnetic resonance imaging and ultrasonography in staging early prostate cancer. N Engl J Med 323:621–626, 1990.
6. Schnall MD, Imai Y, Tomaszewski J, et al: Prostate cancer: Local staging with endorectal surface coil MR imaging. Radiology 178:797–802, 1991.

8. RADIONUCLIDE STUDIES

Donald R. Bodner, M.D., and David Levy, M.D.

1. What is meant by the term "nuclear renogram"?
A nuclear renogram is the activity-vs.-time graph that is generated from the kidney after administration of a radionuclide. Studies are performed to document such factors as differential function of each kidney, renal perfusion, renal obstruction, and rejection.

2. Which radioactive nuclide is most commonly used in nuclear medicine?
Technetium (Tc) 99m is the most commonly used nuclide. It is ideal for examinations taking less than 24 hours, because it has a half-life of 6 hours. The common agents used today for nuclear renograms include Tc 99m diethyltriamine pentaacetic acid (DTPA), Tc 99m MAG3, dimercaptosuccinic acid (DMSA), and [131]iodine (131-I) hippurate.

3. In an adult with suspected atherosclerotic vascular disease and renal insufficiency, which agent is most helpful in assessing renal blood flow?
DTPA is best used in a dynamic fashion for vascular imaging. Analysis is based on observing the intensity and symmetry of kidney visualization. Peak activity in the kidney should be no more than 3 seconds after peak activity is noted in the aorta.

4. In a child with a history of pyelonephritis, what is the most useful agent in assessing renal parenchyma scarring?
DMSA provides detailed anatomic imaging, because it accumulates in the kidneys over several hours. Delayed views show better images of the renal cortex. DMSA is also helpful for interval imaging of the renal cortex.

5. What agents can be used in chronic renal failure?
123-I or 131-I hippurate is the recommended agent, because renal concentration may occur with as little as 3% of normal renal function. Technetium compounds may be preferred when renal vascular problems are suspected, and MAG3 may prove superior to hippurate.

6. When is MAG3 the preferred radionuclide?
MAG3 imaging sequence is similar to DTPA and is often used in the pediatric population, because considerably less uptake in the liver and spleen allows more accurate assessment of renal function.

7. When should Lasix (furosemide) be given during a Lasix renogram?
Lasix should be given when the suspected kidney has the peak number of counts of the radionuclide in the collecting system.

8. What is meant by a superscan noted on a bone scan of a patient with prostate cancer?
A superscan refers to extensive bony involvement of the axial skeleton, which results in intense uptake of the radionuclide in the bone and no uptake by the kidneys.

9. What other nuclear tests are available to the urologist?
Testicular blood flow studies may be performed to aid in the differential diagnosis of testicular torsion and epididymitis. Bone scans are used commonly in the work-up of metastatic

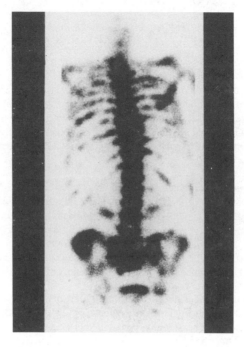

Positive bone scan in metastatic carcinoma of the prostate.

disease of the prostate and other urologic malignancies. Metaiodobenzylguanidine (MIBG) is a tracer that identifies sympathetic activity and may be helpful in localizing ectopic pheochromocytomas.

BIBLIOGRAPHY

1. Croft BY, Joyce JN, Teates CD: Nuclide studies: In Gillenwater JY, Grayhack JT, Howards SS, Duckett JW (eds): Adult and Pediatric Urology, 2nd ed. St. Louis, Mosby, 1991, pp 189–213.
2. Foreman J: The role of radionuclide studies in urologic patient management. Probl Urol 3:531–547, 1989.

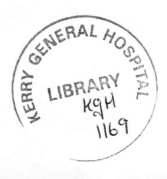

9. RENAL MASS EVALUATION

Andrew C. Novick, M.D.

1. How are renal masses usually detected?

Suggestive symptoms such as abdominal or flank pain, hematuria, or a palpable flank mass on physical examination may prompt radiographic evaluation for a renal mass. An increasing number of renal masses, however, are currently being detected in asymptomatic patients who undergo a noninvasive abdominal imaging study, such as ultrasonography or CT, for an unrelated reason. As many as 50% of all renal cell carcinomas are being detected incidentally in this manner.

2. What is the differential diagnosis of a renal mass in an adult?

1. Benign renal cyst
2. Abscess
3. Hematoma
4. Infarct
5. Vascular malformation
6. Benign mesenchymal tumor
7. Renal pseudotumor
8. Metastatic carcinoma
9. Angiomyolipoma
10. Oncocytoma
11. Transitional cell carcinoma
12. Renal cell carcinoma

3. Which radiographic tests are helpful in establishing the diagnosis of a renal mass?

The available imaging modalities include intravenous pyelography (IVP), ultrasonography, CT, MRI, and renal arteriography. Occasionally, percutaneous aspiration of a renal cyst or percutaneous biopsy of solid renal mass may provide usual diagnostic information.

4. Compare the relative merits of ultrasound, IVP, CT, and MRI in evaluating a renal mass.

IVP with or without nephrotomography can detect many renal masses but may not always distinguish solid from cystic lesions. IVP will also fail to demonstrate small anterior or posterior masses that do not distort the architecture of the kidney.

Ultrasonography is reliable in differentiating solid tissue from fluid and can reliably establish the diagnosis of a simple renal cyst. It can also allow the diagnosis of an angiomyolipoma by the characteristic increased echogenicity produced by fat.

CT scanning is the single most important radiographic test for delineating the nature of a renal mass. CT, with and without contrast administration, is recommended to take full advantage of the enhancement characteristic of highly vascular renal parenchymal tumors. Solid masses with areas of negative CT attenuation numbers (Hounsfield units) indicative of fat are diagnostic of angiomyolipoma. In approximately 10% of renal masses, CT is indeterminate and additional tests or surgical exploration are needed to establish a definitive diagnosis.

MRI offers no diagnostic advantage over ultrasound or CT in characterizing the nature of a renal mass. Because ultrasound and CT are considerably less expensive and easier to obtain, MRI is not recommended for primary evaluation of a renal mass.

5. Explain the difference between a simple renal cyst and a complex renal cyst.

A **simple renal cyst** is a benign lesion and appears as a round, well-marginated mass on ultrasound or CT with a thin smooth wall. A simple renal cyst is anechoic on ultrasound; on CT it demonstrates a low density (< 20 Hounsfield units) with no contrast enhancement.

A **complex renal cyst** has one or more features that may be indicative of malignancy, such as internal septations, calcium in the cyst wall or septum, high density or heterogeneous internal appearance, irregular margin, or areas with contrast enhancement on CT scan. Complex cysts with thin septa or calcium in the cyst wall or septum are most likely benign; however, the other listed features are more suggestive of renal cell carcinoma.

6. What is a renal pseudotumor?

An area of normal renal parenchyma that gives the appearance of a solid renal mass. A renal pseudotumor may represent a hypertrophied column of Bertin, an area of segmental renal hypertrophy, or an unusually shaped kidney. The diagnosis can be established with a technetium dimercaptosuccinic acid (DMSA) renal scan, which will demonstrate increased uptake of isotope with a pseudotumor and decreased uptake of isotope with a cystic or solid renal mass.

7. Is arteriography useful in evaluating a renal mass?

There are relatively few indications for arteriography during the diagnostic evaluation of a renal mass. Most renal cell carcinomas demonstrate neovascularity, while metastatic renal tumors and transitional cell carcinomas are relatively avascular. However, 15–20% of renal cell carcinomas are also avascular. Currently, the major value of arteriography is as an adjunct to surgery in selected patients.

8. When should percutaneous aspiration of a renal cyst or percutaneous biopsy of a renal mass be performed?

If a renal cyst remains equivocal after CT scanning, **aspiration** of fluid from it is occasionally helpful. The presence of abnormal cytologic findings or blood in the aspirate is suggestive of malignancy and may indicate a need for surgical exploration. **Percutaneous biopsy** of a solid renal mass is indicated when a metastatic lesion, abscess, or infected cyst is suspected. Routine biopsy of solid renal masses is not recommended due to a high incidence of false-negative findings in patients with renal cell carcinoma.

9. Outline the appropriate evaluation for an indeterminate renal mass observed on IVP in an asymptomatic patient.

If a mass is demonstrated on IVP, the next step is an ultrasound study. If this demonstrates a simple renal cyst, further evaluation is usually unnecessary. The demonstration of fat within a solid mass on ultrasound indicates an angiomyolipoma. Other solid or complex cystic masses require further evaluation with a CT scan. Contrast enhancement of a solid mass on CT scanning indicates renal cell carcinoma until proven otherwise, although approximately 10% of such masses may prove to be benign (an oncocytoma or adenoma). An indeterminate renal mass on a CT scan may be evaluated further with arteriography or percutaneous biopsy. With this approach, it is currently possible to establish the diagnosis of a renal mass in most patients.

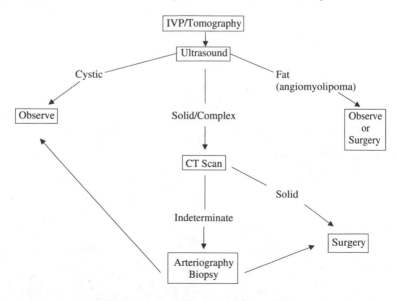

BIBLIOGRAPHY

1. Bosniak MA: Problems in the radiologic diagnosis of renal parenchymal tumors. Urol Clin North Am 20:217, 1993.
2. DeKernion JB, Beidegrun A: Renal tumors. In Walsh PC, Retik AB, Stamey TA, Vaughn ED Jr (eds): Campbell's Urology, 6th ed. Philadelphia, W. B. Saunders, 1992.
3. Levine E: Malignant renal parenchymal tumors in adults. In Pollack HM (ed): Clinical Urography. Philadelphia, W. B. Saunders, 1990.
4. Williams RD: Renal, perirenal and ureteral neoplasms. In Gillenwater JY, Grayhack JT, Howards SS, Duckett JW (eds): Adult and Pediatric Urology, 2nd ed. St. Louis, Mosby, 1991.

10. ABDOMINAL MASSES IN CHILDREN

Jack S. Elder, M.D.

1. In a newborn, what is the most common cause of an abdominal mass?
Hydronephrosis, usually secondary to a ureteropelvic junction obstruction.

2. What is the second most common cause of an abdominal mass in the neonate?
Multicystic kidney.

3. How common are tumors as causes for an abdominal mass in a neonate?
Tumors account for approximately 12% of neonatal abdominal masses.

4. What types of neoplasms occur in neonates that may result in an abdominal mass?
The most common tumors in the newborn include neuroblastoma, mesoblastic nephroma, and sacrococcygeal teratoma. Less common tumors include gastric teratoma, leiomyosarcoma, and hepatoma.

5. Of solid renal tumors in neonates, how common is Wilms' tumor?
Wilms' tumor is extremely uncommon in the newborn. A solid renal tumor is much more likely to be a mesoblastic nephroma.

6. From 1 month to 1 year of age, what are the two most common causes of an abdominal mass?
Hydronephrosis accounts for 40% and tumor for 40%.

7. In children more than 1 year old, what is the most common cause of an abdominal mass?
Tumor.

8. In a neonate, what is the most common cause of hydronephrosis?
Ureteropelvic junction obstruction.

9. What are three other causes of hydronephrosis in the neonate?
Ureterovesical junction obstruction, ectopic ureterocele, and posterior urethral valves.

10. In neonates, what proportion of abdominal masses are caused by genitourinary disorders?
Approximately 75% are caused by genitourinary masses in neonates.

11. What is the initial radiologic examination of choice in children with an abdominal mass? What information does it provide?
Ultrasonography is the initial radiologic study. This test often identifies the organ from which the mass is originating and shows whether it is fluid-filled or solid.

12. If ultrasonography identifies hydronephrosis, what is the next test that should be performed?
A voiding cystourethrogram should be performed to determine whether there is vesicoureteral reflux. In addition, the study may show whether there is a ureterocele or, in a boy, posterior urethral valves.

13. At what age is neuroblastoma more common than Wilms' tumor?
Neuroblastoma is more common in children < 2 years of age, whereas Wilms' tumor is more common in children > 2 years of age.

14. What is aniridia? What is its significance?
Aniridia is developmental absence of most of the iris. Spontaneous aniridia is associated with Wilms' tumor.

15. What is the significance of microcephaly?
Microcephaly is associated with posterior urethral valves and also occurs in Beckwith-Wiedemann syndrome.

16. In which syndrome is macroglossia common?
It is common in Beckwith-Wiedemann syndrome, in which renal and adrenal tumors are also common.

17. What is the significance of hemihypertrophy?
In children with hemihypertrophy, Wilms' tumor is more common.

18. Webbing of the neck is a sign of what syndrome?
It is a sign of Turner's syndrome, in which a horseshoe kidney is the most common renal anomaly.

19. What is the meaning of respiratory distress or pneumothorax in a neonate with an abdominal mass?
These conditions are commonly associated with severe obstructive renal disorders, most commonly posterior urethral valves and urethral atresia.

20. What is the significance of bright pink or bluish subcutaneous nodules in the newborn?
They may indicate the presence of disseminated neuroblastoma.

21. What is the typical appearance of a multicystic kidney on ultrasonography?
This condition consists of multiple cysts of varying sizes without overlying renal parenchyma.

22. What is the significance of hypertension in a child with an abdominal mass?
It may be indicative of neuroblastoma, congenital mesoblastic nephroma, and less commonly Wilms' tumor, hydronephrosis, or multicystic kidney.

23. Describe the two types of polycystic kidneys. What are the ultrasound findings in each type?
Polycystic kidneys may be autosomal recessive or autosomal dominant. The autosomal recessive form, also termed infantile, is more common in neonates. In this type, ultrasound shows enlarged, severely echogenic kidneys because there are numerous tiny cysts. In infants with autosomal dominant polycystic kidney disease (also termed the adult form), the kidneys are enlarged and contain multiple large cysts of varying sizes. In some cases hepatic cysts also occur.

24. What is the significance of hematuria in a newborn with an abdominal mass?
Hematuria may be indicative of renal vein thrombosis.

25. What is the most likely diagnosis of an abdominal mass in a female neonate if there is also a bulging interlabial mass?
Hydrocolpos secondary to an imperforate hymen.

26. What is the significance of stippled calcification in a retroperitoneal solid mass?
Approximately 50% of patients with neuroblastoma have stippled calcification.

27. Which tumor is more likely to be fixed rather than mobile, neuroblastoma or Wilms' tumor?
Neuroblastoma.

28. Which abdominal masses are most likely to be mobile?
Masses in the ovaries, mesentery, and intestine.

29. Name the two primary causes of masses arising from the female genital system.
Hydrocolpos and ovarian cysts.

30. How often are the kidneys palpable in the neonate?
Both kidneys are usually palpable in the neonate.

31. If a renal mass with multiple cysts is detected on ultrasound, there is contralateral vesicoureteral reflux, and a renal scan shows that the mass has no function, what is the most likely diagnosis?
Multicystic kidney.

32. If the mass is found to be in the anterior abdomen, what are the most likely diagnoses?
Duplication anomaly of the gastrointestinal tract, mesenteric cyst, and intestinal atresia.

BIBLIOGRAPHY

1. Elder JS, Duckett JW: Perinatal Urology. In Gillenwater JY, Grayhack JT, Howards SS, Duckett JW (eds): Adult and Pediatric Urology, 2nd ed. St. Louis, Mosby, 1991, pp 1711–1810.
2. Elder JS, Klacsmann PG, Sanders RC, et al: Clinicopathological conference: Flank mass in a neonate. J Urol 126:94, 1981.
3. Gore RM, Shkolnik A: Abdominal manifestation of pediatric leukemias: Sonographic assessment. Radiology 143:207, 1982.
4. Kaplan GW, Brock WA: Abdominal masses. In Kelalis PP, King LR, Belman AB (eds): Clinical Pediatric Urology, 2nd ed. Philadelphia, W. B. Saunders, 1985, pp 57–75.
5. Parrott TS, Woodard JR: Urologic surgery in the neonate. J Urol 116:506, 1976.
6. Selzman AM, Elder JS: Contralateral vesicoureteral reflux in children with a multicystic kidney. J Urol, 1994, in press.

11. EVALUATION OF ACUTE SCROTAL SWELLING IN CHILDREN

Jonathan H. Ross, M.D.

1. List six causes of acute scrotal swelling in children.
Spermatic cord torsion (testicular torsion), torsion of the appendix testis, epididymo-orchitis, hernia, hydrocele, and testis tumor. The last three usually do not present acutely but may on occasion.

2. What are the physical findings suggestive of testicular torsion?
An extremely tender testis that is high-riding is typical of testicular torsion. The cremasteric reflex is often absent, the cord is thick or difficult to distinguish, and elevation of the testis offers no relief (as it may in epididymitis). Although these findings are typical or suggestive of testicular torsion, their absence does not exclude the possibility.

3. Explain the difference between intravaginal and extravaginal torsion.
Typically, testicular torsion is intravaginal—it occurs within the tunica vaginalis. Thus, on exposure of the testicle, the hydrocele sac is opened (the tunica vaginalis) and the torsed cord and testis are inside. In newborns, the tunica vaginalis is not adherent to the surrounding dartos fascia. Hence, the testis and processus vaginalis and tunica vaginalis can torse as a unit (extravaginal torsion). Because the tunica vaginalis becomes adherent to the dartos fascia within the first weeks of life, extravaginal torsion does not occur beyond the newborn period.

4. Do any anatomical features predispose to testicular torsion?
Yes (or I wouldn't have asked the question). The "bell-clapper deformity" results from a variation in the way in which the tunica vaginalis reflects on the testis. This anatomic variant can be detected on physical examination and predisposes to testicular torsion. In patients with a bell-clapper deformity, the testes have a horizontal lie with the long axis oriented in the anteroposterior direction. The variant is bilateral, explaining the risk of metachronous contra-lateral torsion in patients who have experienced a testicular torsion.

5. How is testicular torsion treated surgically?
Bilateral scrotal orchidopexy. Through a scrotal incision, the torsed testis is detorsed and, if viable, fixed to the scrotal wall at three points. Contralateral orchidopexy is also performed because of the high risk of metachronous contralateral torsion.

6. Does testicular torsion always present as a single acute event?
No. Patients with recurrent testicular pain and swelling who have a bell-clapper deformity may be suffering from intermittent torsion. In this condition, the testis torses, resulting in symptoms, but spontaneously detorses within a short time. In patients with a convincing history and the bell-clapper deformity, bilateral scrotal orchidopexy should be considered.

7. What is the "blue dot" sign?
A torsed appendix testis has a bluish hue when viewed through the scrotal skin. A "blue dot" at the upper pole of the testis on physical examination suggests the diagnosis. In the absence of a blue dot, the diagnosis may still be made if scrotal tenderness is isolated to a hard nodule at the upper pole of the testis in the absence of other findings suggesting spermatic cord torsion.

8. How is appendiceal torsion treated?
Nonsteroidal anti-inflammatory drugs (most commonly ibuprofen). The pain usually resolves within 1–2 weeks.

9. What laboratory test is essential in a patient with acute scrotal swelling?
Urinalysis. Significant pyuria is extremely suggestive of epididymitis.

10. What radiographic study should be obtained in a young boy with epididymitis?
Renal ultrasound. Because an ectopic ureter in boys inserts in the wolffian duct structures (e.g., the seminal vesicle or vas), it may present with epididymitis. An ectopic ureter can be detected by hydroureteronephrosis on ultrasound.

11. Which radiographic studies can distinguish testicular torsion from other causes of scrotal swelling?
Radionuclide testicular scan and color-flow Doppler ultrasound. On a radionuclide scan, a torsed testis will appear photopenic. In contrast, epididymo-orchitis results in increased blood flow and, therefore, increased radionuclide. False-positive studies may result from abscess formation or an associated hydrocele. False-negative studies may occur due to scrotal wall hyperemia or, in old torsion, from the inflammatory response. Doppler ultrasonography will demonstrate an absence of blood flow to the testis, although because the intratesticular vessels are small, reliable detection may be difficult. Both studies are very operator dependent, and their availability differs among institutions.

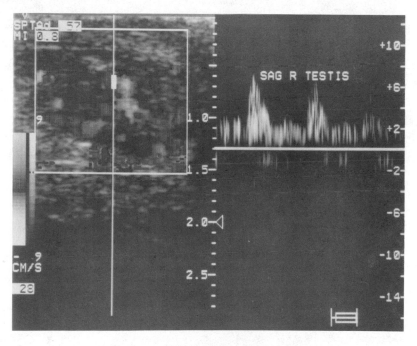

Doppler ultrasound of the testis in a 5-year-old boy with acute testicular pain and swelling demonstrates excellent pulsatile blood-flow consistent with epididymo-orchitis.

12. Name the definitive way to diagnosis testicular torsion.
Surgical exploration. Because time is essential, immediate exploration is indicated in any patient suspected of having testicular torsion. Waiting for a nuclear scan or ultrasound to confirm the diagnosis is inappropriate. Radiographic studies should be reserved for patients who are thought to have a low likelihood of testicular torsion. As with appendicitis, occasional negative explorations are to be expected and are far better than a delayed exploration in a boy who has a torsion.

13. How long before a torsed testicle is no longer salvageable?
Most testicles explored within 6 hours of the onset of symptoms are salvaged. Most testicles explored after 24 hours are not. However, the history is often unreliable. Therefore, the decision of whether to perform an orchidopexy or orchiectomy is based primarily on the appearance of the testis at exploration.

14. In a child with acute scrotal swelling after minor trauma, what is the most important consideration in the differential diagnosis?
A testis tumor may present in this way due to hemorrhage into the tumor.

15. Pus in the scrotum of a young boy should suggest what diagnosis?
Appendicitis. Admittedly, this is a zebra, but it is important to realize that, particularly in infancy, the scrotum is the window to the peritoneum. In many newborns (especially premature infants), the processus vaginalis is patent. Thus, intraperitoneal processes can spread to the scrotum. Other examples are hydroceles in infants with ascites and hard scrotal masses due to dystrophic calcification in infants with meconium peritonitis.

BIBLIOGRAPHY

1. Barada JH, Weingarten JL, Cromie WJ: Testicular salvage and age-related delay in the presentation of testicular torsion. J Urol 142:746–748, 1989.
2. Bartsch G, Frank S, Marberger H, Mikuz G: Testicular torsion: Late results with special regard to fertility and endocrine function. J Urol 124:375–378, 1980.
3. Bartsch G, Mikuz G, Ennemoser O, Janetschek G: Testicular torsion. In Resnick MI, Kursh ED (eds): Current Therapy in Genitourinary Surgery. St. Louis, Mosby, 1992, pp 436–440.
4. Cass AS, Cass BP, Veeraraghaven K: Immediate exploration of the unilateral acute scrotum in young male subjects. J Urol 124:829–832, 1980.
5. Dresner M: Torsed appendage diagnosis and management: Blue dot sign. Urology 1:63–66, 1973.
6. Gislason T, Noronha RFX, Gregory JG: Acute epididymitis in boys: A 5-year retrospective study. J Urol 124:533–534, 1980.
7. Kass EJ, Stone KT, Cacciarelli AA, Mitchell B: Do all children with an acute scrotum require exploration? J Urol 150:667–669, 1993.
8. Kogan SJ: Acute and Chronic Scrotal Swellings. In Gillenwater JY, Grayhack JT, Howards SS, Duckett JW (eds): Adult and Pediatric Urology, 2nd ed. St. Louis, Mosby, 1991, pp 2189–2215.
9. Skoglund RW, McRoberts JW, Ragde H: Torsion of the testicular appendages: Presentation of 43 new cases and a collective review. J Urol 104:598–600, 1970.
10. Steinhardt GF, Boyarsky S, Mackey R: Testicular torsion: Pitfalls of color Doppler sonography. J Urol 150:461–462, 1993.
11. Williams CB, Litvak AS, McRoberts JW: Epididymitis in infancy. J Urol 121:125–126, 1979.

12. EVALUATION OF ACUTE RENAL FAILURE

Stuart M. Flechner, M.D.

1. What is acute renal failure?

Acute renal failure can be defined as any sudden decline in renal function. The degree of renal dysfunction is directly proportional to the decrease in the glomerular filtration rate (GFR) measured in mL/min.

2. How often does acute renal failure occur?

Up to 5% of all hospitalized patients and up to 20% of all patients treated in intensive care units are estimated to experience some degree of acute renal failure. It is associated with increased mortality when it accompanies other potentially life-threatening conditions.

3. How does acute renal failure differ from chronic renal failure?

As compared to chronic renal failure, acute renal failure is usually reversible and limited if the offending cause is identified and proper treatment is instituted. Acute renal failure can lead to permanent renal injury or chronic renal failure in certain circumstances.

4. How does one know if a patient has acute renal failure?

When a sudden decline in renal function has occurred sufficient to raise the level of nitrogenous waste products in the blood above established laboratory control values. This sometimes may also be accompanied by a diminished urine output of < 30 cc/hr in an adult.

5. What is the most accurate test for acute renal failure?

The most accurate measurement of renal function is the GFR. However, its determination can be cumbersome because it requires the use of agents that are removed from the circulation only by filtration at the glomerulus. The clearance of the sugar inulin and certain radioisotopes can be used to accurately measure the GFR.

6. What is the best clinical test to determine if acute renal failure has occurred?

Creatinine clearance. Creatinine is an endogenous product of muscle catabolism produced at a fairly constant rate of about 1 mg/min in an average-sized adult. The clearance of creatinine from the blood approximates the GFR and can be measured on a timed basis such as over 12 or 24 hours. It is calculated by using the formula: UV/P, where U is the urinary concentration of creatinine, V is the rate of urine production over a timed interval, and P is the blood concentration of creatinine. Approximately 80% of creatinine clearance is due to GFR and about 20% is due to renal tubular secretion. Therefore, the result is not as precise as the clearance of an agent removed by GFR alone. Clinically, this becomes important only at low levels of renal function, when tubular secretion may account for a relatively greater percentage of the creatinine clearance.

7. Do other factors affect the serum creatinine?

Body size. Because creatinine is a product of muscle catabolism, large muscular males produce more than small females.

Age. The aging kidney also loses GFR, which results in a higher relative creatinine level.

Trauma. Skeletal muscle injury may raise the serum creatinine, while GFR remains constant.

Drugs. Certain drugs, such as cephalosporins, cimetidine, and trimethoprim, interfere with filtration or tubular secretion and can elevate the serum creatinine.

Despite these other factors, a rising serum creatinine is rare in patients with normal kidney function and remains the best indicator of acute renal failure. In the complete absence of kidney function, the level rises about 1–2 mg/dl/day.

8. Does one have to collect urine for 24 hours?

Renal function can be monitored serially by determining the serum creatinine level alone. The relationship of serum creatinine to creatinine clearance (by inference to the GFR) follows a hyperbolic curve (see figure below). A healthy adult with a serum creatinine concentration of 1 mg/dl has a GFR of about 120 cc/min; a serum creatinine of 2 mg/dl, a GFR of about 60 cc/min, a serum creatinine of 4 mg/dl, a GFR of about 30 cc/min, etc. It is important to note that when the creatinine doubles from 1 to 2 mg/dl, about 50% of renal function has been lost. This steep part of the curve often masks the degree of renal dysfunction present, as the creatinine may remain below 2 mg/dl.

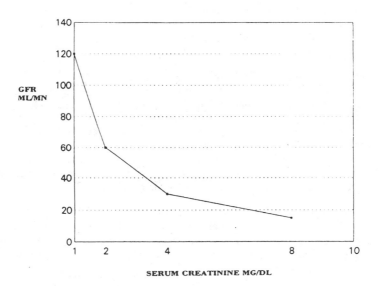

SERUM CREATININE MG/DL

9. Are there other abnormalities associated with acute renal failure?

Yes. Clinical signs and symptoms may include hypertension, fluid overload, congestive heart failure, pericarditis, nausea, vomiting, weakness, lassitude, encephalopathy, and bleeding. Also a number of metabolic abnormalities result from the loss of GFR.

Most Frequent Blood Abnormalities in Acute Renal Failure

INCREASE	DECREASE
Serum creatinine	Serum bicarbonate (acidosis)
Blood urea nitrogen	Free calcium
Serum potassium	Red blood cell mass
Serum phosphorus	Platelet function
Serum magnesium	

10. What causes acute renal failure?

A myriad of insults either alone or in combination can result in kidney dysfunction. For classification they are best thought of as **prerenal**—a decrease in the amount of blood delivered to the kidney; **renal**—a malfunction of the kidney parenchyma; and **postrenal**—obstruction to the flow of urine.

11. Which processes lead to prerenal azotemia?

These insults account for 50–70% of all cases of acute renal failure and produce decreased renal perfusion pressure, resulting in the constriction of the afferent arterioles. These events decrease glomerular capillary pressure and the formation of the glomerular filtrate. To compensate, the tubules avidly reabsorb salt and water, resulting in oliguria.

Prerenal azotemia results from a depletion in the extracellular fluid volume, decreased cardiac output, or direct renal vasoconstriction. Volume loss can result from dehydration, hemorrhage, over-diuresis, burns, diarrhea, sepsis, or sequestration such as crush injuries or pancreatitis. Cardiac output can drop from cardiomyopathy, arrhythmia, coronary artery disease, or cardiogenic shock. Interestingly, volume overload eventuating in congestive heart failure will result in decreased renal perfusion as well. Direct renal vasoconstriction can be precipitated by sepsis, liver disease, and drugs.

Reversible prerenal azotemia can be caused by both angiotensin-converting enzyme (ACE) inhibitors and nonsteroidal anti-inflammatory agents (NSAIDs). ACE inhibitors decrease levels of angiotensin II, resulting in lowered renal perfusion pressure, dilation of the efferent arteriole, and, therefore, lower glomerular capillary filtration pressure. Patients with preexisting renal artery stenosis are particularly susceptible. NSAIDs inhibit the enzyme cyclooxygenase, causing depletion of renal vasodilatory eicosanoids and resulting in afferent arteriolar constriction.

12. Which processes lead to renal azotemia?

These insults account for 20–30% of all cases of acute renal failure, and the most common is acute tubular necrosis (so named for the histopathologic finding of necrotic and regenerating renal tubules with intact basement membranes). Predisposing factors that result in acute tubular necrosis are prolonged prerenal azotemia, nephrotoxic drugs, and pigmenturia. Prolonged prerenal hypoperfusion is the most frequent event. Nephrotoxic drugs such as aminoglycoside antibiotics, iodinated radiographic contrast agents, cisplatin, amphotericin B, and pentamidine are commonly given to hospitalized patients. Patients with diabetes or myeloma are especially susceptible. Pigmenturia caused by intravascular hemolysis or traumatic rhabdomyolysis can lead to acute tubular necrosis.

Other forms of renal azotemia can result from disorders of large and/or small renal blood vessels, including thrombi, emboli, malignant hypertension, hemolytic uremic syndrome, and various forms of vasculitis. Acute glomerulonephritis and interstitial nephritis due to drug allergy or infection may result in acute renal failure.

13. Which processes lead to postrenal azotemia?

These insults are the least common causes of acute renal failure, accounting for < 10% of all cases. Obstructive uropathy can be caused by any process that blocks the flow of urine from the distal tubules to the end of the urethra. Within the kidney, stone crystals or myeloma proteins can obstruct urine flow. Above the bladder, obstruction to both renal collecting systems or ureters is required. Stones, tumors, clots, fungus balls, extrinsic cancerous lesions, fibrosis, or surgical injuries are the more common etiologies. Benign and malignant prostatic disease represent the major cause of obstruction below the bladder.

14. How does one begin to diagnosis the patient with acute renal failure?

The most reliable way to distinguish among the various causes of prerenal, renal, and postrenal azotemia is to take a careful history and do a careful physical examination, highlighting recent clinical events and drug administration. The most recent vital signs, daily weights, and serial intake and output recordings are essential. Bladder catheterization may be required in the anuric patient and may be diagnostic of lower tract obstruction as well as provide urine for culture and sediment evaluation. Complete anuria is uncommon and usually signifies severe postrenal obstruction or bilateral vascular occlusion.

15. What should one look for in the history?

1. Which drugs have been given, how frequently, and at what doses?
2. Does the patient describe irritative or obstructive voiding symptoms, hematuria, a history of stones, trauma, or previous episodes of acute renal failure?

3. Has there been a history of cardiac disease or those disorders that cause extracellular fluid volume loss (diarrhea, vomiting, burns, etc.)?

4. Has the urinary tract or abdominal vasculature been instrumented or operated upon?

5. Does the patient have rashes or fevers suggesting allergy?

6. Is there a history of cancer or use of chemotherapy?

16. What findings are suggestive on physical examination?

Prerenal causes may be entertained if volume depletion (negative intake/output or weight loss) is present. Cardiac dysfunction with signs and symptoms of congestive failure (pulmonary edema, peripheral edema, ventricular gallop, jugular venous distention) can also be suggestive. Flank pain, suprapubic distention, and incontinence can suggest obstructive causes. Harsh abdominal bruits or a palpable aortic aneurysm suggest vascular causes. Skin rashes or ecchymoses suggest vasculitis.

17. Is examination of the urine helpful?

Yes. Pyuria points to an infectious or inflammatory etiology, and hematuria suggests stones, trauma or, urinary tract tumors. Well-formed red blood cell (RBC) casts are diagnostic of glomerulonephritis, and specific crystals (uric acid, cysteine, etc.) suggest urinary calculi. A large amount of urinary protein suggests glomerular injury.

A spot urine sodium measurement can help to distinguish prerenal azotemia from acute tubular necrosis. In the prerenal state, the kidney avidly retains salt and water to compensate for decreased perfusion. This produces a sodium concentration generally < 30 mEq/L and a fractional sodium excretion of < 1%. Injured and regenerating tubules found in acute tubular necrosis are unable to reabsorb salt and water efficiently, resulting in concentrations above these levels. Spot urine chemistries are not usually helpful in cases of postrenal obstruction.

Culture of the urine can be diagnostic in cases of bacterial or fungal infection.

Urine Findings in Acute Renal Failure

CAUSES OF AZOTEMIA	URINE SEDIMENT	FRACTIONAL Na EXCRETION AND Na CONCENTRATION
Prerenal	Rare hyaline casts, usually normal	<1%, <30 mEq/L
Renal		
Tubular necrosis	Tubular epithelial cells granular casts	>1%, >30 mEq/L
Interstitial nephritis	Pyuria with white blood cell casts, eosinophils	Similar to tubular necrosis, nondiagnostic
Glomerulonephritis	Proteinuria, high molecular weight; RBCs and RBC casts	Similar to prerenal, nondiagnostic
Vascular disorders	RBCs may be present	Similar to prerenal nondiagnostic
Postrenal		
Stones	Crystals, fragments, hematuria, pyuria	Nondiagnostic
Tumors	Malignant cytology	Early disease may be similar to prerenal
Extrinsic compression	May be normal	Late disease may be similar to postrenal

18. Are blood tests helpful in making the diagnosis?

The hemogram can provide supportive information. Leukocytosis may be present in septic patients, and eosinophilia suggests an allergic interstitial disease. Abnormal RBC morphology and hemolysis can point to the hemolytic uremic syndrome. Low platelet counts suggest hemolytic uremic syndrome or thrombotic thrombocytopenic purpura. Sickled RBCs are pathognomonic for sickle cell disease.

19. When are radiographic tests helpful?

If diminished renal perfusion is suspected, an **isotope renal scan** can document the presence of renal blood flow as well as differences between the two kidneys. If more specific anatomic information is required, a **renal arteriogram** and/or **renal venogram** will precisely define stenoses, occluded segments, aneurysms, etc. of the renal vasculature. In cases where postrenal obstruction is suspected, an **excretory urogram** or an **ultrasound** examination of the kidneys is useful. Most cases of hydronephrosis can be determined by these tests. More definitive anatomic information can be provided by a CT scan or MRI examination of the abdomen and pelvis.

20. Is any one test most reliable in determining the cause of acute renal failure?

No. The history and physical examination should direct the clinician to one of several possibilities. If other methods are nondiagnostic, the renal biopsy (either percutaneous or open) can provide definitive information as to vascular, tubular, or glomerular pathology.

21. Can acute renal failure be prevented?

Not always. However, certain measures can diminish renal injury if instituted promptly. Dehydration, especially in the elderly, is a universal problem. Replacement of fluids in cases of burns, trauma, surgery, lymphatic loss, and infection is essential. Likewise, inducing diuresis with loop diuretics, volume expansion, and mannitol can be helpful in cases due to pigmenturia, contrast agents, myeloma, crystalluria, and nephrotoxins. The use of known nephrotoxic drugs should be monitored, and dose adjustments made as indicated by the level of renal function. Nephrotoxic agents should be avoided in high-risk patients.

22. How is acute renal failure treated?

The key to effective treatment is making the correct diagnosis. Removal of an offending drug, restoring euvolemia, normalizing cardiac performance, and relieving obstruction are the essential remedies.

Nonoliguric renal failure is easier to manage than oliguric renal failure. Therefore, diuretics may be helpful. Ensuring adequate nutrition is also helpful. Other abnormalities such as hyperkalemia, hyperphosphatemia, acidosis, and anemia should also be corrected. Some suggest that low doses of dopamine may improve renal perfusion. When obstruction cannot be promptly relieved, a percutaneous nephrostomy tube can temporarily relieve more distal obstruction and restore metabolic imbalance. Ultimately, if acute renal failure is severe causing systemic metabolic toxicity, temporary hemodialysis or peritoneal dialysis is required.

BIBLIOGRAPHY

1. Davidman M, et al: Iatrogenic renal disease. Arch Intern Med 151:1809–1810, 1991.
2. Gurwitz JH, et al: Nonsteroidal anti-inflammatory drug associated azotemia in the very old. JAMA 264:471–473, 1990.
3. Hou SH, et al: Hospital acquired acute renal insufficiency: A prospective study. Am J Med 74:242–245, 1983.
4. Kaufman J, et al: Community acquired acute renal failure. Am J Kidney Dis 17:191–194, 1991.
5. Levinsky NG, Alexander EA, et al: Acute renal failure. In Brenner B, Rector F (eds): The Kidney. Philadelphia, W. B. Saunders, 1991, pp 1181–1236.
6. Shusterman N, et al: Risk factors and outcome of hospital acquired acute renal failure. Am J Med 83:65–68, 1987.
7. Weinberger HD, Andersen RJ: Prevention of acute renal failure. J Crit Care 6(2):95–99, 1991.

13. EVALUATION OF HYDRONEPHROSIS IN CHILDREN

Robert Kay, M.D.

1. Is hydronephrosis the same as upper tract obstruction?
No. Hydronephrosis, which is the dilatation of the urinary tract, may be seen with obstruction, vesicoureteric reflux, or nonobstructive uropathy such as megacalycosis.

2. In children, hydronephrosis is best detected by what test?
Without question, **screening ultrasound** is the best test to anatomically define the kidney. It is noninvasive, inexpensive, and very accurate and involves no radiation in determining the presence or absence of hydronephrosis.

3. Can ultrasound determine the level of obstruction?
An experienced ultrasonographer can determine the level of obstruction. The presence of a dilated ureter suggests lower urinary tract obstruction. Conversely, if no ureter is seen, it is unlikely that the obstruction is beyond the ureteropelvic junction. Other tests, such as a renal scan or retrograde pyelogram, may be needed to confirm the initial suspicion.

4. How is a retrograde or antegrade pyelogram helpful in evaluating obstruction?
Routinely, these may not be needed, but in certain cases, they may be very helpful. Although neither test is a functional test for obstruction, each can define the level of obstruction. A retrograde pyelogram may visualize the most distal level of obstruction. Its disadvantage is in neonatal boys because of the need of urethral manipulation. An antegrade pyelogram may be helpful in neonatal boys or other unique situations.

5. What is the best way to determine if obstruction is present?
If a cystogram has ruled out reflux, a provocative test may be used to assess the functional status of the kidney. If urine transport is impeded, then obstruction is present. This can be tested by overloading the kidney by diuresis and examining with a diuretic intravenous pyelogram or by diuretic renal scan. The kidney may be stressed by a pressure perfusion test (Whitaker test) in which the kidney is stressed by a fluid overload and pressures are measured. An increase in pressure suggests an obstruction.

6. What is the normal washout in a kidney during a diuretic renal scan?
A normal kidney has a characteristic pattern in which initially, there is an increase of the renal isotope as the kidney excretes the isotope into the collecting system followed by rapid clearance of the isotope. When measuring the clearance, the half-life of the renal isotope should be < 10–15 minutes. If the half-life is > 20 minutes, obstruction is likely. Of course, these results must be correlated to the clinical state and other studies.

7. Can false-positive test results occur in the diuretic renal scan?
A flat curve might be seen because of poor renal function and an inability to respond to the diuretic. It may also be seen in severe levels of obstruction. The bladder needs to be drained to rule out an overlapping bladder with isotope as well as bladder causes of obstructive uropathy.

8. What leads to false-negative test results in the diuretic renal scan?
The test may be read as normal if the cursor is not over the area of concern. For example, if distal obstruction is present, the pelvis may appear to clear, but the ureter may be the problem and it needs to be monitored. Also, the test needs to be interpreted carefully in solitary kidneys and neonates.

9. Why was the pressure perfusion test developed?

Originally, the test was created to distinguish obstructed ureters from nonobstructed ureters in valve patients. Some patients with severe posterior urethral valves have severe hydroureteronephrosis which may persist following the oblation of the valves. The test was described by Whitaker in 1973 to confirm his hypothesis that most of these urinary systems were dilated but not obstructed.

10. What is the normal pressure of the urinary system?

Most kidneys have a pressure of 7 cm H_2O or less. The range of normal is up to 15 cm H_2O with perfusion.

11. At what perfusion rate is the Whitaker test done?

To stress the system to superphysiologic levels, a rate of 10 ml/min is used.

12. Obstruction is indicated by what pressure?

Intrarenal pressures > 22 cm H_2O are felt to represent obstruction. This is a subtracted pressure, with the bladder pressure eliminated.

13. Are other tests used in assessing the functional state of obstruction?

Real-time ultrasonography and color-flow Doppler with calculated vascular resistance.

14. If in utero hydronephrosis is noted, when should the kidney be evaluated?

A baby with in utero hydronephrosis should have an ultrasound on day 1 or 2. However, caution must be used in interpretation. Physiologic dilatation, rehydration, and a low urinary output secondary to low levels of neonatal glomerular filtration rate may give erroneous results. If the child is not seriously ill or if there is no evidence of urethral valves, the infants should be placed on prophylactic antibiotics and a repeat sonogram done at 1 month of age. At this time, the glomerular filtration rate will have reached normal levels, dehydration will have resolved, and the physiologic dilatation of the neonate may have disappeared. If hydronephrosis is still present, further evaluation with a voiding cystourethrogram and renal scan should be done.

15. What size of the renal pelvis in the newborn is considered abnormal?

The renal pelvis > 12 mm is usually indicative of significant dilatation and probable abnormalities.

BIBLIOGRAPHY

1. Chung S, Majd M, Rushton HG, Belman AB: Diuretic renography in the evaluation of neonatal hydronephrosis: Is it reliable? J Urol 150:765, 1993.
2. Dejter SW, Gibbons MD: The fate of infant kidneys with fetal hydronephrosis but initially normal postnatal sonography. J Urol 142:661, 1989.
3. Homsy YL, Saad F, Laberge I, et al: Transitional hydronephrosis of the newborn and infant. J Urol 144:579, 1990.
4. Kass EJ, Majd M, Belman AB: Comparison of the diuretic renogram and the pressure perfusion study in children. J Urol 134:92, 1985.
5. Koff SA, Thrall JH, Keyes JW: Diuretic radio-nuclei urography: A non-invasive method for evaluating nephroureteral obstruction. J Urol 122:451, 1979.
6. O'Reilly PH: Investigation of obstructive uropathy. In O'Reilly PH, George NJ, Weiss RM (eds): Diagnostic Techniques in Urology. Philadelphia, W. B. Saunders, 1990.
7. Palmer JM, Lindfords KK, Ordorica RC, Marder DM: Diuretic Doppler sonography in postnatal hydronephrosis. J Urol 146;605, 1991.
8. Weiss RM: Obstructive uropathy: Pathophysiology and diagnosis. In Kelalis PP, King LR, Belman AB (eds): Clinical Pediatric Urology, 3rd ed. Philadelphia, W. B. Saunders, 1992, pp 664–682.
9. Whitaker RH: Methods of assessing obstruction in dilated ureters. Br J Urol 45:15, 1973.

14. IMPOTENCE

Drogo K. Montague, M.D. and Milton M. Lakin, M.D.

1. What is impotence?
Impotence (the preferred term is erectile dysfunction) is the persistent inability to obtain or maintain a penile erection adequate for coitus.

2. How common is erectile dysfunction?
Erectile dysfunction affects approximately 20 million men in the United States.

3. Describe two types of erectile dysfunction?
Psychogenic erectile dysfunction occurs primarily for psychological reasons. **Organic erectile dysfunction** is secondary to organic disease. Whereas erectile dysfunction may be exclusively psychogenic in origin, organic erectile dysfunction is often associated with varying degrees of psychological factors.

4. How do the relative frequencies of psychogenic and organic erectile dysfunction vary with age?
The incidence of erectile dysfunction is relatively low in young men but progressively increases with age. In men under age 35, psychogenic erectile dysfunction is probably more common than organic erectile dysfunction. In contrast, in men over age 50, erectile dysfunction is more likely to be organic rather than psychogenic.

5. What are the organic causes of erectile dysfunction?
The term **IMPOTENCE** itself is a useful mnemonic:*

			Examples
I	=	Inflammatory	Prostatitis
M	=	Mechanical	Peyronie's disease
P	=	Postsurgical	Radical prostatectomy
O	=	Occlusive vascular	Atherosclerosis
T	=	Traumatic	Pelvic fracture
E	=	Endurance factors	Chronic renal failure
N	=	Neurogenic	Multiple sclerosis
C	=	Chemicals	Antihypertensive drugs
E	=	Endocrine	Diabetes mellitus

*Modified from Smith AD: Urol Clin North Am vol 8:83, 1981.

6. List the ten elements in the evaluation of a man with erectile dysfunction.

1. Sexual history
2. Medical history
3. Psychologic evaluation
4. Physical examination
5. Blood studies
6. Nocturnal penile tumescence
7. Duplex ultrasonography
8. Cavernosometry
9. Cavernosography
10. Penile arteriography

7. Are there any conditions likely to be confused with erectile dysfunction?
Men with premature ejaculation or hypoactive sexual desire (low libido) may be mistakenly thought to have problems obtaining or maintaining erections.

8. What is nocturnal penile tumescence (NPT)?
NPT is a test to help differentiate psychogenic from organic erectile dysfunction. Because penile rigidity and not just tumescence is required for coitus, NPT testing should record

both penile tumescence and rigidity. With some exceptions, NPT in men with psychogenic erectile dysfunction is normal, whereas in men with organic erectile dysfunction it is either absent or impaired.

9. How are vasoactive drugs used in the diagnostic evaluation of erectile dysfunction?
Vasoactive drugs such as papaverine, phentolamine, or prostaglandin E_1 promote cavernosal arterial dilatation and cavernosal smooth muscle relaxation. These drugs are injected into the penile corpora cavernosa at the time of duplex ultrasonography, cavernosometry, cavernosography, and penile arteriography to evaluate the arterial and veno-occlusive components of erectile function.

10. How is duplex ultrasonography used in the diagnostic evaluation of erectile dysfunction?
Duplex ultrasonography is used to evaluate the cavernosal arteries and thus the arterial inflow into the corpora cavernosa of the penis. After the intracavernosal injection of vasoactive drugs, a duplex ultrasound scanner images the cavernosal arteries and determines the velocity of blood flow through these vessels.

11. What are cavernosometry and cavernosography?
These test are also performed after intracavernosal injection of vasoactive drug to evaluate the veno-occlusive mechanisms of the corpora cavernosa. Cavernosometry measures intracavernosal pressures while saline flow rates needed to obtain and maintain full erection are determined. In cavernosography, contrast is infused into the corpora cavernosa, and radiographic imaging is performed to document pathways of any venous leakage from the corpora.

12. List the treatments for erectile dysfunction.
1. Sex therapy
2. Medical therapy
3. Vacuum erection devices
4. Intracavernosal injection therapy
5. Penile prosthesis implantation
6. Arterial revascularization
7. Penile venous ligation
8. Combined therapy

13. What is sex therapy?
Sex therapy, which is most commonly used to treat psychogenic erectile dysfunction, involves treatment, whenever possible, for both the man and his sexual partner. Couple education and behavioral therapy are used in an attempt to reestablish normal sexual function.

14. How is medical therapy used in the treatment of erectile dysfunction?
1. **Withdrawal of offending medication.** When the onset of erectile dysfunction is associated with the administration of a new medication, it is appropriate, whenever possible, to select another drug with less potential to affect erectile function.
2. **Hormonal therapy.** Men with hypogonadism and erectile dysfunction may benefit from parenteral testosterone administration. Men with erectile dysfunction and hyperprolactinemia can usually be treated successfully with the oral medication bromocriptine. Significant hypogonadism or hyperprolactinemia in men with erectile dysfunction is, however, rather infrequent.

15. Describe how vacuum erection devices are used to treat erectile dysfunction.
Vacuum erection devices have three parts: an acrylic chamber which fits over the penis, a vacuum pump which is attached to this chamber, and an elastic constriction ring which is applied to the base of the chamber. The patient applies a water-soluble lubricant to his penis and to the inside of the opening to the chamber. He inserts his penis into the chamber and presses the chamber base against his body to create a tight seal. The pump is then used to create a vacuum inside the chamber, which results in an erection-like state. The constriction ring is transferred from the outside of the device to the base of the penis (to maintain the erection), the chamber is removed, and the patient has coitus.

16. What is intracavernosal injection therapy?
The injection of vasoactive drugs (papaverine, phentolamine, and prostaglandin E_1) is useful not only for the diagnosis of erectile dysfunction but also for its treatment. Men using this treatment are taught to inject these drugs into the corpora prior to coitus.

17. What is a penile prosthesis?
Penile prostheses are devices that are surgically implanted into the corpora to produce an erection-like state. There are two types of penile prostheses:

　　1. **Nonhydraulic penile prostheses** are paired rod-like devices that are implanted into the corpora cavernosa to create a permanent penile rigidity, which enables the recipient to have coitus.

　　2. **Hydraulic (inflatable) penile prostheses** consist of paired penile cylinders, a pump, and a fluid reservoir. An erection is created by pumping fluid from the reservoir to the cylinders. Penile flaccidity is achieved by activating a release mechanism that returns cylinder fluid to the reservoir.

18. How successful is penile arterial revascularization?
Various procedures have been developed to treat erectile dysfunction secondary to arterial insufficiency. In young men with traumatic arterial occlusion, these procedures are successful in approximately 70% of cases. In older men with atherosclerotic arterial disease, they are much less successful and seldom performed.

19. How successful is penile venous ligation surgery?
Penile venous resection and ligation has been used to treat erectile dysfunction resulting from impairment of the corporeal-venous occlusive mechanism. Short-term (1–3 years) success rates generally range from 50–60%.

20. What is combined therapy?
Combined sex therapy and medical or surgical treatment of organic erectile dysfunction. By using couple sex therapy to provide education and reduce performance anxiety while medical or surgical treatment is used to correct or compensate for organic factors, it is often possible to achieve optimal treatment results.

BIBLIOGRAPHY

1. Carson CC: Implantation of semi-rigid rod penile prostheses. Urol Clin North Am 1:61–70, 1993.
2. Fuchs AM, Mehringer CM, Rajfer J: Anatomy of penile venous drainage in potent and impotent men during cavernosography. J Urol 141:1353–1365, 1989.
3. Hatzichristou D, Goldstein I: Penile microvascular arterial bypass surgery. Atlas Urol Clinic North Am 1:39–60, 1993.
4. Jarow JP, Pugh VW, Routh WD, Dyer RB: Comparison of penile duplex ultrasonography to pudendal arteriography. Invest Radiol 28:806–810, 1993.
5. Lakin MM, Montague DK: Surgical treatment of the patient with erectile dysfunction: Clinical evaluation and diagnostic techniques. Atlas Urol Clin North Am 1:9–19, 1993.
6. Lakin MM, Montague DK, Vanderbrug-Medendorp S, et al: Intracavernous injection therapy: Analysis of results and complications. J Urol 143:1138–1141, 1990.
7. Lewis RW: Venous surgery in the patient with erectile dysfunction. Atlas Urol Clin North Am 1:21–38, 1993.
8. Lowe MA, Schwartz AN, Berger RE: Controlled trial of infusion cavernosometry in impotent and potent men. J Urol 146:783–758, 1991.
9. Morale A, Condra M, Reid K: The role of nocturnal penile tumescence monitoring in the diagnosis of impotence: A review. J Urol 143:441–445, 1990.
10. Mulcahy JJ: Implantation of hydraulic penile prostheses. Atlas Urol Clin North Am 1:71–92, 1993.
11. Salvatore FT, Sharman GM, Hellstrom WJG: Vacuum constriction devices and the clinical urologist: An informed selection. Urology 38:323–327, 1991.
12. Virag R, Shoukry K, Floresco J, et al: Intracavernous self-injection of vasoactive drugs in the treatment of impotence: eight-year experience in 615 cases. J Urol 145:287–293, 1991.

15. INFERTILITY

Allen D. Seftel, M.D.

1. Define infertility.
Infertility is the inability of a couple to conceive after 1 year of unprotected intercourse.

2. Which partner usually is the cause of the infertility?
Roughly 50% of infertility is due to male factor problems and roughly 50% to female issues.

3. What usually causes male factor infertility?
The most common identifiable cause of male factor infertility is the **varicocele.** While present in approximately 15% of the total population, varicoceles are found in roughly 40% of men with male factor infertility.

4. What is a varicocele?
A varicocele is a dilated vein or set of veins in the pampiniform plexus in the spermatic cord.

5. How does a varicocele cause infertility?
It is believed that the varicocele does not permit efficient blood flow out of the scrotum. Testicles which sit in the scrotum are approximately 2° lower than body temperature and depend on an efficient inflow and outflow system to maintain that temperature. Just as in your automobile's cooling system, the coolant must circulate to maintain the temperature and prevent overheating. If there is stagnation of blood due to an inefficient exit mechanism (i.e., varicose vein), then there may be pooling of blood, an increase in temperature, and an adverse effect on spermatogenesis.

Specifically, the varicocele most commonly causes a "stress" pattern on semen analysis. This would be characterized by a low sperm count (< 20,000,000 sperm/ml), low sperm motility (< 50% motile sperm), and a low sperm morphology (< 15% normal forms using strict criteria developed by Kruger).

6. Are there common characteristics of men with varicoceles?
Most frequently, varicoceles are asymptomatic. On occasion, a varicocele can be large and easily identified by visual inspection (this is called grade 3). Occasionally, they cause pain or a heaviness or fullness in the scrotal area. Grade 2 and grade 1 varicoceles, often referred to as subclinical varicoceles, are not readily identifiable by visual inspection but are seen during physical examination.

7. How does one identify a varicocele?
Examine the patient in a warm room in the standing position. Grade 3 varicoceles are easily identifiable. Grade 1 and 2 varicoceles are identified by placing your right hand on the patient's left spermatic cord and asking the patient to perform a Valsalva maneuver. With the increased abdominal pressure, there may be a rush of blood through this venous plexus. This is a grade 2 varicocele. If this rush of blood is not felt, then a office Doppler can be used to detect the rush of blood. If the rush of blood is heard only with the Doppler, then it is a grade 1 varicocele. A similar procedure is carried out on the right.

8. Are varicoceles unilateral or bilateral?
Historically varicoceles have been thought to occur most commonly on the left side. However, now they are often found to be bilateral. An exclusively right-sided varicocele is unusual.

9. How is a varicocele managed?
Historically they have been repaired surgically by various approaches.

1. **Inguinal approach.** The inguinal canal is opened similar to a hernia repair, and the varicose veins are ligated or excised in that portion of the inguinal canal.

2. **Retroperitoneal approach.** An incision is made near the anterior superior iliac spine, the muscles are retracted, and the veins are ligated as they exit the internal ring.

3. **Subinguinal approach.** A small incision is made inferior to the external ring and the veins are ligated at that site.

4. **Laparoscopic approach.** Through laparoscopic techniques, the veins are ligated high in the retroperineum.

5. **Interventional radiologic approach.** In a minimally invasive technique, the veins are embolized by access through the femoral vein, the vein is cannulated in the retrograde fashion, and then it is embolized by either coils or other embolization material.

10. How successful is varicocele ligation?

Approximately 95% of surgical cases are successful, meaning that varicocele does not recur. Seventy percent of men who have a successful repair will have an improvement in sperm parameters, usually a marked increase in sperm count, sperm motility, and morphology.

11. What are the other common causes of male factor infertility?

Hypogonadotropic hypogonadism is a deficiency of the luteinizing (LH) and follicle-stimulating hormones (FSH), which are important in testosterone and sperm production, respectively. This disorder is manifested by low LH, FSH, and serum testosterone levels. These patients may have severely low sperm counts or may be totally azoospermic.

A blocked exit of sperm from the genital tract will produce infertility and can result from the congenital absence of the vas deferens, which is commonly seen in men with cystic fibrosis, or from a blocked ejaculatory duct. Also possible is retrograde ejaculation in individuals who are diabetic as well as inability to ejaculate in individuals with spinal cord injury. Testicular failure may be due to maturation arrest, in which there is incomplete maturation of the sperm in the testicle. In germinal cell aplasia, also known as Sertoli-cell-only syndrome, the germ cells are absent from the testicle. Finally, other uncommon causes of male factor infertility include occupational exposure or other medical syndromes such as Noonan or Klinefelter syndrome.

12. Does testicular cancer cause infertility?

Men who have testicular cancer who undergo radiation therapy to the abdomen after orchiectomy or retroperitoneal lymph node resection or who have chemotherapy for their malignancy may have impairment of sperm production as a consequence. It is imperative that men with testicular cancer bank sperm prior to the orchiectomy and other adjuvant therapies. In addition, these men may be subfertile prior to therapy.

13. Can any infectious diseases cause infertility?

Prostatitis and other urinary tract infections may predispose to male factor infertility by unknown mechanisms. Other systemic infectious diseases, such as tuberculosis, may cause vasal or epididymal obstruction.

14. What systemic diseases affect fertility?

Leukemia and lymphomas may involve testicular tissue and be associated with male factor infertility. Any type of chemotherapy given systemically for any malignancy may impair spermatogenesis. Thus, any young man facing chemotherapy should be counseled about banking sperm for future use.

15. What is the cardinal sign of testicular failure?

An elevation in serum FSH, usually 1–2 and often 3 times normal.

16. How does the physician treat azoospermia?

If the FSH is elevated, as above, then artificial insemination with donor sperm or adoption are options. If the FSH is normal, then reconstructive surgery (most often an epididymo-vasostomy) is performed. Microscopic sperm aspiration from the epididymis is performed in men with absent vasa. This is combined with in vitro fertilization.

17. How does the physician treat ejaculatory failure?
Vibratory or electroejaculation.

18. How is retrograde ejaculation treated?
A sample of the first urine after ejaculation is obtained and the sperm processed for intrauterine insemination. The patient is asked to take an oral alkalization agent such as sodium bicarbonate prior to ejaculation.

BIBLIOGRAPHY

1. Anguiano A, Oates RD, Amos JA: Congenital bilateral absence of the vas deferens: A primarily genital form of cystic fibrosis. JAMA 267:1994–1997, 1994.
2. Lipschultz LI (ed): Male Infertility. Urol Clin North Am 21(3):1994.
3. Lipshultz LI, Howards SS (eds): Infertility in the Male. New York, Churchill Livingstone, 1991.

16. NEUROGENIC BLADDER

Donald R. Bodner, M.D.

1. What is the role of the autonomic nervous system in micturition?
The autonomic nervous system consists of the parasympathetic and sympathetic nervous systems. The parasympathetic innervation to the bladder originates in the S2–S4 nerve roots and travels via the pelvic nerve or nervi eregentes. These nerve fibers stimulate the cholinergic fibers in the bladder and are responsible for bladder contraction, which produces bladder emptying. The sympathetic innervation to the bladder originates in the thoracolumbar portion of the spinal cord (T10–L2) and richly supplies the bladder neck and proximal urethra. Stimulation of the sympathetic nervous system causes contraction of the alpha fibers in the bladder neck, which closes the bladder neck and relaxes the bladder body, resulting in urinary storage.

2. What is the role of the somatic nervous system in micturition?
The somatic nervous system provides voluntary control to the striated muscle of the external urinary sphincter. Voluntary relaxation of the external sphincter is required to initiate the sacral reflex arc and micturition. The striated sphincter is also responsible for voluntarily stopping the urinary stream.

3. What is the role of the brainstem in normal micturition?
The micturition control center is located in the brainstem. Inhibitory signals are sent from the brainstem when micturition is not appropriate. Typically, stretch receptors from the bladder send signals to the spinal cord when the bladder is full. Were it not for inhibitory signals from the brainstem, urinary urge incontinence would occur, as in patients who suffer a stroke.

4. At what vertebral level does the spinal cord end in the adult?
In the adult the spinal cord ends between the L1 and L2 vertebral levels. Thus a severe injury, such as a burst fracture to the L1 or L2 vertebral body that causes spinal cord injury, may injure the cauda equina or the S2–S4 nerve roots, resulting in a lower motor neuron injury and a flaccid bladder.

5. What is meant by spinal shock?
Spinal shock is a loss of muscle reflexes below the level of spinal cord injury that may last for a period of hours to several months or longer after injury. The bladder initially may have low pressure and no detrusor contraction; then, like the muscles of the lower extremity, it may become spastic.

6. How do the bladder and sphincter function after a complete spinal cord injury above the level of the sacral reflex arc?
With filling of the bladder, stretch receptors send signals to the spinal cord that the bladder is distended, and reflex contractions of the bladder occur. The striated sphincter may become spastic and contract instead of relaxing as the detrusor contracts, thus resulting in bladder outlet obstruction (detrusor–sphincter dyssynergia). This obstruction prevents effective bladder emptying and results in high-pressure voiding with residual urine. Over time, this condition may result in hydronephrosis, vesicoureteral reflux, and eventually renal failure, if not treated.

7. What type of bladder dysfunction is seen in diabetes?
Typically, one thinks of a sensory neurogenic bladder in diabetes. Individuals with longstanding diabetes may not sense that the bladder is full. Persons without diabetes report the first sensation to void on a cystometrogram at approximately 125 cc and become quite uncomfortable at

400–500 cc. Diabetics may not sense that the bladder is full until quite large volumes have accumulated. Treatment consists of timed voiding. Patients must go to the bathroom to void every 3–4 hours by their watch. They are instructed to double-void to ensure that the bladder is empty. If this approach is not effective, treatment consists of intermittent self-catheterization.

8. What urologic manifestations are seen in multiple sclerosis?

Multiple sclerosis is unique in that the voiding problems change with time as the disease changes. The most common finding is uninhibited bladder contractions. Bladder-sphincter dyssynergia also may be seen.

9. What are the urologic manifestations of stroke?

Patients who have had strokes may experience acute urinary retention, and after recuperation the typical finding is urinary urge incontinence. Patients void with a normal bladder pressure, bladder-sphincter synergy, and low postvoid residuals. The pathology in stroke is the loss of inhibitory signals from the brainstem. Treatment consists of anticholinergic medication.

10. What is the most consistent urodynamic finding in patients with neurogenic voiding dysfunction secondary to disc disease?

Detrusor areflexia is the most consistent urodynamic finding in patients with neurogenic voiding dysfunction secondary to disc disease. Most disc protrusions compress the spinal cord at the L4–L5 or L5–S1 disc spaces. Patients generally complain of low back pain with radiation along the path of the involved nerve and difficulty with voiding or urinary retention.

11. What is autonomic dysreflexia? How is it treated?

Autonomic dysreflexia is unopposed sympathetic discharge in patients with spinal cord injury at the level of T6 or above. With distention of the bladder or bowel or a painful stimulus to the lower extremity, autonomic dysreflexia may be triggered. The patient experiences headache, sweating and piloerection. The patient is noted to be hypertensive and bradycardic. Treatments consists of eliminating the noxious stimuli (such as draining the bladder) and placing the patient in a sitting position. If the blood pressure does not come down, medications such as nifedipine or nitroprusside should be used. Untreated autonomic dysreflexia may result in cerebral vascular accidents.

12. What are the goals in the treatment of the neurogenic bladder?

The goals are to maintain kidney function, to prevent infection, and, if possible, to achieve continence. Clean, intermittent catheterization with selective use of anticholinergic medication to lower bladder pressure and to prevent uninhibited bladder contraction is a mainstay of treatment.

BIBLIOGRAPHY

1. De Groat WC: Anatomy and physiology of the lower urinary tract. Urol Clin North Am 20:383–401, 1993.
2. Barrett DM, Wein AJ: Voiding function: Diagnosis, classification and management. In Gillenwater JY, Grayhack JT, Howards SS, Duckett JW: Adult and Pediatric Urology, 2nd ed. St. Louis, Mosby, 1991, p 1001.

II. Benign and Malignant Tumors of the Genitourinary Tract

17. RENAL CELL CARCINOMA

Andrew C. Novick, M.D.

1. What is the prevalence of renal cell carcinoma (RCC)?

In the United States, approximately 27,000 new cases of RCC are detected each year. It accounts for 3% of all adult malignancies and 85% of all primary malignant renal tumors.

2. What is the etiology of RCC?

The etiology of RCC is unknown, with cigarette smoking being the only known risk factor. There is an increased incidence of RCC in patients with von Hippel–Lindau disease, horseshoe kidneys, adult polycystic kidney disease, and acquired renal cystic disease from uremia.

3. Explain the staging systems for patients with RCC.

There are two primary staging systems for renal cell carcinoma. The **Robson system** is simple and easy to use, but the staging categories do not always relate directly to prognosis; for example, stage 3 disease includes isolated renal vein involvement, which carries a good prognosis, as well as lymph node involvement, which is associated with poor survival. The **tumor-node-metastasis** (TNM) system is more detailed in classifying the extent of tumor involvement.

Staging of Renal Cell Carcinoma

	ROBSON STAGE	TNM STAGE
Small tumor, minimal distortion	I	T1
Large tumor, renal distortion	I	T2
Perirenal fat involvement	II	T3a
Renal vein involvement	IIIa	T3b
Infradiaphragmatic vena caval involvement	IIIa	T3c
Invading adjacent structures	IVa	T4a
Superior vena caval involvement	IIIa	T4b
No nodes involved	I, II	N0
Single node involvement	IIIb	N1
Multiple nodes involved	IIIb	N2
Fixed nodes involved	IIIb	N3
Distant metastases	IVb	M1

4. What are the signs and symptoms of RCC?

The most common presenting signs and symptoms are gross or microscopic hematuria, abdominal or flank pain, and a palpable abdominal mass. These findings, the classic triad, will be present in 10–15% of patients. Patients with metastatic disease may present with symptoms of lung or bone metastasis, such as dyspnea, cough, or bone pain. RCC may also be associated with paraneoplastic syndromes such as erythrocytosis, hypercalcemia, hypertension, and nonmetastatic hepatic dysfunction.

5. If the diagnostic evaluation of a renal mass indicates RCC, how do you proceed?
Studies are necessary for clinical staging of the tumor and in preparation for surgery. Routine clinical staging studies include a history and physical examination, complete blood count, renal and hepatic function tests, urinalysis, chest x-ray, and a CT scan of the abdomen and pelvis. A radionuclide bone scan is indicated in patients with bone pain or an elevated serum alkaline phosphatase level. When abdominal CT scanning suggests inferior vena caval involvement, additional imaging with either MRI or contrast inferior venacavography is necessary to establish the presence and extent of vena caval involvement. Renal arteriography is indicated in patients undergoing a complicated partial nephrectomy and in patients with a known vena caval tumor thrombus; in the latter group, if arteriography demonstrates an arterialized tumor thrombus, preoperative angioinfarction can facilitate extraction of the thrombus at surgery.

6. How is a localized unilateral RCC treated?
Surgical excision is the only curative form of treatment for RCC. **Radical nephrectomy** is the treatment of choice for patients with a localized unilateral RCC and a normal-functioning opposite kidney. Radical nephrectomy involves removal of the entire kidney outside Gerota's fascia. The adrenal gland also must be removed if the upper portion of the kidney is involved with malignancy. The benefit of performing a regional lymphadenectomy is controversial.

The 5-year survival rate following radical nephrectomy for Robson stage I RCC is 70–80%. This rate is reduced in the presence of perinephric fat involvement (60–70%), renal vein involvement (50–60%), vena caval involvement (40–50%), extension to regional lymph nodes (5–20%), invasion of adjacent organs (0–5%), and distant metastases (0–5%).

7. When should a nephron-sparing operation (partial nephrectomy) be done for localized RCC?
Nephron-sparing surgery is indicated in patients with localized RCC present bilaterally or in a solitary kidney, since radical nephrectomy would necessitate immediate renal replacement therapy. In recent years, the indications for this surgery have expanded to include other patients in whom preservation of renal function is clinically relevant. Examples of this are patients with unilateral RCC and a functioning but impaired contralateral kidney or patients with unilateral RCC and a contralateral kidney whose function is potentially threatened by a concomitant urologic or systemic disorder. For patients with low-stage RCC, the long-term results of nephron-sparing surgery are comparable to those of radical nephrectomy. The major disadvantage is the risk of postoperative local tumor recurrence, which is seen in 6–10% of patients.

8. What is the approach to RCC involving the inferior vena cava?
For patients with nonmetastatic RCC and inferior vena cava (IVC) involvement, 5-year survival rates of 47–68% have been reported following complete surgical excision. The presence of lymph node or distant metastases in such patients carries a dismal prognosis that is not appreciably altered by radical surgical extirpation. There is a palliative role for surgery in some patients with metastasis who experience severe disability from intractable edema, ascites, cardiac dysfunction, or associated local symptoms such as abdominal pain or hematuria.

When performing radical nephrectomy with removal of an IVC thrombus, it is essential to obtain control of the IVC above the thrombus to prevent intraoperative embolization of a tumor fragment. When the thrombus extends above the diaphragm, a combined thoracic and abdominal surgical approach is necessary. In such cases, adjunctive cardiopulmonary bypass with deep hypothermic circulatory arrest allows extensive IVC thrombi to be completely and safely removed.

9. What are the indications for nephrectomy in patients with metastatic RCC?
Nephrectomy has a palliative role in patients with metastatic RCC who experience severe disability from associated local symptoms, although some patients in this category can be managed with percutaneous renal angioinfarction. In patients with RCC and a solitary resectable metastasis, surgical excision of the primary and metastatic lesion is warranted based on reported

5-year survival rates of 30–35%. Many biologic response modifier protocols to treat metastatic RCC currently require preliminary removal of the primary tumor; however, the advantage of routine preliminary nephrectomy in this setting is not established.

10. How frequently do metastases occur in RCC? How are they treated?

Approximately one-third of patients with RCC have metastatic disease at the time of diagnosis, and an additional 30–50% develop metastatic disease within 5 years. Currently, approximately 11,000 patient deaths occur per year from metastatic RCC in the United States.

Until recently, the treatment for metastatic RCC was relatively ineffective. Various hormonal and cytotoxic chemotherapeutic agents, used individually or in combination, have yielded response rates of < 15%. RCC is not sensitive to radiation therapy, although this modality can provide palliation for patients with symptomatic metastatic lesions. More recently, adoptive immunotherapy with biological response modifiers, such as inferon-α and interleukin-2, has shown promise with response rates as high as 30–40%. However, this form of therapy is investigational and requires further evaluation.

BIBLIOGRAPHY

1. Aso Y, Homma Y: A survey on incidental renal cell carcinoma in Japan. J Urol 137:340, 1992.
2. Figlin RA, Abi-Aad AS, Belldegrun A, deKernion JB: The role of interferon and interleukin-2 on the immunotherapeutic approach to renal cell carcinoma. Semin Oncol 18(5):102, 1991.
3. Fowler JE Jr: Nephrectomy in metastatic renal cell carcinoma. Urol Clin North Am 14:749–756, 1987.
4. Licht M, Novick AC: Nephron-sparing surgery for renal cell carcinoma. J Urol 149:1, 1993.
5. Novick AC, Kaye M, Cosgrove DM, et al: Experience with cardiopulmonary bypass and deep hypothermic circulatory arrest in the management of retroperitoneal tumors with large vena caval thrombi. Ann Surg 212:472, 1990.
6. Robertson CN, Marston WM, Pass HI, et al: Preparative cytoreductive surgery in patients with metastatic renal cell carcinoma treated with adoptive immunotherapy with interleukin-2 or interleukin-2 plus lymphokine activated killer cells. J Urol 144:614, 1990.
7. Robson CJ, Churchill BM, Anderson W: The results of radical nephrectomy for renal cell carcinoma. J Urol 101:297, 1969.
8. Skinner DG, Colvin RB, Vermillion CD, et al: Diagnosis and management of renal carcinoma: A clinical and pathologic study of 309 cases. Cancer 28:1165, 1971.
9. Skinner DG, Pritchett TR, Lieskovsky G, et al: Vena caval involvement by renal cell carcinoma: Surgical resection provides meaningful long-term survival. Ann Surg 210:387, 1989.
10. Thompson IM, Peek M: Improvement in survival of patients with renal cell carcinoma: The role of serendipitiously detected tumor. J Urol 140:487, 1988.
11. Tolia BM, Whitmore WF Jr: Solitary metastasis from renal cell carcinoma. J Urol 114:836, 1975.
12. Tosaka A, Ohya K, Yamada K, et al: Incidence and properties of renal masses and asymptomatic renal cell carcinoma detected by abdominal ultrasonography. J Urol 144:1097, 1990.
13. Williams RD: Renal, perirenal and ureteral neoplasms. In Gillenwater JY, Grayhack JT, Howards SS, Duckett JW (eds): Adult and Pediatric Urology, 2nd ed. St. Louis, Mosby, 1991.

18. PHEOCHROMOCYTOMA

David A. Goldfarb, M.D.

1. What is a pheochromocytoma?

Pheochromocytoma is a tumor derived from chromaffin cells that is associated with pathologic secretion of catecholamines (norepinephrine and epinephrine).

2. Where are they located?

About 90% are located in the adrenal gland; 10% may be extra-adrenal. Most extra-adrenal pheochromocytomas are associated with sympathetic ganglia in the retroperitoneum, but tumors may be found anywhere in the midline in association with the sympathetic chain from the bladder to the base of the skull. Extra-adrenal tumors are often called paragangliomas.

3. Who gets pheochromocytoma?

Most occur in middle-aged adults, but 10% occur in children, in whom they are more likely to be multiple or extra-adrenal. Ten percent occur in patients with multiple endocrine neoplasia (MEN) syndrome.

4. What syndromes are associated with pheochromocytoma?

- MEN (type 2) is composed of pheochromocytoma (often bilateral) in combination with medullary thyroid cancer and hyperparathyroidism.
- MEN (type 3) is pheochromocytoma (often bilateral) in combination with medullary thyroid cancer, mucosal neuromas, thickened corneal nerves, alimentary tract ganglioneuromatosis, and marfanoid habitus.
- Neurofibromatosis
- von Hippel–Lindau disease

5. What is the rule of 10%?

Ten percent of tumors are:
Extra-adrenal
Malignant
Associated with MEN syndromes
Bilateral
Pediatric

6. What are the symptoms?

The symptoms are those of excessive catecholamine secretion and include the classic triad of headaches, sweating, and palpitations. Pheochromocytoma, however, can present with various nonspecific symptoms, including tremors, nausea, dyspnea, fatigue, dizziness, and chest or abdominal pain. An increasing number of patients are being diagnosed without any symptoms other than the incidental finding of an adrenal mass on x-ray evaluation for an unrelated complaint.

7. What are the physical findings?

The most common physical finding is hypertension, which may be sustained or paroxysmal. There may be orthostatic hypotension. Other signs of catecholamine excess include tachycardia, tremor, lean body habitus, and Raynaud's phenomenon. A mass may be noted in the abdomen. There may be signs of a familial syndrome.

8. Who should be evaluated?

Priority for evaluation should be given to patients with:
- Headaches, sweating, and palpitations
- Incidental adrenal mass

- Hypertensive crisis with surgery, anesthesia, or parturition
- Family history of pheochromocytoma

9. How is pheochromocytoma diagnosed?

The diagnosis is based on the finding of excessive catecholamines or their metabolites in blood and/or urine. Resting plasma catecholamines are measured first. Values >2000 pg/ml confirm the diagnosis, and values <500 pg/ml are normal. Values between 500 and 2000 pg/ml are equivocal, and further evaluation with urinary tests or pharmacologic tests is needed. A 24-hour urine collection for metanephrines is the most accurate of the urinary tests. Other 24-hour urinary tests which may show elevated results include vanillylmandelic acid and urinary free catecholamines. To optimize the identification of patients with pheochromocytoma, both plasma and urine testing is recommended.

10. What is pharmacologic testing?

In the hypertensive patient with equivocal plasma catecholamine levels, the clonidine suppression test helps to differentiate between pheochromocytoma and essential hypertension. Clonidine suppresses plasma catecholamines to <500 pg/ml in essential hypertension but has no effect in pheochromocytoma. In patients with equivocal plasma catecholamines and mild hypertension, the glucagon stimulation test is used as a provocative test. It will result in an increase in catecholamines in patients with pheochromocytoma but not with other causes of hypertension. The glucagon stimulation test has the risk of causing severe hypertension but can be performed while patients are on certain antihypertensive medications (calcium channel blockers).

11. How are pheochromocytomas localized?

1. **CT scan of the abdomen or pelvis** is the most common test for localization. It is an excellent initial examination because 97% of tumors are located below the diaphragm and 90% are intra-adrenal.

2. **Magnetic resonance imaging** (MRI) has the advantage of improved soft tissue characterization. Pheochromocytoma has a characteristically high signal intensity on the T2-weighted images. MRI has an improved sensitivity for the identification of multifocal and extra-adrenal disease.

3. **I-Metaiodobenzylguanidine** (MIBG) is a radiopharmaceutical analog of guanethidine that accumulates in pheochromocytomas. Although the sensitivity of MIBG is lower than that for MRI, MIBG scintigraphy can image the whole body. It is useful in cases in which localization is difficult. It can also confirm that an adrenal mass seen on CT is a pheochromocytoma.

12. Describe the preoperative regimen.

The goal of preoperative management is to prevent cardiovascular morbidity due to severe hypertension. The standard medical preparation has been to treat patients with the noncompetitive α-adrenergic blocker, phenoxybenzamine, for 4 weeks before surgery. The newer α-blocking agents, such as prazosin, terazosin, and doxazosin, may also be used, as well as various calcium channel blockers. Occasionally, β-blocking drugs are used to control cardiac arrhythmias. In these cases, α-blockade should be in place first to avoid a paradoxical hypertensive crisis. In addition to medications, many of these patients are volume depleted and require vigorous intravenous hydration the day before surgery.

13. What is the surgical management?

All patients should be maintained with arterial and central venous catheters for hemodynamic monitoring. Rapidly acting vasoactive agents, such as nitroprusside, nitroglycerin, and phentolamine, should be readily available to deal with cardiovascular lability. There should be close communication between surgical and anesthetic teams.

The operative approach depends on the location of the tumors. Traditionally, a transperitoneal approach (subcostal incision) has been used. At exploration, the paravertebral sympathetic chains should be palpated to the level of the aortic bifurcation to identify any new tumors that have escaped radiologic detection. Palpation of the contralateral renal gland is recommended for similar reasons. A steep rise in blood pressure associated with such an exploration is taken as evidence of multifocal tumor. After exploration, pheochromocytomas should be removed with a minimal amount of manipulation, and early ligation of the main adrenal vein should be performed.

Recently, this traditional surgical approach with complete exploration has been challenged in light of the increased accuracy of contemporary imaging techniques (CT, MRI, MIBG). Some groups have advocated selective use of extraperitoneal approaches, such as a flank incision.

14. What is the postoperative management?
Hypotension is a common problem, due to the release from catecholamine-induced vasoconstriction. It should be managed primarily by volume repletion, not vasoconstrictors. Hypoglycemia is occasionally observed and blood glucose should be routinely monitored.

15. What about follow-up?
These patients can develop recurrent or metastatic disease. Blood pressure should be monitored yearly. Repeat biochemical evaluation should be conducted in patients in whom hypertension persists after surgery or recurs at some point in follow-up.

BIBLIOGRAPHY

1. Bravo EL: Pheochromocytoma: New concepts and future trends. Kidney Int 40:544–556, 1991.
2. Greene JP, Gray AT: New perspectives in pheochromocytoma. Urol Clin North Am 16:487–503, 1989.
3. Manger WM, Gifford RW: Pheochromocytoma: Current diagnosis and management. Cleve Clin J Med 60:365–378, 1993.
4. Sheps SG, Jiang NS, Klee GG, vanHeerden JA: Recent developments in the diagnosis and treatment of pheochromocytoma. Mayo Clin Proc 65:88–95, 1990.

19. PRIMARY ALDOSTERONISM

David A. Goldfarb, M.D.

1. Define primary aldosteronism.
It is a secondary cause of hypertension characterized by excessive and unregulated secretion of aldosterone.

2. What are its causes?
An adrenal cortical adenoma is present in 60–80% of cases, whereas bilateral adrenal hyperplasia is responsible for 20–40% of cases. This distinction is important because adenomas respond to surgery, whereas hyperplasia is treated medically.

3. What are the signs and symptoms?
Hypertension is a central feature of the disease. Other symptoms are nonspecific and may include polyuria, nocturia, proximal muscle weakness, and headaches (bitemporal).

4. List the biochemical features of primary aldosteronism.
Hypokalemia
High plasma aldosterone
Low plasma renin activity
Metabolic alkalosis

5. Who should be screened for the disease?
Hypertensive patients with:
- Spontaneous hypokalemia (serum K+ <3.5 mEq/L)
- Moderately severe hypokalemia after conventional diuretic therapy (serum K+ <3.0 mEq/L)
- Refractory hypertension

6. How do you screen for primary aldosteronism?
1. **Hypokalemia** occurs with inappropriate kaliuresis (24-hr urine K^+ >30 mEq, serum K^+ <3.5 mEq/L).

2. **Plasma renin activity** (PRA) is usually low (<1.0 ng/ml/hr), although there is a large overlap with levels seen in essential hypertension. A PRA <3.0 ng/ml/hr after 4 hours of upright posture suggests primary aldosteronism.

3. **Plasma aldosterone** (PA) is physiologically quite variable and is neither sensitive nor specific for the disease. However, a PA/PRA ratio >20 suggests primary aldosteronism.

If several of these features are identified in a hypertensive patient, confirmatory testing should be pursued.

7. How is the diagnosis confirmed?
The best way to confirm the diagnosis of primary aldosteronism is to demonstrate nonsuppressible aldosterone secretion during prolonged salt repletion. This can be accomplished in the outpatient setting by adding 10–12 gm of sodium chloride to the patient's diet for 5–7 days. Then, a 24-hour urine collection for aldosterone and sodium should be obtained. A urinary sodium >250 mEq suggests adequate salt repletion. Urinary aldosterone > 14 µg/24 hr indicates primary aldosteronism.

8. What are the localization procedures?
Computed tomographic (CT) scan of the adrenals should be the first imaging study, as it can identify 90% of adenomas. Sometimes the adenomas are small (<1.0 cm) and beyond the resolution of CT. Bilaterally enlarged adrenals suggest hyperplasia.

Scintigraphy with radiolabeled iodocholesterol (NP59) is a noninvasive test to differentiate between adenoma and hyperplasia. Unilateral concentration of NP59 suggests adenoma, whereas symmetric activity suggests hyperplasia.

Adrenal vein sampling for aldosterone can be performed if the results of CT or NP59 scintigraphy are ambiguous. This is the *most accurate* localization technique. An ipsilateral/contralateral aldosterone concentration ratio of >10:1 implies the presence of an adenoma.

9. Are there any biochemical clues to differentiate adenoma from hyperplasia?
Severe spontaneous hypokalemia (<3.0 mEq/L), plasma 18-OH-corticosterone >100 mg/dl, and anomalous postural decrease in plasma aldosterone are associated with adenoma (but are not present in all cases).

10. What are the indications for surgery?
A patient with biochemical evidence of primary aldosteronism and a unilateral adenoma.

11. Which patients are treated medically?
Those with bilateral hyperplasia or patients with adenoma who are unsuitable surgical candidates.

12. What surgical approach should be used?
An extraperitoneal approach should be used, as these tumors are benign and frequently small. Either a posterior or flank approach can be used, depending on the experience and preference of the surgeon. The posterior approach is the most direct to the adrenal gland.

13. What medications are used to treat primary aldosteronism?
Spironolactone, because it is a potassium-sparing diuretic. Triamterene or amiloride may also be used.

14. Can these tumors be malignant?
Adrenal cortical carcinoma causing only primary aldosteronism is rare, accounting for <1% of these cancers.

BIBLIOGRAPHY

1. Bravo EL: Primary aldosteronism. Urol Clin North Am 16:481–486, 1989.
2. Bravo EL: Primary aldosteronism: New approaches to diagnosis and management. Clev Clin J Med 60:379–386, 1993.
3. Geisinger MA, Zelch MG, Bravo EL, et al: Primary hyperaldosteronism: Comparison of CT, adrenal venography and venous sampling. AJR 141:299–302, 1983.
4. Novick AC: Surgery for primary hyperaldosteronism. Uron Clin North Am 16:535–545, 1989.
5. Novick, AC, Straffon RA, Kaylor W, Bravo EL: Posterior transthoracic approach for adrenal surgery. J Urol 141:254–256, 1989.
6. Young WF, Hogan MJ, Klee GG, et al. Primary aldosteronism: Diagnosis and treatment. Mayo Clin Proc 65:96–110, 1990.

20. ADRENAL CORTICAL ADENOMA AND CARCINOMA

Andrew C. Novick, M.D.

1. What is meant by a functioning adrenal cortical adenoma or carcinoma? What clinical syndromes do they cause?

Adrenal cortical adenomas and carcinomas may be nonfunctioning or functioning. The term *functioning* refers to metabolically active tumors which produce excessive amounts of adrenal cortical hormones. The most common clinical syndromes associated with a functioning adrenal cortical *adenoma* are primary hyperaldosteronism or Cushing's syndrome. The most common clinical syndrome associated with a functioning adrenal cortical *carcinoma* is Cushing's syndrome, although many patients also have evidence of virilization. Feminization occasionally occurs in men with an adrenal cortical carcinoma, whereas aldosterone-secreting adrenal cortical carcinomas are rare.

2. What is Cushing's syndrome?

Cushing's syndrome is caused by excessive adrenal secretion of corticosteroid with a resulting characteristic clinical presentation of truncal obesity, buffalo hump, virilization in the female, impotence or gynecomastia in the male, increased bruising and striae, hypertension, osteoporosis, peripheral extremity muscle wasting, and variable mental aberrations. Cushing's syndrome may be due to a pituitary adenoma (Cushing's disease, 70%), an ectopic ACTH-producing tumor (10%), or primary adrenal cortical tumor (20%).

3. How do you determine if Cushing's syndrome is due to a primary adrenal tumor?

In all cases of Cushing's syndrome, the plasma cortisol level is elevated with loss of normal diurnal variation. In patients with true Cushing's disease due to a pituitary adenoma, the plasma cortisol level is suppressed by administration of exogenous dexamethasone. Those cases of Cushing's syndrome that do not suppress with dexamethasone have either an independently functioning adrenal cortical tumor or an extra-adrenal ACTH-producing tumor. The differentiation between these two conditions is made by measurement of the plasma ACTH, which is high in the latter and low in the former.

4. Which radiographic imaging tests are useful in evaluating a suspected adrenal cortical tumor?

Most adrenal cortical adenomas and carcinomas can be detected with a noninvasive imaging study such as **CT, MRI, or ultrasonography.** These imaging modalities can demonstrate masses as small as 1 cm within the adrenal gland and can detect tumor spread into adjacent organs, regional lymph nodes, or the inferior vena cava.

Arteriography adds little diagnostic information to the above studies and is of value primarily in delineating the vascular supply of a large tumor before surgery. Intravenous pyelography and adrenal venography are no longer useful screening or diagnostic studies in this condition. Some centers continue to employ iodocholesterol scanning to detect small functioning adrenal cortical tumors.

5. In a patient with Cushing's syndrome due to a primary adrenal tumor, how can you determine if the underlying lesion is an adenoma or carcinoma?

ADRENAL CORTICAL ADENOMA	ADRENAL CORTICAL CARCINOMA
Lesion size <6 cm	Lesion size >6 cm
Pure Cushing's syndrome present	Mixed hormonal pattern (i.e., Cushing's and virilization or feminization)
	Markedly elevated 17-ketosteroids
Low signal intensity from tumor on T2-weighted MRI	Hyperintense signal from tumor on T2-weighted MRI

6. Describe the treatment of Cushing's disease.
The primary treatment for Cushing's disease of pituitary origin is **transsphenoidal hypophysectomy,** which is currently successful in about 80–90% of patients. The remaining 10–20% in whom this form of treatment is ineffective require **bilateral surgical adrenalectomy** with subsequently corticosteroid replacement therapy.

7. What is the treatment for Cushing's syndrome due to a primary adrenal cortical tumor?
Surgical adrenalectomy. Small adenomas may be removed through an extraperitoneal surgical incision. Adrenal lesions which are large or potentially malignant are removed transabdominally through either a bilateral subcostal or thoracoabdominal incision.

8. How common is adrenal cortical carcinoma?
Adrenal cortical carcinoma is an uncommon malignancy, with an incidence of 1–2 cases/million population/year.

9. What is the clinical presentation of patients with an adrenal cortical carcinoma?
Approximately 50% of adrenal cortical carcinomas are functioning with symptoms related to excessive adrenal cortical steroid production. The remaining 50% are nonfunctioning tumors, and these patients present with nonspecific symptoms such as abdominal pain, abdominal mass, fatigue, and weight loss. More than half of patients with adrenal cortical carcinoma have regional or distant tumor spread when the diagnosis is established. This is presumably due to the large number of patients with nonfunctioning tumors as well as the remote anatomical location of the adrenal gland deep in the retroperitoneum, which renders it inaccessible to physical examination.

10. Describe the treatment options for patients with an adrenal cortical carcinoma?
Currently, **complete surgical excision** is the only effective form of therapy for patients with adrenal cortical carcinoma. These tumors are not sensitive to radiotherapy, and the results with cytotoxic chemotherapy have been disappointing. Some studies have suggested that survival of patients with metastatic adrenal cortical carcinoma can be prolonged with surgical adrenalectomy followed by adjuvant administration of mitotane (o,p'-DDD).

11. How successful is treatment for adrenal cortical carcinoma?
The prognosis for patients with adrenal cortical carcinoma is relatively poor. In a large series of 82 patients from the Cleveland Clinic, the overall 3- and 5-year survival rates were 37.5% and 25.1%, respectively. The only factor influencing patient survival was the presence of localized (i.e., surgically resectable) disease at initial diagnosis; in these patients, the 3- and 5-year survival rates after excision were 57% and 43.9%, respectively. The 5-year survival rates for patients with regional or metastatic disease were 12.5% and 5.5%, respectively. In patients with regional or metastatic disease, there was no difference in survival among those who received mitotane, cytotoxic chemotherapy, radiation therapy, or none of these treatment methods.

BIBLIOGRAPHY

1. Bellegrun A, Hussain S, Seltzer SE, et al: Incidentally discovered mass of the adrenal gland. Surg Gynecol Obstet 163:203, 1986.
2. Bodie B, Novick AC, et al: Cleveland Clinic experience with adrenal cortical carcinoma. J Urol 141:257, 1989.
3. Brown D, Schumacher OP: Adjuvant therapy, o,p'-DDD in the treatment of metastatic adrenocortical carcinoma. Clin Res 27:626A, 1979.
4. Gold EM: The Cushing's syndrome: Changing views of diagnosis and treatment. Ann Intern Med 90:829, 1979.
5. Guz B, Straffon R, Novick AC: Operative approaches to the adrenal gland. Urol Clin North Am 16:527, 1989.
6. Lipsett MB, Hertz R, Ross GT: Clinical and pathophysiologic aspects of adenocortical carcinoma. Am J Med 35:374, 1963.
7. Mitty HA, Cohen BA: Adrenal imaging. Urol Clin North Am 12:771, 1985.
8. Nader S, Hickey RC, Sellin RV, Samaan NA: Adrenal cortical carcinoma: A study of 77 cases. Cancer 52:707, 1983.
9. Novick AC, Libertino J (eds): Adrenal surgery. Urol Clin North Am 16(Aug):1989.

21. TRANSITIONAL CELL CARCINOMA OF THE RENAL PELVIS

Andrew C. Novick, M.D.

1. How common is transitional cell carcinoma (TCC) of the renal pelvis?
TCC of the renal pelvis comprises 5–7% of all renal malignancies, and the incidence of bilaterality is 2–4%. Renal pelvic TCC comprises only 3–4% of all urothelial malignancies. Approximately 30–50% of patients with renal pelvic TCC subsequently develop TCC of the bladder.

2. What signs and symptoms are caused by renal pelvic TCC?
Gross hematuria is the most common presenting symptom and is seen in 70–90% of patients. **Flank pain** may result from ureteral obstruction caused by the tumor or associated blood clots. **Irritative voiding symptoms** are present in 5–10% of patients. **Systemic symptoms** of anorexia, weight loss, and weakness are uncommon and are usually associated with metastatic disease. Approximately 10% of patients present with a **flank mass** due to hydronephrosis or a large tumor.

3. How is the diagnosis of renal pelvic TCC established?
The standard diagnostic regimen for renal pelvic TCC is radiographic evaluation with intravenous pyelography (IVP), retrograde pyelography, and selective upper urinary tract cytology studies. If retrograde pyelography is not possible (as in patients with an existing urinary diversion), percutaneous nephrostomy with antegrade pyelography can provide radiographic access to the involved kidney. Occasionally, angiography is indicated to differentiate renal cell carcinoma, which is typically hypervascular, from an invasive TCC, which has a characteristic pruned-tree appearance as a result of encasement of vessels.

When a filling defect is seen upon IVP or retrograde pyelography, ultrasonography can distinguish a tumor from a calculus. A thin-cut computed tomography (CT) scan obtained with and without intravenous contrast can also make the distinction. When the diagnosis remains in doubt following these studies, ureteropyeloscopy with or without biopsy of the renal pelvis can establish the diagnosis with a high degree of accuracy.

4. Describe the staging system for TCC of the renal pelvis.
The staging of renal pelvic TCC is analogous to that of bladder TCC and is determined by the presence of invasion through the thin muscle wall of the renal pelvis or extension into surrounding structures. The criteria for TNM stages are essentially those of bladder TCC, except that T2 and T3A (superficial and deep muscle invasion) cannot be differentiated in the thin muscle layer of the collecting system. Tumor grade and stage correlate closely with survival.

Staging of Renal Pelvic TCC

	BATATA SYSTEM	TNM SYSTEM
Confined to mucosa	O	T_aT_{is}
Invasion of lamina propria	A	T1
Invasion of muscularis	B	T2
Extension into fat or renal parenchyma	C	T3
Spread to adjacent organs	D	T4
Lymph node spread	D	N+
Distant metastases	D	M+

5. What is the treatment for localized renal pelvic TCC?
In patients with localized unilateral renal pelvic TCC and a normal-functioning opposite kidney, **nephroureterectomy** is the treatment of choice for several reasons: the multifocal nature of renal

pelvic TCC, the high attendant risk of ipsilateral recurrence, the low incidence of contralateral renal involvement, and the anatomically thin wall of the renal pelvis which may favor local invasion and metastatic spread at an early stage. For patients with low-grade noninvasive renal pelvic TCC, the 5-year survival rate following nephroureterectomy is 75–90%.

6. When is conservative or nephron-sparing surgery indicated?

A conservative surgical approach for localized renal pelvic TCC is indicated in selected patients with malignancy present bilaterally or in a solitary kidney or in patients with two kidneys but marginal renal function. The available nephron-sparing surgical options in these patients include partial nephrectomy, open pyelotomy with tumor excision and fulguration, percutaneous endoscopic tumor resection, or ureteropyeloscopic resection. Following a nephron-sparing procedure, a topical chemotherapeutic agent, such as BCG, may be instilled directly into the renal pelvis as an added measure to prevent tumor recurrence.

7. How should patients with metastatic disease be managed?

Patients should receive cisplatin-based chemotherapy analogous to patients with metastatic bladder TCC. The involved kidney is removed if there are significant associated local symptoms or if there is a complete response to chemotherapy. Radiation therapy is generally not effective.

BIBLIOGRAPHY

1. Batata M, Grabstald H: Upper urinary tract urothelial tumors. Urol Clin North Am 3:79, 1976.
2. Catalona WJ: Urothelial tumors of the urinary tract. In Walsh PC, Retik AB, Stamey TA, Vaughan ED (eds): Campbell's Urology, 6th ed. Philadelphia, W. B. Saunders, 1992.
3. Guz B, Streem S, Novick AC, et al: Role of percutaneous nephrostomy in patients with upper tract transitional cell carcinoma. Urology 37:331, 1991.
4. Huffman JL, Bagky D, Lyon E, et al: Endoscopic diagnosis and treatment of upper tract urothelial tumors: A preliminary report. Cancer 55:1422, 1985.
5. Smith AD, et al: Percutaneous management of renal pelvic tumors: A treatment option in selected cases. J Urol 137:852, 1987.
6. Streem S, Pontes E, Novick AC, et al: Ureteropyeloscopy in the evaluation of upper tract filling defects. J Urol 136:383, 1986.
7. Studer UE, et al: Percutaneous BCG perfusion of the upper urinary tract for carcinoma in situ. J Urol 142:975, 1989.
8. Ziegelbaum M, Novick AC, Streem SB, et al: Conservation surgery for transitional cell carcinoma of the renal pelvis. J Urol 138:1146, 1987.

22. WILMS' TUMOR

Sandip Vasavada, M.D., and Jack S. Elder, M.D.

1. Who is Wilms' tumor named after?
The tumor is named after Max Wilms, who characterized the tumor in 1899, although Rance first described it in 1914.

2. What percentage of all solid malignancies does Wilms' tumor represent?
Wilms' tumor accounts for approximately 8% of all solid childhood malignancies. Wilms' tumor represents > 80% of all genitourinary cancers in children < 15 years old.

3. What is the typical age of patients with Wilms' tumor?
More than 90% of all Wilms' tumor cases are noted prior to age 7, with a peak incidence between ages 3 and 4.

4. Describe the major pathologic event thought to account for the development of Wilms' tumor.
Wilms' tumor arises from abnormal proliferation of metanephric blastema without differentiation into glomeruli and tubules. The majority of Wilms' tumors are thought be nonhereditary. Patients with bilateral or familial tumors and those associated with aniridia or genitourinary anomalies present at a younger age and their tumors are thought to be hereditary in origin.

5. What are the microscopic characteristics of Wilms' tumor?
The tumor is triphasic, consisting of a blastemal component ("nephrogenic" cells with a tubuloglomerular pattern), a stromal component, and an epithelial component, which may contain mature tubules or be primitive in appearance.

6. The Wilms' tumor suppressor gene has been localized to which chromosome?
The short arm of the eleventh chromosome (11p13).

7. How do patients with Wilms' tumor typically present?
More than 90% of patients with Wilms' tumor have a palpable smooth abdominal or flank mass, 33% have abdominal pain, and 30–50% exhibit microscopic or gross hematuria. Approximately 50% are hypertensive.

8. What is the differential diagnosis of a childhood abdominal mass?

Renal masses	Nonrenal causes
Wilms' tumor	Mesenteric and choledochal cysts
Multicystic dysplastic kidney	Intestinal duplication cysts
Hydronephrosis	Splenomegaly
Polycystic kidney	Neuroblastoma
Congenital mesoblastic nephroma	Rhabdomyosarcoma
	Lymphoma
	Hepatoblastoma

9. Name some common anomalies associated with Wilms' tumor.
Approximately 15% of patients with Wilms' tumor will exhibit associated anomalies including hemihypertrophy, Beckwith-Wiedemann syndrome, aniridia, musculoskeletal anomalies, neurofibromatosis, and a wide spectrum of genitourinary anomalies such as hypospadias, cryptorchidism, renal duplication, ectopia, and fusion anomalies.

10. What is the WAGR syndrome?
The WAGR syndrome consists of Wilms' tumor, aniridia, genitourinary anomalies, and mental retardation.

11. What is the Beckwith-Wiedemann syndrome?
Beckwith-Wiedemann syndrome consists of visceromegaly involving the adrenal cortex, kidney, liver, pancreas, and gonads. Other findings include hemihypertrophy, omphalocele, mental retardation, microcephaly and macroglossia. Neoplasm develops in approximately 10% of cases.

12. Describe the role of imaging studies in the diagnosis of Wilms' tumor.
Ultrasound shows that the abdominal mass is solid and arising from the kidney. It also allows one to image the renal vein and inferior vena cava to assess whether a tumor thrombus is present. An intravenous pyelogram (IVP) or CT scan should be obtained to image the contralateral kidney and assess renal function. A chest x-ray or CT scan of the chest should be done to check for pulmonary metastases. The role of MRI and MR angiography have yet to be determined.

13. What does nonvisualization of the kidney on IVP suggest?
Nonvisualization suggests complete obstruction of the collecting system (renal pelvis or ureter) with tumor, severe obstruction of the renal vein, or massive parenchymal replacement of the kidney with tumor. Approximately 10% of Wilms' tumors are not visualized.

14. What are the unfavorable pathologic subtypes of Wilms' tumor?
Recognition of unfavorable histologic features has allowed clinicians to identify an important prognostic factor. Although unfavorable subtypes account for only 10% of Wilms' tumors, they are responsible for 60% of tumor deaths. Unfavorable subtypes include anaplastic tumor, rhabdoid tumor, and clear cell sarcoma. The rhabdoid tumor is the most lethal, and many consider this variant to be a sarcoma not of metanephric origin. These tumors tend to metastasize to the brain. Clear cell sarcoma ("bone metastasizing renal tumor of childhood") also is thought to be a separate tumor from Wilms' tumor.

15. Name the favorable types of Wilms' tumor.
Favorable tumors include any lesions that do not contain unfavorable elements. Specific favorable subtypes include multilocular cyst, congenital mesoblastic nephroma, and rhabdomyo-sarcoma tumor (not rhabdoid tumor).

16. Describe a congenital mesoblastic nephroma.
Congenital mesoblastic nephroma is a renal tumor that presents in early infancy. This tumor often has a male predilection. Grossly, it is a massive, firm tumor that contains interlacing bundles of whitish tissue resembling a leiomyoma. When completely excised, it has a benign course and no further treatment is necessary.

17. What are nephrogenic rests? Nephroblastomosis? What is their relationship to Wilms' tumor?
Wilms' tumor is not congenital. It has been speculated that precursors of Wilms' tumor are present that undergo transformation in the two-step process of tumor induction. It has been postulated that nephrogenic elements that persist beyond the end of nephrogenesis at 36 weeks might be these precursors. These lesions have been found in 1% of infant autopsies and 30–40% of kidneys containing a Wilms's tumor.

   Nephrogenic rests are abnormally persistent nephrogenic cells that can be induced to form a Wilms' tumor. Nephrogenic rests have been subdivided into perilobar (peripheral) and intralobar (central) rests. Perilobar rests are often smooth and well defined, with a distribution at the lobar periphery. Intralobar rests, on the contrary, are irregular, usually single, and are distributed randomly throughout the renal lobe. Perilobar rests often contain predominantly blastemal cells early, whereas intralobar rests often are composed of primarily of stromal cells. Perilobar nephrogenic rests are identified in 17% of Wilms' tumors and intralobar rests in 22% of Wilms' tumors.

Nephroblastomatosis refers to a diffuse pattern of nephrogenic rests or their derivatives.

18. How is Wilms' tumor staged?

National Wilms' Tumor Staging System

Stage I:	Tumor limited to kidney and completely excised. The surface of the renal capsule is intact. Tumor was not ruptured before or during removal. There is no residual tumor apparent beyond the margins of resection.
Stage II:	Tumor extends beyond the kidney but is completely removed. There is regional extension of the tumor, i.e., penetration through the outer surface of the renal capsule into perirenal soft tissue. Vessels outside the kidney substance are infiltrated or contain tumor thrombus. The tumor may have undergone biopsy or there has been local spillage of tumor confined to the flank. There is no residual tumor apparent at or beyond the margins of excision.
Stage III:	Residual nonhematogenous tumor confined to abdomen. Any one or more of the following occur: a. Lymph nodes on biopsy are found to be involved in the hilus, the periaortic chains, or beyond. b. There has been diffuse peritoneal contamination by tumor, such as by spillage or tumor beyond the flank before or during surgery, or by tumor growth that has penetrated through the peritoneal surface. c. Implants are found on the peritoneal surfaces. d. The tumor extends beyond the surgical margins either microscopically or grossly. e. The tumor is not completely resectable because of local infiltration into vital structures.
Stage IV:	Hematogenous metastases. Deposits beyond stage III, e.g., lung, liver, bone, and brain.
Stage V:	Bilateral renal involvement at diagnosis. An attempt should be made to stage each side according to the above criteria on the basis of extent of disease before biopsy.

19. What are the most important prognostic determinants in children with Wilms' tumor?
Histopathology (favorable or unfavorable) and tumor stage.

20. What are the most common sites of metastasis for Wilms' tumor?
The lungs are the most common metastatic site for Wilms' tumor. The liver is the second most common site, followed by bone and brain.

21. Describe the preferred initial surgical approach to Wilms' tumor.
All patients should be explored through a transverse supraumbilical transperitoneal incision. The contralateral (normal) kidney is mobilized and inspected carefully to be absolutely certain that it is not involved. Any suspicious area should be biopsied. If the normal kidney contains Wilms' tumor, the patient should be managed as a stage V (bilateral Wilms' tumor) patient. Next, resectability of the tumor is determined.

Important points to stress include gentle handling of the tumor to avoid spillage of tumor cells. NWTS-III patients with intraoperative tumor spill had a > sixfold increase in abdominal relapse. The adrenal gland is taken with the kidney if the tumor involves the upper pole. A lymph node sampling is important for staging, but formal lymph node dissection does not improve survival.

22. What if the tumor is unresectable?
Preoperative chemotherapy should be administered followed by renal exploration.

23. Which chemotherapeutic agents are most effective in children with Wilms' tumor?
Actinomycin D, vincristine, and doxorubicin.

24. What is the role of radiation therapy in Wilms' tumor?
The first National Wilms' Tumor Study (NWTS-I) showed that there was no survival advantage for routine radiotherapy in patients who were given actinomycin D for at least 15 months. NWTS-III showed that radiation therapy conferred no additional benefit in patients with stage II

tumors either. In stage III 1000 cGy is as effective as higher doses. If the lungs or liver are involved, those areas should be radiated also.

25. What are the treatment plans following radical nephrectomy in children with Wilms' tumor?

Stage I:	Actinomycin D plus vincristine for 18–24 weeks.
Stage II:	Actinomycin D plus vincristine for 18–65 weeks.
Stage III:	Actinomycin D, vincristine and doxorubicin for 24–65 weeks plus radiation therapy. Half of these patients (stages I–III) receive their chemotherapy in a pulsed/intensive manner.
Stage IV:	Radiation therapy plus actinomycin D, vincristine, and doxorubicin for 65 weeks.

26. What is the initial treatment in a child with suspected Wilms' tumor who presents with pulmonary metastases?
If the tumor is resectable, radical nephrectomy.

27. What is the survival for children with stages I, II, III, and IV Wilms' tumor with favorable histology following treatment by the NWTS protocol?
I: 97%; II: 92%; III: 84%; IV: 83% (data from NWTS-III).

28. What is the survival for children with stages I–III, unfavorable histology, and stage IV, unfavorable histology?
I–III, unfavorable histology: 68%; IV, unfavorable histology: 55%.

29. Describe some common toxicities associated with Wilms' tumor therapy.
As a result of the chemotherapeutic effect on the bone marrow, hematologic toxicity occurs relatively frequently. Similarly, hepatic toxicity frequently occurs as a result of the liver's inclusion in the radiotherapy field and from chemotherapeutic agents. Renal effects of radiation often cause azotemia, microhematuria, and chronic nephritis. Late orthopedic complications have been reported in as many as 30% of patients receiving radiation therapy, and are most severe with children under 2 years of age are treated with high-dose radiation therapy. Vertebral hypoplasia and scoliosis are the most common complications. Myocardial damage may result from doxorubicin. Ovarian failure may result following radiation therapy.

30. What is the incidence of secondary neoplasms following treatment for Wilms' tumor?
Approximately 17% of patients develop a secondary neoplasm following radiotherapy, with a peak incidence 15–19 years following diagnosis.

31. What is the approximate incidence of bilateral Wilms' tumor?
It is 5%, synchronous accounting for 4% and metachronous for 1%.

32. What is the optimal therapy for bilateral Wilms' tumor?
Previously bilateral Wilms' tumor was managed with a primary surgical approach, whereby a nephrectomy was performed in the more involved kidney and, if feasible, a contralateral partial nephrectomy was performed. Recently the preferred approach has been to perform an initial biopsy, to confirm the diagnosis, to determine whether the tumor is favorable or unfavorable, and to start chemotherapy. Surgical exploration with definitive tumor resection is performed after significant reduction in the tumor burden has occurred. Overall, patients with bilateral Wilms' tumor necessitate close follow-up, as late recurrences have been documented.

BIBLIOGRAPHY

1. Banner MP, Pollack HM, Chatten J, Witzleben C: Multilocular renal cysts: Radiologic-pathologic correlation. AJR 136:239, 1981.
2. Beckwith JB, Palmer NF: Histopathology and prognosis of Wilms' tumor. Cancer 41:1937, 1978.

3. Beckwith JB, D'Angio GJ: Anaplastic Wilms' tumor: Clinical and pathological studies. J Clin Oncol 3:513–520, 1985.
4. Blute ML, Kelalis PP, Offord KP, et al: Bilateral Wilms' tumor. J Urol 138:968–973, 1987.
5. D'Angio GJ, Breslow W, Beckwith JB, Evans A, et al: Treatment of Wilms' tumor: Results of the Third National Wilms' Tumor Study. Cancer 64:349–360, 1989.
6. D'Angio GJ, Evans AE, Breslow N, et al: The treatment of Wilms' tumor: Results of the National Wilms' Tumor Study. Cancer 38:633, 1976a.
7. D'Angio GJ, Evans AE, Breslow N, et al: The treatment of Wilms' tumor: Results of the Second National Wilms' Tumor Study. Cancer 47:2302, 1981.
8. D'Angio GJ, Evans AE, Breslow N, et al: Results of the Third National Wilms' Tumor Study (NWTS-3): A preliminary report [Abstract 723]. Proc Am Assoc Cancer Res 25:183, 1984.
9. D'Angio GJ, Tefft M, Breslow N, et al: Radiation therapy of Wilms' tumor: Results according to dose, field, post-operative timing and histology. Int J Radiat Oncol Biol Phys 4:769, 1978.
10. de Lorimier AA, Belzer FO, Kountz SL, Kushner JO: Treatment of bilateral Wilms' tumor. Am J Surg 122:275, 1971.
11. Green DM, Norkool P, Breslow NE, et al: Severe hepatic toxicity after treatment with vincristine and dactinomycin using single-dose or divided dose schedules: A report from the National Wilms' Tumor Study. J Clin Oncol 8:1525–1530, 1990.
12. Jones B: Metachronous bilateral Wilms' tumor. Am J Clin Oncol 5:545, 1982.
13. Keating MA, D'Angio GJ: Wilms' tumor update: Current issues in management. Dialogues Pediatr Urol 11:1–8, 1988.
14. Pendergrass TW: Congenital anomalies in children with Wilms' tumor. Cancer 37:403, 1976.
15. Ritchey ML, Haase GM, Shochat S: Current management of Wilms' tumor. Semin Surg Oncol 9:502–509, 1993.
16. Sotelo-Avila C, Gonzales-Crussi F, deMello D, et al: Renal and extrarenal rhabdoid tumors in children: A clinicopathologic study of 14 patients. Semin Diagn Pathol 3:151, 1986.
17. Zuppan C, Beckwith JB, Luckey D: Anaplasia in unilateral Wilms' tumor: A report from the National Wilms' Tumor Study Pathology Center. Hum Pathol 19:1199–1209, 1988.

23. NEUROBLASTOMA

Jonathan H. Ross, M.D.

1. How common is neuroblastoma?
Neuroblastoma is the most common extracranial solid tumor of childhood, with an annual incidence of approximately 1/100,000 children. The median age at diagnosis is 22 months, and 80% of children are diagnosed at < 4 years of age.

2. Where in the body do neuroblastomas occur?
These tumors are of neural crest cell origin and can occur anywhere in the neuroectodermal chain. Approximately 50% arise in the adrenal medulla, and most of the others occur along the sympathetic chain in the abdomen or mediastinum.

3. Describe the histologic appearance.
Neuroblastomas are one of the ''small blue tumors of childhood.'' They occur in sheets of lobules of cells. Pseudorosettes of one or two layers of neuroblasts surrounding pink material (neuropil) are a characteristic feature seen in approximately 30% of cases.

4. Are ganglioneuroblastomas a type of neuroblastoma?
Sort of. Ganglioneuroma is a benign tumor that occurs most commonly in young adults. It is composed of mature neural elements (as opposed to neuroblasts). Ganglioneuroblastomas are tumors composed of neuroblastic elements and benign foci of ganglioneuroma. The relative preponderance of these elements occurs in a spectrum from tumors closely resembling ganglioneuromas to those that are nearly indistinguishable from neuroblastoma. While the relative amount of neuroblastic tissue in a given tumor probably affects the prognosis, the presence of any immature elements makes the tumor potentially malignant.

5. How do neuroblastomas present?
Neuroblastomas may present with various symptoms due to the primary lesion or metastases. Unlike patients with Wilm's tumor, patients with neuroblastoma often have systemic findings at the time of presentation. The most common presenting signs and symptoms are fever, abdominal pain or distension, abdominal mass, weight loss, anemia, bone pain, and/or proptosis and periorbital ecchymoses (due to retro-orbital metastases).

6. How is neuroblastoma staged?
Although there is no universally accepted staging system for neuroblastoma, several factors seem to be most important, including the local extent of tumor beyond the organ of origin or across the midline, the completeness of surgical resection, the status of regional lymph nodes, and the presence and specific location of metastatic deposits. The international staging system suggested by Broeder et al. and used by the Children's Cancer Study Group is shown here.

Staging System for Neuroblastoma

Stage 1	Tumor confined to organ of origin with grossly complete excision
Stage 2A	Unilateral tumor with gross residual after resection
Stage 2B	Unilateral tumor with positive ipsilateral lymph nodes
Stage 3	Tumor crossing the midline or positive contralateral lymph nodes
Stage 4	Metastatic disease beyond regional lymph nodes
Stage 4S	Unilateral tumor with or without positive ipsilateral lymph nodes with metastatic disease limited to the liver, skin, and/or bone marrow

7. What is the significance of stage 4S disease?
Stage 4S reflects a unique expression of metastatic neuroblastoma. These patients are generally < 1 year of age, have relatively localized primary tumors, and metastases limited to the liver, skin, and

bone marrow. These tumors have a tendency to resolve with little or no treatment. The survival rate for these patients in one study was 77%, compared to 6% for those with standard stage 4 disease.

8. Describe the appropriate radiographic work-up of the primary tumor in a patient with neuroblastoma.

Ultrasound is the most frequent first study in the evaluation of a child with an abdominal mass. Either **computed tomography** (CT) or **magnetic resonance imaging** (MRI) is obtained to further characterize and stage the lesion. Both studies will detect extension beyond the midline and hepatic involvement. However, MRI better displays the relationship of the tumor to the great vessels and is able to detect intraspinal extension without invasive myelography. The latter capability is more important for neuroblastomas arising in the sympathetic chain than it is for adrenal neuroblastomas. CT offers the advantage of detecting calcification in most neuroblastomas. Because calcification is rare in Wilm's tumor, this capability may be particularly important for large suprarenal tumors for which the organ of origin is uncertain.

9. Describe the metastatic evaluation.

The most common metastatic sites at presentation are regional and distant lymph nodes, bone marrow, cortical bone, liver, and skin. Preoperative radiographic evaluation of **lymphatic spread** is inaccurate. Because lymphatic involvement will ultimately be detected at surgical exploration, invasive studies, such as lymphangiography, are not routinely performed. **Bone marrow metastases** are best detected by aspiration biopsy and trephine biopsy at two sites—usually both iliac crests. Immunostaining of aspirates with monoclonal antibody has further improved the sensitivity of this technique. Bony metastases are evaluated by ^{99}Tc-MDP (technetium 99 and methylene diphosphate) bone scan and a conventional skeletal survey. **Liver metastases** are detected on the MRI or CT scan used to evaluate the primary tumor. **Lung metastases** are uncommon, and a chest x-ray is adequate for detecting pulmonary involvement.

10. Why do we measure urinary catecholamine metabolites?

In addition to radiographic evaluation, all patients undergo a 24-hour urine collection for measurement of catecholamine metabolites. Urinary homovanillic acid (HMA) and/or vanillylmandelic acid (VMA) levels are elevated in more than 90% of patients with neuroblastoma. The diagnosis of neuroblastoma is confirmed either by histologic evaluation of a tumor biopsy or by a positive bone marrow in conjunction with elevated urinary HMA and VMA levels.

11. What is an MIBG scan?

Metaiodobenzylguanidine (MIBG) is an amine precursor that is concentrated in neuroblastomas and other neuroendocrine tumors. MIBG scans are very sensitive for detecting neuroblastomas. They also may be helpful occasionally in distinguishing a neuroblastoma from a Wilms' tumor or in detecting residual or recurrent disease.

12. List three biochemical markers of prognostic significance in neuroblastoma.

The urinary ratio of VMA/HMA, serum ferritin, and serum neuronspecific enolase. In disseminated disease, there is an inverse relation between the VMA/HMA ratio and survival. Elevated levels of ferritin and neuron-specific enolase are associated with a poor prognosis.

13. The amplification of which oncogene is associated with a poor prognosis?

The N-*myc* oncogene. A strong correlation has been found between amplification of this oncogene and poor outcome. In a study of 89 patients, 18-month progression-free survival was 70%, 30%, and 5% for patients whose tumors had 1, 3–10, and > 10 N-*myc* copies, respectively.

14. How is treatment selected for patients with neuroblastoma?

Many different treatment protocols are available for children with neuroblastoma. Treatment is generally based on a risk assessment that considers tumor stage, grade, and biochemical and genetic risk factors. Patients with low-stage favorable tumors may be treated with surgical excision alone. Patients with higher risk tumors require adjuvant multiagent chemotherapy and sometimes radiotherapy as well. Patients with very aggressive tumors are candidates for newer modalities, such as autologous bone marrow transplantation.

15. How are patients with stage 4S disease treated?
Patients with 4S disease generally do well without treatment. These patients, who are good surgical risks, undergo an initial exploration to ensure that the stage assignment is correct (e.g., to ensure negative contralateral lymph nodes). The primary tumor is resected only if this can be accomplished safely. Patients are treated with low-dose irradiation and oral cyclophosphamide if massive liver involvement is present.

16. What is the general outlook for patients with neuroblastoma?
Unfortunately, despite intense research, adjunctive measures have had little impact on patient survival. Those children with favorable tumors (a minority) do well without treatment beyond surgical excision, and those with unfavorable tumors do poorly despite the addition of radiation or chemotherapy.

17. Can neuroblastomas regress spontaneously?
Yes. The evidence for this comes from two sources. First, autopsy studies reveal an incidence of "neuroblastoma in situ" in fetuses and infants that is 40 times the incidence of clinically apparent neuroblastoma. Presumably, most "neuroblastomas in situ" regress. However, recent evidence suggests that what has previously been referred to as "neuroblastoma in situ" may represent a normal stage in adrenal development and not have any direct relation to neuroblastoma itself. The second line of evidence supporting spontaneous regression comes from the behavior of stage 4S tumors. Clearly, many of these tumors become inactive despite incomplete surgical extirpation.

BIBLIOGRAPHY

 1. Brodeur GM, Castleberry RP: Neuroblastoma. In Pizzo PA, Poplak DG (eds): Principals and Practice of Pediatric Oncology, 2nd ed. Philadelphia, J. B. Lippincott, 1993, pp 739–767.
 2. Brodeur GM, Nakagawara A: Molecular basis of clinical heterogeneity in neuroblastoma. Am J Pediatr Hematol Oncol 14:111–116, 1992.
 3. Brodeur G, Seeger R, Barrett A, et al: International criteria for diagnosis, staging, and response to treatment in patients with neuroblastoma. J Clin Oncol 6:1874–1881, 1988.
 4. Cheung N-K: Immunotherapy: Neuroblastoma as a model. Pediatr Clin North Am 38:425–441, 1991.
 5. Evans AE, Baum E, Chard R: Do infants with stage IV-S neuroblastoma need treatment? Arch Dis Child 56:271–274, 1981.
 6. Evans AE, D'Angio DJ, Newton WA, Randolph JA: A proposed clinical staging for children with neuroblastoma: Children's Cancer Study Group A. Cancer 27:374–378, 1971.
 7. Finkelstein JZ, Krailo MD, Lenarsky C, et al: 13-Cis-retinoic acid (NSC 122758) in the treatment of children with metastatic neuroblastoma unresponsive to conventional chemotherapy: Report from the Children's Cancer Study Group. Med Pediatr Oncol 20:307–311, 1992.
 8. Johnson FL, Goldman S: Role of autotransplantation in neuroblastoma. Hematol Oncol Clin North Am 7:647–662, 1993.
 9. Joshi VV, Cantor AB, Brodeur GM, et al: Correlation between morphologic and other prognostic markers of neuroblastoma: A study of histologic grade, DNA index, N-myc gene copy number, and lactic dehydrogenase in patients in the Pediatric Oncology Group. Cancer 71:3173–3181, 1993.
10. Look AT, Hayes FA, Shuster JJ, et al: Clinical relevance of tumor cell ploidy and N-myc gene amplification in childhood neuroblastoma: A Pediatric Oncology Group study. J Clin Oncol 9:581–591, 1991.
11. Mastrangelo R, Lasorella A, Iavarone A, et al: Critical observations on neuroblastoma treatment with 131-I-metaiodobenzylguanidine at diagnosis. Med Pediatr Oncol 21:411–415, 1993.
12. Ng YY, Kingston JE: The role of radiology in the staging of neuroblastoma. Clin Radiol 47:226–235, 1993.
13. Ninana J: Neuroblastoma. In Plowman PN, Pinkerton CR (eds): Pediatric Oncology: Clinical Practice and Controversies. London, Chapman & Hall, 1992, pp 351–377.
14. Pizzo PA, Poplack DG, Horowitz ME, et al: Solid tumors of childhood. In DeVita VT Jr, Hellman S, Rosenberg SA (eds): Cancer: Principles and Practice of Oncology. Philadelphia, J. B. Lippincott, 1993, pp 1738–1791.
15. Seeger RC, Brodeur GM, Sather H, et al: Association of multiple copies of the N-myc oncogene with rapid progression of neuroblastomas. N Engl J Med 313:1111–1116, 1985.

24. BENIGN TUMORS OF THE KIDNEY

Eric A. Klein, M.D.

1. What is the most common benign renal mass lesion?
A simple cyst, which may be single or multiple, unilateral or bilateral, and typically ranges from a few millimeters to several centimeters in diameter. Most simple cysts are found incidentally on abdominal or renal imaging studies, are asymptomatic, and require no treatment. Occasionally, a cyst may become very large and cause pain or obstruction of the collecting system.

2. Describe the radiographic characteristics of simple cysts.
On **renal ultrasound,** simple cysts are smooth-walled, sharply demarcated from surrounding parenchyma, and anechoic and exhibit posterior acoustic shadowing. On **intravenous urography,** cysts usually show a mass effect and may distort the renal outline or collecting system. On **computed tomography** (CT), cysts are thin-walled, sharply demarcated, and fluid-filled with a tissue attenuation similar to water. On **angiography,** simple cysts are avascular.

3. What is a renal cortical adenoma?
As originally described by Bell, these are small (<3 cm), well-circumscribed solid tumors comprising uniform clear or acidophilic cells with uniform histology. Adenomas are almost always asymptomatic, found incidentally, and often multifocal.

4. How can a renal adenoma be distinguished from a small renal cell carcinoma?
In clinical practice, these lesions are indistinguishable. Both adenomas and small renal cell carcinomas appear radiographically as solid tumors, but even benign-appearing renal cortical tumors < 3 cm can metastasize. The diagnosis of adenoma is therefore based solely on pathologic examination. Molecular and cytogenetic studies suggest that adenomas of papillary histology are characterized by a loss of the Y chromosome and trisomy of chromosomes 7 and 17, as compared with renal cell carcinoma which is characterized by a deletion of the short arm of chromosome 3.

5. Describe the appearance and behavior of renal oncocytoma.
Oncocytomas are usually round, well-circumscribed, and brown or tan and may contain a central stellate scar. Histologically they comprise nests, cysts, or tubular aggregates of polygonal cells with granular eosinophilic cytoplasm. Mitoses are rare. Electron microscopy demonstrates an abundance of mitochrondria. Oncocytomas show no tendency to invade surrounding structures or metastasize.

6. Can renal oncocytoma be distinguished clinically or radiographically from renal cell carcinoma?
No. Although increasingly diagnosed as incidental radiographic findings, both tumors may present with hematuria or other symptoms and appear radiographically as solid mass lesions which distort the renal contour and/or collecting system. It has been suggested that the appearance of a central stellate scar on CT or a spoke-wheel pattern of tumor vessels on angiography is suggestive of oncocytoma, but these patterns are rare and nonspecific. Both oncocytoma and renal cell carcinoma can present with multiple and bilateral synchronous tumors, and oncocytoma can occur simultaneously with renal cell carcinoma in the same or contralateral kidney in up to one-third of cases.

7. Can renal oncocytoma be distinguished pathologically from renal cell carcinoma?
Yes. True oncocytomas are low grade, have a characteristically uniform histologic appearance, typically have diploid DNA histograms, lack expression of HLA A,B, and C antigens, and are characterized by loss of the Y chromosome and translocations involving the long arm of chromosome 11. However, many renal cell carcinomas contain "oncocytic" features on histologic examination that could be misleading if the tumor is not adequately sampled. This fact,

along with the frequent coexistence of oncocytoma and renal cell carcinoma in the same or opposite kidney, limits the preoperative use of percutaneous needle biopsy of solid renal masses to establish the diagnosis of oncocytoma.

8. How is renal oncocytoma treated?
Surgical excision, by partial or total nephrectomy.

9. Describe the histologic appearance of angiomyolipoma (renal hamartoma).
These tumors are composed of variable amounts of blood vessels (*angio-*), smooth muscle (*myo-*), and fat (*lipoma*).

10. In what clinical scenarios are angiomyolipomas encountered?
Angiomyolipomas occur sporadically or in association with tuberous sclerosis. Sporadic angiomyolipomas are more commonly right-sided (two-thirds of cases), occur almost exclusively in adult females, and are usually smaller and less frequently bilateral than those seen with tuberous sclerosis. Although increasingly diagnosed incidentally, both types occur with similar symptoms, including abdominal or flank pain, palpable mass, intratumoral hemorrhage, hematuria, anemia, and hypertension.

11. What are the clinical features of tuberous sclerosis?
Tuberous sclerosis is a hereditary syndrome characterized by mental retardation, epilepsy, and adenoma sebaceum. Hamartomas may be found in the brain, eye, heart, lung, and bone. Because of the high incidence and potential morbidity of renal hamartomas, all patients with tuberous sclerosis should be screened with renal ultrasonography or CT scans.

12. How do the renal hamartomas of tuberous sclerosis differ from sporadic angiomyolipomas?
The angiomyolipomas of tuberous sclerosis occur at a younger age, are bilateral in 80% of cases, and tend to be larger at the time of diagnosis. The symptomatic presentations and histologic appearances are similar.

13. Describe the radiographic appearance of angiomyolipoma.
The radiographic appearance of these lesions is determined by their fat content. By ultrasonography, they appear as highly echogenic and hyperechoic renal masses. On CT, angiomyolipomas usually appear as heterogeneous solid tumors which can achieve massive size. The CT hallmark of these tumors is the presence of fat density within the tumor, which usually appears black and measures −40 or below in Hounsfield units. The tumors appear hypervascular on angiography.

14. How is angiomyolipoma treated?
The treatment of angiomyolipoma depends on tumor size, focality, and the presence of symptoms. Because tumors of < 4 cm in diameter are usually asymptomatic, a patient with an isolated tumor of < 4 cm may be observed with yearly CT or ultrasound. Larger asymptomatic tumors may be similarly observed, but if significant growth is observed on follow-up studies, the tumor should be embolized or excised surgically. Large symptomatic tumors should be embolized or excised. Because the diagnosis of angiomyolipoma can usually be suspected preoperatively and because angiomyolipoma is rarely associated with renal cell carcinoma, a nephron-sparing surgical technique is indicated.

15. Are the angiomyolipomas associated with tuberous sclerosis treated differently?
The nephron-sparing approach is particularly important in patients with tuberous sclerosis, in whom both kidneys may be affected by multiple tumors. In these cases, surgery should be delayed until tumors reach > 4 cm or are associated with significant symptoms.

16. What is the clinical presentation of juxtaglomerular tumors?
This tumor causes a syndrome of hypertension, elevated serum renin, and hyperaldosteronism due to a functional renin-secreting tumor of juxtaglomerular cells. The tumors are usually small (< 3 cm), not detectable radiographically, and curable by surgery.

17. What other benign tumors affect the kidneys?

Fibromas, lipomas, myomas, lymphangiomas, and hemangiomas occur rarely and usually as mass lesions on radiographic studies. They may arise from the renal capsule or other stromal elements of the kidney. Because of the uncertainty of clinical diagnosis, the nature of these tumors is usually not established until they are removed surgically.

BIBLIOGRAPHY

1. Bell ET: Renal Disease, 2nd ed. Philadelphia, Lea & Febiger, 1950.
2. Bonavita JA, Pollack HM, Banner MP: Renal oncocytoma: Further observations and literature review. Urol Radiol 2:229–232, 1981.
3. Licht MR, Novick AC, Tubbs RR, et al: Renal oncocytoma: Clinical and biological correlates. J Urol 150:1380–1383, 1993.
4. Maatman TJ, Novick AC, Tancino BF, et al: Renal oncocytoma: A diagnostic and therapeutic dilemma. J Urol 132:878–880, 1984.
5. Meloni A, Bridge J, Sandberg AA: Reviews on chromosome studies in urological tumors: I. Renal tumors. J Urol 148:253–265, 1992.
6. Oesterling J, Fishman EK, Goldman SM, Marshall FF: The management of renal angiomyolipomas. J Urol 135:1121–1125, 1986.
7. Quinn MJ, Hartman DS, Freidman A, et al: Renal oncocytoma: New observations. Radiology 153:49–52, 1984.
8. Steiner MS, Goldman SM, Fishman EK, Marshall FF: The natural history of renal angiomyolipoma. J Urol 150:1782–1786, 1993.
9. Stillwell TJ, Gomez MR, Kelalis PP: Renal lesions in tuberous sclerosis. J Urol 138:477, 1987.
10. Tannenbaum M: Surgical and histopathology of renal tumors. Semin Oncol 10:385–389, 1983.

25. RETROPERITONEAL TUMORS

Elroy D. Kursh, M.D.

1. How common are primary retroperitoneal tumors?

They are rare. In a large series from the United States, retroperitoneal tumors represented 0.16–0.2% of all malignancies. Of all the soft tissue sarcomas, 10–20% are retroperitoneal in origin.

2. What are the pathologic types of primary retroperitoneal tumors?

There are numerous varieties of retroperitoneal neoplasms. Malignant tumors are more common than benign lesions, accounting for 70–80%. Liposarcoma predominates, followed by leimyosarcoma, fibrosarcoma, and neurogenic sarcoma. Malignant fibrous histiocytomas are being diagnosed with increased frequency due to a better understanding the histopathology of this lesion and subsequent reclassification of many tumors previously diagnosed as pleomorphic variants of the above-mentioned neoplasms.

3. Describe the signs and symptoms of a retroperitoneal tumor.

The most common early signs of a retroperitoneal tumor are the insidious development of abdominal enlargement and weight loss, which may be associated with diffuse and often vague abdominal pain and fever. Because of their location in the retroperitoneum, the tumors may become large or even mammoth before they are noticed. Various other symptoms may be associated with retroperitoneal tumors, such as nausea or vomiting, obstipation, leg edema, flank pain, dysuria, and urgency; back pain may occur later in the course of disease from compression or invasion of adjacent organs. Oddly, the patient rarely notes an increase in abdominal girth despite the frequent large size of the mass, which is usually palpable and represents the most constant physical finding, occurring in about 75% of patients.

4. How is the diagnosis of a primary retroperitoneal tumor established?

Radiographic examination confirms the presence of a retroperitoneal mass. Computed tomography (CT) has become the most reliable means of determining the size and consistency of the tumor and the relationship of the neoplasm to contiguous retroperitoneal and intraperitoneal structures.

5. Are any other diagnostic studies indicated?

Because nephrectomy is often required to completely excise the neoplasm (in about 25% of cases), excretory urography is indicated to assess the status of the involved and opposite kidney if the abdominal CT does not yield satisfactory information. Varying degrees of hydronephrosis may be present on the intravenous pyelogram (IVP), and displacement of the kidney is not uncommon. If the patient has symptoms referable to the intestinal tract or the CT scan suggests possible involvement, barium contrast studies of the gastrointestinal tract are indicated. Venography is indicated if there is evidence of venous compression because vena cava resection may be required. Angiography may be helpful, but a normal vascular pattern does not rule out a malignant tumor; this test is often not done today with the superior ability of the CT scan to define the extent of the mass.

6. What is the treatment of primary retroperitoneal tumors?

The only effective treatment is **surgical removal** of the mass. Bowel preparation is indicated preoperatively since complete excision may require bowel resection in up to 20% of cases. Adequate exposure is achieved through an abdominal, transperitoneal route, and if possible excision of the tumor is done well outside the tumor "pseudocapsule." Unfortunately, complete excision is only feasible in about 50% of cases. If complete extirpation of the tumor is feasible, it is preferable to avoid open biopsy because of the risk of implanting the tumor and causing diffuse peritoneal sarcomatosis. Even if all gross disease cannot be removed, every effort should be made to resect as much as possible in order to reduce the bulk of residual disease, which is marked with metallic clips to assist postoperative treatment.

7. What is the prognosis of a primary retroperitoneal tumor?

In the past, 5-year survival figures have been dismal, ranging from 5–20%. Reported 5-year survival rates have gradually increased to approximately 40–50% with more aggressive surgical resection and improved perioperative care. However, there has been little improvement in survival for patients with partial excision. Survival, therefore, is dependent on the fixation of the tumor, the ability to completely resect it, and the tumor grade.

8. Is any other therapy indicated for primary retroperitoneal tumor?

Because of the success of radiotherapy in the soft tissue sarcomas of the extremities, some have advised adjuvant radiotherapy following surgical removal of retroperitoneal sarcomas, but its exact role remains unclear. Postoperative radiation therapy is generally attempted if the tumor cannot be completely resected or pathology reveals positive margins. The role of adjuvant chemotherapy in the treatment of retroperitoneal sarcomas, except for embryonal rhabdomyosarcoma, is unknown because randomized studies have not been published, but it is being attempted more often in partially resected tumors and for metastatic sarcomas.

9. How should patients be followed after a primary surgical extirpation?

Some retroperitoneal sarcomas lend themselves to repeat attempts at removal because of their tendency to recur locally and their slow growth. In these, follow-up CT scans of the abdomen are indicated. Scans are obtained every 3 or 4 months for an arbitrary period of 1–2 years postoperatively and then yearly thereafter for several years. If recurrent tumor is noted, repeat surgical excision is worthwhile and may provide a cure.

BIBLIOGRAPHY

1. Cody HS III, Turnbull AD, Fortner JG, Hajder SI: The continuing challenge of retroperitoneal sarcomas. Cancer 47:2147, 1981.
2. Dalton RR, Donohue JH, Mucha P Jr, et al: Management of retroperitoneal sarcomas. Surgery 106:725, 1989.
3. Kursh ED: Primary retroperitoneal tumors: In Resnick MI, Kursh ED (eds): Current Therapy in Genitourinary Surgery. Toronto, B.C. Decker, 1987, pp 43–44.
4. McGrath PC, Neifeld JP, Lawrence W Jr, et al: Improved survival following complete excision of retroperitoneal sarcomas. Ann Surg 200:200, 1984.
5. Moore SV, Aldrete JS: Primary retroperitoneal sarcomas. The role of surgical treatment. Am J Surg 142:358, 1981.
6. Zhang G, Chen KK, Manivel C, Fraley EE: Sarcomas of the retroperitoneum and genitourinary tract. J Urol 141:1107, 1989.

26. URETERAL TUMORS

Stevan B. Streem, M.D.

1. How do ureteral tumors present?

The most frequent symptoms are hematuria or flank pain associated with obstruction. However, because ureteral tumors are generally slow-growing, the obstruction can be insidious and often painless.

2. Are ureteral tumors usually benign or malignant?

Benign tumors of the ureter are the exception, though children may have fibroepithelial polyps. The vast majority of ureteral tumors are urothelial in origin, and almost all these are transitional cell carcinoma (TCC). Squamous cell carcinoma of the ureter is extremely rare but may occur in association with chronic inflammation or infection.

3. Are the risk factors for TCC of the ureter the same as for TCC of the bladder?

The environmental carcinogens associated with TCC of the bladder appear to place the patient at increased risk for upper tract TCC. In addition, specific risk factors for upper tract TCC have been described, including analgesic abuse, papillary necrosis, and Balkan nephropathy. Cigarette smoking places the entire urothelium at increased risk for TCC.

4. How is the diagnosis of a ureteral tumor made?

Generally, a patient with hematuria undergoes an intravenous pyelogram that reveals a filling defect of the ureter or obstruction. A retrograde study is then often done for better radiographic definition. A tumor is suggested by a persistent intraluminal filling defect.

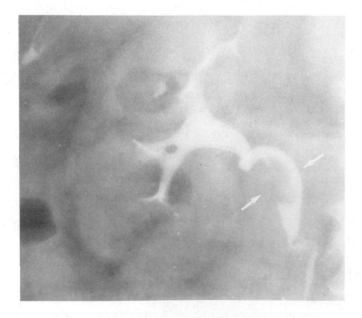

Retrograde pyelogram reveals a proximal ureteral "filling defect" (*arrows*) in this patient with painless hematuria. This subsequently proved to be TCC.

5. Can radiographic studies differentiate a tumor from a benign problem such as a lucent calculus?

Calculi can be distinguished from ureteral tumors by ultrasound or CT. In a search for calculi, the CT should be obtained without intravenous contrast, and "thin-cut" sections should be taken at the level of concern.

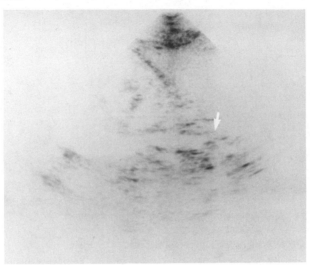

This patient had left-sided obstruction to the level of a proximal ureteral filling defect by intravenous urography. Ultrasound clearly reveals the problem to be a calculus in the proximal ureter. The "defect" is highly echogenic and casts acoustic shadows. This is consistent with a calculus, presumably uric acid.

6. Describe the staging classification for ureteral tumors.

Staging is analogous to that for TCC of the bladder:

Staging System for Ureteral Tumors

UICC	JEWITT	PATHOLOGY
pTa	0	Confined to mucosa
pT_1	A	Confined to lamina propia
pT_2, pT_{3a}	B_1, B_2	Confined to muscularis
pT_{3b}, pT_4, N+	C, D	Periureteral tissue or lymph node involvement

7. Are all parts of the ureter affected with equal frequency?

No. The risk for ureteral TCC increases progressively from the rarely affected proximal ureter to the more frequently involved distal ureter.

8. Is urine cytology helpful?

Cytologic evaluation of voided urine has a relatively high false-negative rate for ureteral tumors. Cytologic accuracy can be improved by examining urine obtained selectively from the involved side at the time of cystoscopy and retrograde studies. Brushing the lesion for cytologic examination can also be done at that time.

9. What is the single most accurate way of diagnosing a ureteral tumor?

If the diagnosis is in doubt, upper tract endoscopy with rigid or flexible ureteroscopes offers a high degree of reliability in diagnosis. During ureteroscopy, biopsy specimens may be obtained to help with preoperative grading and even staging of the tumor. (See figure on top of next page.)

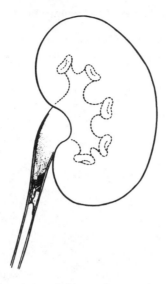

Transureteroscopic biopsy of a ureteral tumor.

10. What is the best treatment for a ureteral tumor?

Because TCC of the ureter can be multifocal, standard definitive treatment (assuming the contralateral kidney is normal) is a nephroureterectomy during which the entire kidney, ureter, and a cuff of the bladder are removed. If the tumor is limited to the distal ureter, a distal ureterectomy with reimplantation is also acceptable and even preferential.

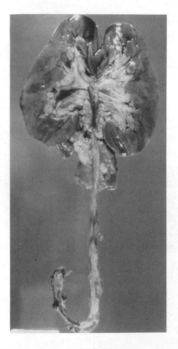

Nephroureterectomy specimen from patient with ureteral TCC.

11. Does a history of TCC of the bladder place the patient at increased risk for ureteral tumors?
Yes. TCC represents urothelial "field change" disease characterized by a tendency to poly-chronotropism (multiple recurrences in time and space). The incidence of upper tract disease in patients with TCC of the bladder is approximately 3%.

12. What about removing just part of the ureter if the tumor is in the proximal or mid-ureter?
The risk of ipsilateral recurrence is highest when ureter is left below the level of the tumor. However, segmental ureterectomy can almost always be justified in the presence of a functionally solitary kidney, significant contralateral renal disease, or bilateral upper tract TCC. Indications for segmental ureterectomy in the presence of a normal contralateral kidney are controversial though some urologists feel segmental ureterectomy is justifiable if the tumor is unifocal, low grade, and low stage.

13. Do radiation or chemotherapy have roles in ureteral carcinoma?
Radiation therapy has marginal proven benefit for upper tract TCC. For invasive disease, combination chemotherapy protocols analogous to those for invasive TCC of the bladder are proving beneficial.

BIBLIOGRAPY

1. Albarran MJ (1902): Cited by Melicow MM, Findlay HV: Primary benign tumors of the ureter: Review of literature and report of a case. Surg Gynecol Obstet 54:680, 1932.
2. Babaian RJ: Primary carcinoma of the upper urinary tract urothelium: An overview. In Crawford ED, Pas S (eds): Current Genitourinary Cancer Surgery. Philadelphia, Lea & Febiger, 1990.
3. Babaian RJ, Johnson DE: Primary carcinoma of the ureter. J Urol 123:357, 1980.
4. Babaian RJ, Johnson DE, Chan RC: Combination nephroureterectomy and postoperative radiotherapy for infiltrative ureteral carcinoma. Int J Radiat Oncol Biol Phys 6:1229, 1980.
5. Batata MA, et al: Primary carcinoma of the ureter: A prognostic study. Cancer 35:1626, 1975.
6. Huffman JL, Bagley DH, Lyon ES, et al: Endoscopic diagnosis and treatment of the upper tract urothelial tumors. Cancer 55:1422, 1985.
7. McCoy JG, Honda H, Reznicek M, et al: Computerized tomography for detection and staging of localized and pathologically defined upper tract urothelial tumors. J Urol 146:1500, 1991.
8. Schmauz R, Cole P: Epidemiology of cancer of the renal pelvis and ureter. J Natl Cancer Inst 523:1431, 1974.
9. Streem SB, Pontes JE, Novick AC, et al: Ureteropyeloscopy in the evaluation of upper tract filling defects. J Urol 136:383, 1986.
10. Vest SA: Conservative surgery in certain benign tumors of the ureter. J Urol 53:97, 1945.
11. Zincke H, et al: Significance of urinary cytology in the early detection of transitional cell cancer of the upper urinary tract. J Urol 116:781, 1976.

27. TRANSITIONAL CELL CARCINOMA OF THE BLADDER

Eric A. Klein, M.D.

1. What is the incidence of transitional cell carcinoma (TCC) of the bladder?
About 50,000 new cases of bladder TCC were diagnosed in the United States in 1994, occurring in a 3:1 male-to-female ratio. TCC is the fourth most common cancer in men and eighth most common in women.

2. What risk factors are associated with bladder TCC?
- Age (peak incidence in seventh decade)
- Occupational exposure to aniline dyes and aromatic amines
- Cigarette smoking (four times increased risk)
- Phenacetin abuse
- Treatment with cyclophosphamide

3. Describe the histologic appearance of normal bladder urothelium.
Normal bladder is lined by transitional cell epithelium which varies from 3–7 cells in thickness. The basal layer rests on a lamina propria basement membrane and is covered by several layers of intermediate cells, with the most superficial layer composed of flat "umbrella" cells. The lamina propria contains a discontinuous muscularis mucosa and is rich in lymphatics. The muscularis propria lies deep to the lamina propria.

4. What proliferative lesions in bladder urothelium can be confused with TCC?

1. Epithelial hyperplasia
2. Atypical hyperplasia
3. Inverted papilloma
4. Cystitis cystica
5. von Brunn's nests
6. Cystitis glandularis
7. Nephrogenic adenoma
8. Squamous metaplasia

5. What is the significance of epithelial and atypical hyperplasia?
Epithelial hyperplasia is a benign proliferation of urothelium in response to inflammation or irritation. **Atypical hyperplasia** is characterized by an increased number of cell layers *and* nuclear atypia with derangement of the umbrella layer. Atypical hyperplasia is preneoplastic.

6. Describe von Brunn's nests and their significance.
von Brunn's nests are islands of benign-appearing urothelium residing in the submucosa and resulting from inward proliferation of the basal cell layer. They are a normal variant of urothelial histology.

7. What are cystitis cystica and cystitis glandularis?
Both are variants of von Brunn's nests with additional histological changes. In **cystitis cystica,** the center of the nest is filled with liquefied material and appears more cyst-like than glandular. In **cystitis glandularis,** the transitional epithelium has undergone glandular metaplasia, and the cells appear columnar with mucin-containing cytoplasm. Cystitis glandularis may appear as a papillary lesion, is often associated with pelvic lipomatosis, and may give rise to adenocarcinoma.

8. Describe inverted papilloma and nephrogenic adenoma and explain their significance.
Both inverted papilloma and nephrogenic adenoma are benign lesions that occur in response to trauma or infection. **Inverted papilloma** is a submucosal proliferative lesion that typically occurs on the trigone and vesical neck and is covered by normal urothelium. **Nephrogenic adenoma** appears raised or papillary and histologically resembles primitive renal collecting tubules.

9. What is squamous metaplasia?

Squamous metaplasia is a benign proliferative and metaplastic lesion in which normal urothelium is replaced by nonkeratinized squamous epithelium. It appears most commonly as whitish plaques on the trigone in women.

10. Bladder cancer most frequently occurs as what histologic type?

Transitional cell carcinoma accounts for > 90% of all bladder cancers. Other histologic subtypes arising from urothelium include adenocarcinoma, squamous carcinoma, and urachal carcinomas.

11. Which nonurothelial tumors occur in the bladder?

- Small cell carcinoma
- Lymphoma
- Sarcomas (typically leiomyosarcoma)
- Pheochromocytoma
- Carcinosarcoma
- Metastatic tumors

12. Explain the staging system for TCC.

TCC is divided into noninvasive (''superficial'') and invasive forms. Noninvasive tumors may appear papillary or flat and do not invade the muscularis propria. Papillary tumors are frondular or more solid-appearing exophytic tumors which project into the bladder lumen. Flat tumors are usually carcinoma-in-situ (CIS), which appears as an erythematous velvety patch comprised of high-grade TCC.

Invasive tumors demonstrate invasion into muscularis propria, are usually solid, and exhibit a sessile growth pattern. Papillary tumors which invade the lamina propria are sometimes called ''superficially invasive.''

Staging System for TCC

STAGE	DEFINITION
Superficial tumors	
Ta	Confined to mucosa
T1	Invasion into lamina propria
TIS	Intraepithelial CIS
Invasive tumors	
T2	Invasion into superficial muscularis propria
T3a	Invasion into deep muscularis propria
T3b	Invasion through muscle into perivesical fat
T4	Invasion into adjacent organs

13. How is TCC graded histologically?

Most systems assign grade based on the degree of cellular anaplasia, although there is no universally accepted scheme. Normal urothelium exhibits a very regular pattern of base-to-surface cellular maturation and polarity. TCC exhibits progressive degrees of disturbance in this orderly array and is graded accordingly. Distinction is usually made between well, moderately, and poorly differentiated tumors which correspond to low, medium, or high grades. Most CIS is considered high grade, although some systems include lower grades.

14. Explain the difference between bladder papilloma and well-differentiated TCC.

Some pathologists distinguish these as separate entities. A **papilloma,** sometimes referred to as a grade 0 tumor, is a papillary lesion with a thin fibrovascular core covered with normal urothelium. A **well-differentiated papillary TCC** is a grade 1 papillary tumor with a thickened urothelium exhibiting mild anaplasia and pleomorphism.

15. What cytogenetic abnormalities have been observed in TCC?
Abnormalities (gains, losses, or rearrangements) of chromosomes 3, 5, 7, 9, and 11 are observed with increased frequency in TCC. Trisomy 7 and deletions of all or part of chromosomes 9 and 11p occur most commonly.

16. What is meant by "field change"?
The common occurrence of multifocal TCC, the high frequency of recurrent tumors at new sites, and the occasional occurrence of concurrent or asynchronous upper tract TCC have suggested that the entire urothelium has a propensity to develop tumors. Presumably this is due to diffuse genetic instability or urothelium which leads to multiple tumor clones. However, some evidence suggests that at least some tumors are derived from a single (monoclonal) source which gives rise to multifocal tumors by implantation, pagetoid spread, or lymphatic spread.

17. How does bladder cancer present?
The most frequent presenting symptom is painless hematuria, especially for noninvasive tumors. Irritative symptoms, including frequency, urgency, and dysuria, are also common and suggest diffuse CIS or invasive cancer. Other symptoms can include flank pain due to ureteral obstruction, pelvic mass, or those due to metastatic disease.

18. What is the natural history of noninvasive TCC? Invasive TCC?
Approximately 70–75% of TCC are superficial, noninvasive tumors at presentation, and most low-grade tumors are destined to remain so. However, most patients, depending upon tumor size, grade, focality, ploidy, and other factors, are prone to multiple recurrences over time and in other bladder sites. About 10–15% of noninvasive tumors, usually those of higher grade and with documented invasion of the lamina propria, progress to muscle invasion.

Most invasive tumors are invasive at the time of diagnosis, and about one-half have occult metastatic disease. Untreated invasive disease predictably results in patient death within about 2 years.

19. What prognostic factors predict an aggressive potential for noninvasive tumors?

Tumor grade*	Ploidy
Tumor stage*	Frequency of recurrence
Presence of CIS*	Marker chromosomes
Lymphatic invasion	Expression of Lewis X antigen
Size	Epidermal growth factor receptor expression
Multifocality	Expression of p53
	Loss of expression of the Rb protein

*Most important prognostic factors.

20. Describe the clinical features of CIS.
CIS may be asymptomatic or produce irritative urinary symptoms (urgency, frequency, bladder pain) which are often confused with prostatism, infection, interstitial cystitis, or neurogenic bladder. CIS occurs more commonly in men and may occur alone or in association with noninvasive papillary or invasive TCC. Symptomatic CIS is typically due to diffuse urothelial involvement. When associated with other tumors, CIS is usually more focal and may surround the base of a high-grade papillary tumor. The occurrence of CIS in conjunction with papillary tumors indicates a higher likelihood of recurrence and progression to invasive disease. Urinary cytology is almost universally positive in the presence of CIS because of tumor cell slough from the basement membrane of the lamina propria.

21. How should patients with suspected TCC be evaluated?
Patients should have a urinary cytology, bimanual examination under anesthesia, diagnostic cystoscopy with tumor biopsy or resection, and an upper tract imaging study. In some patients,

biopsy of the prostatic urethra is also indicated. Flow cytometric and quantitative fluorescent image analysis to detect aneuploid stem lines in bladder wash specimens is still investigative.

22. Should random areas of normal-appearing mucosa be biopsied at resection of noninvasive tumors?

This is controversial. Some urologists believe that the detection of occult dysplasia or focal CIS by this method adds prognostic information and influences treatment decisions. Several studies have shown, however, that routine use of random biopsies is not helpful. A disadvantage of random biopsies is the potential for tumor implantation at the biopsy sites.

23. What is the ideal imaging study in evaluating patients with TCC?

The ideal study should evaluate renal function, test for the presence of renal parenchymal abnormalities, and visualize the upper tract urothelium. This is best achieved with an intravenous urogram, although renal ultrasound and retrograde pyelograms yield similar information but without functional details. A CT scan of the abdomen and pelvis is not indicated in patients with noninvasive tumors because of the low likelihood of extravesical disease. MRI is not capable of distinguishing the depth of tumor invasion. In patients with invasive tumors, a CT scan of the abdomen and pelvis is helpful in determining tumor extent and the presence of macroscopically enlarged lymph nodes, but a "negative" scan does not rule out the presence of microscopic lymphatic metastasis.

24. Can noninvasive bladder TCC cause hydronephrosis?

Usually not. The presence of hydronephrosis is usually due to obstruction of the intramural ureter and is invariably a sign of invasive TCC.

25. How are noninvasive tumors managed?

TCC is initially managed by transurethral resection. In patients with low-grade (1 or 2) Ta tumors, cystoscopy at regular intervals and with repeat resection or fulguration as necessary is usually adequate. In patients with multiple and frequent recurrences and those with grade 3 or T1 tumors at presentation, intravesical immunotherapy or chemotherapy is generally employed.

26. What is the recommended regimen for surveillance cystoscopy following resection of noninvasive TCC?

Historical practice has been to do cystoscopy at 3-month intervals for the first 2 years, then every 6 months for 1–2 years, then yearly, although recent evidence suggests that low-grade tumors can be safely followed with urinary cytology and less frequent cystoscopy.

27. What are the most effective intravesical agents for treating noninvasive TCC?

Immunotherapy with bacille Calmette-Guérin (BCG) is the most active agent for most patients with noninvasive tumors. Mitomycin C is the most active chemotherapeutic agent. Interferon-α, doxorubicin, Epodyl, and thiotepa are also used occasionally.

28. How is CIS treated?

Because natural history of CIS is variable, some patients have an indolent course of multiple recurrences without progression, whereas others progress soon after diagnosis and develop metastatic disease despite early therapy. Current first-line treatment for diffuse CIS is intravesical immunotherapy with BCG, which produces complete responses in up to 70% of patients. Treatment of refractory or recurrent CIS after BCG therapy is still evolving, with some advocating repeat BCG instillation, second-line therapy with another intravesical agent such as mitomycin C or interferon-α, or radical cystectomy. Patients with CIS who fail two courses of intravesical therapy are at high risk for progressive cancer and should undergo cystectomy.

29. What are the goals of intravesical immunotherapy or chemotherapy?

It depends on the stage and grade of the tumor:

STAGE	GOAL
Multiple recurrent low-grade Ta	Prevent or reduce rate of recurrences
Grade 3 and T1	Prevent recurrences and progression to muscle invasion
Diffuse CIS	Eradicate established tumor

30. What are the side effects of BCG?
Local symptoms of bladder irritability are most prominent. Mild systemic symptoms with low-grade fever and myalgias are also common. High or persistent fever (> 24–48 hrs) and/or more severe systemic symptoms require early antituberculous therapy. Several deaths have been attributed to systemic ''BCGosis,'' usually occurring after intravesical administration following traumatic urethral catheterization.

31. Do lasers have a role in the treatment of TCC?
The Nd:YAG laser is an alternative to fulguration of recurrent low-grade noninvasive tumors with the potential advantages of outpatient use without anesthesia, a low risk of infield recurrence, and lower risk of tumor implantation. However, use of the laser without resection or biopsy provides no pathologic or prognostic information and should be restricted to patients with recurrent tumors who are judged to be at low risk of progression.

Photodynamic therapy with a systemic photosensitizer and argon-dye laser is an experimental approach for treating BCG-refractory diffuse CIS and for prophylaxis against recurrent papillary tumors. This method is cumbersome due to cutaneous photosensitivity, uncertainties about light dosimetry, and the development of severe bladder contractures.

32. What is the risk of developing an upper tract TCC after diagnosis of bladder TCC?
Approximately 5%. The frequency with which repeat upper tract screening studies (urogram or retrograde pyelograms) need to be preformed has never been adequately defined. Historical practice has been to perform them at yearly intervals.

33. What is the risk of developing bladder TCC after diagnosis of an upper-tract TCC?
Approximately 40–70%. All patients with upper tract TCC require cystoscopy at the time of diagnosis and at routine intervals thereafter.

34. How is muscle-invasive TCC (stage T2 or greater) treated?
Usually by radical cystectomy. Unfortunately, up to 50% of patients have occult systemic metastasis at the time of presentation and are not cured by cystectomy alone.

35. What are the commonest sites of metastasis from invasive TCC?
1. **Lymphatic metastases:** pelvic lymph nodes, including the obturator nodes, external iliac nodes, paravesical nodes, and common iliac nodes.
2. **Hematogenous metastases:** liver, lung, bone, adrenal, and bowel.

36. What is meant by "radical" rather than "simple" cystectomy?
In men, radical cystectomy implies bilateral pelvic lymphadenectomy and wide excision of the bladder and prostate including the urachal remnant, overlying peritoneum, and vascular pedicles. In selected cases, nerve-sparing cystoprostatectomy with a more limited dissection of the posterior vesical pedicles is indicated and does not compromise cancer control. In women, radical cystectomy implies anterior pelvic exenteration including the uterus, fallopian tubes, ovaries, anterior vaginal wall, and complete removal of the urethra.

37. What is the incidence of unsuspected TCC of the prostate in men undergoing radical cystectomy for invasive tumors?

As high as 45% in one series. The presence of prostatic TCC is best evaluated by deep transurethral and transrectal prostatic biopsies before cystectomy. These should be routinely performed in all candidates for orthotopic bladder replacement to the urethra.

38. How frequently does urethral TCC recur after cystectomy? Should all men have a prophylactic urethrectomy?

Clinical recurrence occurs in only 7–10% of patients, a risk that does not justify routine urethrectomy. However, the presence of TCC invading the prostatic stroma does predict recurrence. These patients *should* undergo prophylactic urethrectomy. All other patients should be followed with serial urethral wash cytologies.

39. Is transurethral resection alone ever curative for invasive TCC?

Only rarely. Patients with small, first-time tumors with only superficial muscle invasion (stage T2) which are completely re-resected after initial resection may be candidates for this. Survival rates equal to those for radical cystectomy have been reported using this approach.

40. What is the role for partial cystectomy for invasive TCC?

Partial cystectomy should be considered in patients with lower grade, unifocal, first-time tumors which are located away from the ureteral orifices and bladder floor and in whom a minimum 2-cm margin of normal tissue can be obtained. Random mucosal biopsies should be obtained at the time of staging evaluation to test for the presence of multifocal dysplasia and/or CIS which, if present, dictate radical rather than partial cystectomy.

41. Are systemic neoadjuvant (precystectomy) or adjuvant (postcystectomy) chemotherapy useful in the treatment of invasive TCC?

Neoadjuvant therapy produces responses in about 50% of patients, but most harbor residual disease in the bladder and require cystectomy. Its effect on survival is being assessed in randomized clinical trials. Several studies have suggested a modest increase in survival in patients with poor prognostic factors (perivesical fat invasion or positive nodes) following adjuvant chemotherapy.

42. What are the most popular forms of urinary diversion after radical cystectomy?

The ileal or Bricker conduit has the longest track record of any single technique. This is the simplest and least prone to major complications of all diversions, but it is limited by the need for an external urinary appliance. Various forms of continent urinary diversion were popularized in the 1980s and are now considered the gold standard in terms of improved patient lifestyle.

43. Describe the advantages and disadvantages of end and loop ileal conduit stomas.

The main advantage of a loop stoma is the ease of obtaining an everted bud above skin level. Both types produce equivalent functional results and complication rates in properly selected patients. End stomas are more prone to ischemic complications.

44. Name the four most important factors in obtaining good postoperative results from an ileal conduit stoma.

1. Patient education
2. Planned preoperative stomal site selection
3. Creation of an everted stomal bud without mesenteric ischemia
4. Postoperative support from enterostomal therapists.

45. Describe the jejunal conduit syndrome.

This syndrome consists of hyponatremia, hypochloremia, hyperkalemia, and acidosis resulting from the increased absorptive capacity of jejunum (versus ileum). It occurs in patients with jejunal conduits and is related to the length of the conduit and/or impaired renal function.

46. What are the most popular forms of continent urinary diversions?
Continent cutaneous diversions include the Indiana and Kock pouches and their variations. These have internal reservoirs with a valve mechanism to prevent continuous efflux of urine. They require the patient to perform clean intermittent catheterization several times daily to empty.

Orthotopic diversions to the urethra have been used in men and women. These pouches may be formed from ileum, colon, or both and are anastomsed to the urethra. This form of urinary diversion most closely approximates normal voiding, although about 10% of patients require intermittent catheterization to empty completely.

47. How should patients with metastatic or locally unresectable tumors be treated?
With platinum-based combination chemotherapy. The most commonly used regimen is MVAC (methotrexate, vinblastine, doxorubicin, and cisplatin), but CMV (MVAC without the doxorubicin) and CISCA (cisplatin, doxorubicin, and cyclophosphamide) have been used with similar response rates.

BIBLIOGRAPHY

1. Bretton PR, Herr HW, et al: Intravesical BCG therapy for in situ transitional cell carcinoma involving the prostatic urethra. J Urol 141:853, 1989.
2. Catalona WJ, Ratliff TL: BCG and superficial bladder cancer: Clinical experience and mechanism of action. Surg Annu 22:363, 1990.
3. Chechile G, Klein EA, Bauer L, et al: Functional equivalence of end and loop ileal conduit stomas. J Urol 147:582, 1992.
4. Droller MJ: Treatment of regionally advanced bladder cancer. Urol Clin North Am 19:685–693, 1992.
5. Hardeman SW, Soloway MS: Urethral recurrence following radical cystectomy. J Urol 144:666, 1990.
6. Herr HW: Conservative management of muscle-infiltrating bladder cancer: Prospective experience. J Urol 138:1162, 1987.
7. Herr HW, Laudone VP, Badlalmaent RA: BCG therapy alters the progression of superficial bladder cancer. J Clin Oncol 6:1450, 1988.
8. Klein EA, Montie JE, Montague DK, Straffon RA: Jejunal conduit urinary diversion. J Urol 135:244, 1986.
9. Klein EA, Rogatko A, Herr HW: Management of local BCG failures in superficial bladder cancer. J Urol 147:601, 1992.
10. Lamm DL: Long-term results of intravesical therapy for superficial bladder cancer. Urol Clin North Am 19:573–580, 1992.
11. Lieskovsky G, Skinner DG: Role of lymphadenectomy in the treatment of bladder cancer. Urol Clin North Am 11:709, 1984.
12. Rowland RG, Mitchell ME, Bihrle R, et al: Indiana continent urinary reservoir. J Urol 137:1136, 1987.
13. Skinner DG, Lieskovsky G, Boyd SD: Continent urinary diversion. J Urol 141:1323, 1989.
14. Spruck CH, Ohneseit PF, Gonzalez-Zulueta M, et al: Two molecular pathways to transitional cell carcinoma of the bladder. Cancer Res 54:784, 1994.
15. Sternberg CN, Yagoda A, Scher HI, et al: MVAC for advanced transitional cell carcinoma of the urothelium. J Urol 139:461, 1988.
16. Tsai YC, Nichols PW, Hiti AL, et al: Allelic losses of chromosomes 9, 11, and 17 in human bladder cancer. Cancer Res 50:44, 1990.
17. Wood DP, Montie JE, Pontes JE, et al: Transitional cell carcinoma of the prostate in cystoprostatectomy specimens removed for bladder cancer. J Urol 141:346, 1989.
18. Wood DP, Montie JE, Pontes JE, et al: The role of magnetic resonance imaging in the staging of bladder cancer. J Urol 140:741, 1988.
19. Zabbo A, Montie JE, et al: Management of the urethra in men undergoing radical cystectomy for bladder cancer. J Urol 131:267, 1984.

28. CARCINOMA OF THE PROSTATE

Martin I. Resnick, M.D.

1. List the different types of prostate cancer. Which one is most common.
Several histologic types of prostate cancer have been identified and include adenocarcinoma, transitional cell carcinoma, carcinosarcoma, and sarcoma. Greater than 90% of patients have adenocarcinoma which has several variations including neuroendocrine, endometrioid, and mucinous types.

2. What is the prevalence of carcinoma of the prostate in the United States?
Carcinoma of the prostate is the most common malignancy diagnosed in American men. Approximately 30% of men over 50 years of age have histologic evidence of carcinoma of the prostate. This percentage rises as the population ages.

3. What are the estimated incidence and death rate?
The American Cancer Society estimates that 200,000 new cases of carcinoma of the prostate will be diagnosed and 38,000 men will die of the disease in 1994.

4. Which men typically are at greater risk for developing carcinoma of the prostate?
Blacks have a higher risk of developing carcinoma of the prostate than whites. Additionally, they have a higher mortality from the disease. The stage of the disease is usually more advanced at time of diagnosis in blacks.

Men with one **first-degree relative** with carcinoma of the prostate have a 2-fold increased chance of developing the disease, and this increases to 9-fold if two first-degree relatives are affected. These familial predilections predominant in younger men with the disease.

5. In which portion of the prostate does cancer typically form?
Approximately 70% of adenocarcinomas originate in the peripheral zone of the prostate, 20% occur in the transition zone, and 10% in the central zone. Cancers in the fibromuscular stroma usually result from invasion by tumors arising in other zones, particularly the transition zone.

6. What symptoms are associated with carcinoma of the prostate?
In the early stages, patients have no symptoms related to the malignancy. Many may have symptoms similar to those of benign prostatic hyperplasia (e.g., nocturia, urinary urgency, weakness of the urinary stream). In patients with advanced disease, particularly bony metastases, skeletal pain may be a presenting symptom.

7. Describe the typical physical findings.
On digital rectal examination, prostate carcinomas are typically palpable as discrete, hard nodules. In patients with localized tumors, these nodules can be 0.5–1.0 cm in size, and with more advanced disease the entire prostate may be involved. With the increased use of tumor markers and prostate biopsy, more men are being diagnosed with carcinoma of the prostate who have no palpable abnormalities.

8. What is PSA? How is it used?
Prostate-specific antigen (PSA) is produced by both normal and malignant prostate epithelial cells. PSA is a serine protease of the kallikrein family and is associated with semen. Serum levels of PSA are elevated in many but not all men with cancer of the prostate but also in some men with benign prostatic hyperplasia. The marker is used in monitoring patients who have been treated for carcinoma of the prostate. Its use in screening and early detection remains controversial.

9. Why is acid phosphatase measured?

Acid phosphatase is an enzyme that hydrolyzes phosphate in an acid environment. Prostate-specific acid phosphatase is the first tumor marker that was associated with cancer of the prostate. It is produced by the epithelial cells and is elevated in approximately two-thirds of men with metastatic disease. With the introduction of PSA, the enzymatic assay for prostatic acid phosphatase now has limited use but remains helpful in staging patients with confirmed carcinoma of the prostate.

10. How is the diagnosis of carcinoma of the prostate usually established?

Patients with elevations in PSA and/or palpable abnormalities of the prostate are usually evaluated with ultrasonography and ultrasound-directed biopsies. If abnormalities are noted, these specific areas are biopsied, but if not, systematic or sextant biopsies of the prostate are obtained to establish a diagnosis. These biopsies are usually performed transrectally, and cores of tissue are obtained.

11. What are the different stages of carcinoma of the prostate?

TNM Classification System of Prostate Carcinoma

Primary tumor (T)	
TX	Primary tumor cannot be assessed
T0	No evidence of primary tumor
T1	Clinically inapparent tumor not palpable or visible by imaging
T1a	Tumor incidental histologic finding in ≤5% of tissue resected
T1b	Tumor incidental histologic finding in >5% of tissue resected
T1c	Tumor identified by needle biopsy (e.g., because of elevated PSA)
T2	Palpable tumor confined within prostate
T2a	Tumor involves half of a lobe or less
T2b	Tumor involves more than half of a lobe, but not both lobes
T2c	Tumor involves both lobes
T3	Tumor extends through the prostatic capsule
T3a	Unilateral extracapsular extension
T3b	Bilateral extracapsular extension
T3c	Tumor invades seminal vesicle(s)
T4	Tumor is fixed or invades adjacent structures other than seminal vesicles
T4a	Tumor invades external sphincter, bladder neck, and/or rectum
T4b	Tumor invades levator muscles and/or is fixed to pelvic wall
Lymph node (N)	
NX	Regional lymph nodes cannot be assessed
N0	No regional lymph nodes metastasis
N1	Metastasis in single lymph node, ≤ 2 cm in greatest diameter
N2	Metastasis in single lymph node, > 2 cm but ≤ 5 cm in greatest dimension, or multiple lymph nodes, none > 5 cm in greatest dimension
N3	Metastasis in a lymph node, > 5 cm in greatest dimension
Distant metastasis (M)	
MX	Presence of distant metastasis cannot be assessed
M0	No distant metastasis
M1	Distant metastasis present
M1a	Nonregional lymph nodes
M1b	Bone
M1c	Other sites

12. Is a bone scan useful in diagnosis?

A bone scan is a radionuclide study useful in detecting bone metastases. With the introduction of PSA, its use is limited and it is more commonly obtained in patients with significant elevation of PSA (> 20 ng/dl) or the presence of bone pain.

13. What is Gleason's sum?

Gleason's sum is based on the pattern of cells comprising the carcinoma. Two regions of the prostate are viewed, each being graded 1–5. A total of the patterns comprise a Gleason's sum—i.e., 2–10. Tumors may be classified as well differentiated (2,3,4), moderately differentiated (5,6,7) or poorly differentiated (8,9,10).

14. What is a radical prostatectomy?

A surgical procedure used for treating patients with carcinoma of the prostate. The procedure involves removing the prostate and seminal vesicles, with anastomosis of the urethra to the bladder. The procedure can be performed through a retropubic or perineal approach.

15. How is radiation therapy used?

Radiation therapy can be administered by external beam or placement of interstitial seeds. External sources include cobalt, linear accelerated, protons, and neutrons. Interstitial seeds include gold-198, iodine-125, and iridium-192.

16. What is salvage prostatectomy?

Salvage prostatectomy is used in patients in whom radiation therapy has failed. A radical prostatectomy is performed to accomplish cure in these patients.

17. What is the purpose of endocrine therapy?

The malignant prostatic cell, like the normal hyperplastic cell, requires testosterone for growth. Endocrine therapy is directed at reducing the circulating levels of testosterone available to the prostate and/or interfering with the metabolism of testosterone within the prostate epithelial cells. Atrophy and death of prostatic cells occur and tumor progression is reduced.

18. How do LH/RH analogs function?

Luteinizing hormone-releasing hormone (LH/RH) analogs reduce circulating LH levels and subsequently interfere with the secretion of testosterone by the Leydig cells of the testicle. Castrate levels of testosterone are obtained in patients treated with these agents.

19. What does total androgen blockade do and how is it carried out?

Total androgen blockade attempts not only to interfere with testosterone produced by the testicle either with castration or an LH/RH analog, but also to interfere with the action of other circulating androgens, particularly those produced by the adrenal gland. Antiandrogens (e.g., flutamide) are effective in interfering with the binding of dihydrotestosterone to a specific cytoplastic receptor. Combination therapy is what is referred to as total androgen blockade.

BIBLIOGRAPHY

1. Andriole GL, Catalona WJ: Advanced Prostate Carcinoma. Urol Clin North Am 18(1), 1991.
2. Das S, Crawford ED: Cancer of the Prostate. New York, Marcel Dekker, 1993.
3. Fitzpatrick JM, Krane RJ: The Prostate. Edinburgh, Churchill Livingstone, 1989.
4. Lepor H, Lawson RK: Prostate Diseases. Philadelphia, W. B. Saunders, 1993.
5. Paulson DF: Prostatic Disorders. Philadelphia, Lea & Febiger, 1989.
6. Smith JA: Early Detection and Treatment of Localized Carcinoma of the Prostate. Urol Clin North Am 17(6), 1990.

29. BENIGN PROSTATIC HYPERPLASIA

Martin I. Resnick, M.D.

1. Describe the anatomic relationship of the prostate to adjacent structures.
Superiorly, the prostate is attached to the bladder neck, and inferiorly it is bound by the urogenital diaphragm. Posteriorly, the prostate is next to the rectum, and to its anterior lies the pubus, to which the prostate is attached by the puboprostatic ligaments. The dorsal venous complex lies between the prostate and the pubus, and Denonvilliers' fascia, a reflection of the peritoneum, lies between the prostate and rectum. Laterally, the prostate is bound by the levator muscles.

2. What does the prostate do?
The specific function of the prostate has not been fully clarified, but it provides the bulk of the ejaculate. The secretions of the prostate include nutrients for sperm cells and proteases which function to liquefy the ejaculate. It is likely that many other functions have not been identified.

3. What are the zones of the prostate?
The prostate comprises the peripheral, central, and transition zones. The anterior fibromuscular stroma is devoid of glandular structures.

4. Describe the histologic components of the prostate.
The prostate is composed of stromal and epithelial elements. Organized acinar glands compose the epithelial components which make up a ductal system that drains into the urethra. The fibromuscular stromal component is made up of smooth and skeletal elements that interact with the epithelial structures.

5. How is testosterone metabolized in the prostate?
Free testosterone enters the prostate cell by passive diffusion and is reduced by 5α-reductase to dihydrotestosterone. Dihydrotestosterone becomes bound to a specific receptor and is translocated into the nucleus where it stimulates the expression of specific RNA synthesis and thus directs cellular activity.

6. Are the zones of the prostate associated with specific diseases?
Benign hyperplasia of the prostate has its origin in the transition zone. The peripheral zone gives rise to most carcinomas of the prostate, and the central zone tends to be devoid of specific disease processes.

7. What is the prevalence of benign prostatic hyperplasia (BPH)?
Histologic BPH begins to be detected in men in their early 30s. The prevalence of the disease continues to rise and approaches 90% in men at age 80 years. Symptoms secondary to prostatic enlargement and bladder outlet obstruction increase, and significant symptoms are present in approximately one-fourth of men by the seventh decade of life.

8. List the symptoms associated with BPH.

OBSTRUCTIVE SYMPTOMS	IRRITATIVE SUMPTOMS	OTHER SYMPTOMS
Weakness of urinary stream	Urinary urgency	Hematuria
Hesitancy	Frequency	Urinary tract infection
Terminal dribbling	Nocturia	Urinary retention
Intermittency	Incontinence (at times)	Renal failure (in severe
Sensation of incomplete bladder		obstruction)
emptying		
Straining to urinate (at times)		

9. What is meant by symptom score?
Various symptom scores have been developed that quantitate the subjective symptoms associated with BPH. Specific symptoms (e.g., nocturia, urinary frequency, urinary urgency) are graded and a total score is derived which relates to the severity of the patient's symptoms. Treatment decisions and assessment of outcomes are based on symptom scores. The most commonly used symptom score was developed by the American Urological Association.

10. What are the potential consequences of untreated BPH?
In addition to the significant symptoms that develop, BPH can result in the development of bladder calculi and associated symptoms, urinary retention, hydronephrosis, and in severe cases chronic, renal failure. Several of these conditions respond to treatment (e.g., urinary retention and bladder stones), but others may be permanent (renal failure) and may not respond to removal of the obstructing prostate.

11. When should patients with BPH be treated?
Increasingly, it appears that the severity of symptoms are directing the need for treatment. Patients with mild symptoms can be observed. However, those with moderate to severe symptoms require some form of therapy. Other indications for treatment relate to the complications associated with BPH, such as chronic urinary tract infection, bladder calculi, urinary retention, hydroureteronephrosis, and renal failure.

12. What diagnostic studies are useful in evaluating BPH?
In addition to a symptom score, specific studies such as measurement of residual urine and urinary pressure-flow studies are helpful in establishing the diagnosis of BPH and in assessing its severity.

13. What is finasteride? How does it work?
Finasteride is a 5-α reductase inhibitor that is used in the treatment of patients with symptomatic BPH. Interfering with the conversion of testosterone to dihydrotestosterone, finasteride typically shrinks the prostate gland by approximately 25% over 3 months. Symptomatic improvement follows, though patients must be maintained on the medication for at least 1 year.

14. Why are alpha-blocking agents effective in treating patients with BPH?
α-Receptors are located in the trigone of the bladder and fibromuscular stroma of the prostate. The fibromuscular stroma is composed in part of smooth muscle, and these, in addition to those located in the bladder neck, relax under α-blockade. Studies have demonstrated that prostates with a greater density of smooth muscle have a greater response to α-blockade.

15. What is a simple prostatectomy?
A simple prostatectomy is performed in patients with symptomatic BPH and involves removing the hyperplastic tissue located within the transition zone. A simple prostatectomy can be performed by transurethral resection or an open procedure, via either a suprapubic or retropubic approach.

16. List the potential complications of transurethral resection of the prostate.

Intraoperative Complications	*Postoperative Complications*
Hemorrhage	Uretral stricture
Hyponatremia (due to absorption of irrigating fluid)	Bladder neck contracture
	Incontinence
	Retrograde ejaculation

17. What is a transurethral incision of the prostate?

Transurethral incision of the prostate involves incising the prostatic urethra in an attempt to reduce urethral resistance and relieve voiding symptoms. The procedure is most efficacious in patients with small prostates and is associated with less morbidity than transurethral prostatic resection.

18. Are other forms of therapy available for treating patients with BPH?

New forms of therapy are being developed, including balloon dilation of the prostatic urethra and use of prostatic stents. Other forms of therapy include hyperthermia, thermotherapy, and more recently, high-temperature radio frequency ablation of prostatic tissue.

BIBLIOGRAPHY

1. Hinman F Jr: Benign Prostatic Hypertrophy. New York, Springer Verlag, 1983.
2. Lepor H: Controversies and advances in treatment of benign prostatic hyperplasia. Probl Urol 5:1991.
3. Lepor H, Lawson RK: Prostate Diseases. Philadelphia, W. B. Saunders, 1993.
4. Lepor H, Walsh PC: Benign Prostatic Hyperplasia. Urol Clin North Am 17(3):1990.

30. SQUAMOUS CELL CARCINOMA OF THE PENIS

Kurt H. Dinchman, M.D.

1. What is the most common form of carcinoma of the penis?
Squamous cell carcinoma.

2. What is carcinoma in situ of the penis?
Carcinoma in situ of the penis, also referred to as erythroplasia of Queyrat or Bowen's disease, may precede and progress to invasive squamous cell carcinoma of the penis.

3. How is circumcision related to the incidence of penile carcinoma?
Squamous cell carcinoma of the penis is rare among men who were circumcised at infancy. Development of squamous cell carcinoma of the penis in uncircumcised men is attributed to chronic irritative effects of smegma and chronic bacterial infection that may be related to smegma in men with poor hygiene.

4. Has the human papilloma virus (HPV) been implicated in penile cancer?
Recent studies have shown that men with HPV and genital herpetic infections have a higher incidence of penile carcinoma.

5. What is the most common presenting manifestation of squamous cell carcinoma?
Squamous cell carcinoma usually presents as a persistent sore or ulcer of the glans and/or the foreskin. The sores are usually painless; for this reason, patients may delay seeking treatment.

6. What are the most common premalignant lesions of the penis?
- Leukoplakia
- Erythroplasia of Queyrat
- Balanitis xerotica obliterans
- Buschke-Löwenstein tumor

7. How is carcinoma of the penis staged?
Accurate assessment of stage is important in determining the type of therapy that the patient requires. Initial diagnosis should be made by an excisional biopsy, which allows accurate assessment of the depth of invasion. The status of inguinal lymph nodes should be assessed by careful physical examination. CT scan of the abdomen and pelvis is also required to assess the status of the pelvic and abdominal lymph nodes.

8. What is the most commonly used staging system for carcinoma of the penis?
The most commonly used staging system is the Jackson staging system. Stage 1 refers to tumors confined to the glans and prepuce; stage 2, to tumors extending into the shaft of the penis; stage 3, to tumors with inguinal metastases that are amenable to surgery; and stage 4, to inoperable inguinal metastases or distant metastases.

9. How is the primary lesion treated in squamous cell carcinoma of the penis?
Removal of the cancer by partial or total penectomy is standard therapy. Partial penectomy requires a 2-cm margin of normal cancer-free penile shaft for effective removal of tumor. For extensive lesions approaching the penoscrotal junction, total penectomy should be performed with excision of both corpora and creation of a perineal urethrostomy. Small lesions involving the foreskin may be managed with circumcision alone; however, diligent postoperative follow-up is required because of the high rate of recurrence.

10. What is the most important factor in the prognosis of penile carcinoma?
The most important factor is the presence of inguinal metastases.

11. What is the current recommendation for treatment of Jackson stages 1 and 2 without inguinal lymphadenopathy?
The current recommendation is local excision of the lesion with a wide tumor-free margin and examination of inguinal lymph nodes every 3–4 months for approximately 24 months.

12. What is the current recommendation for treatment of Jackson stages 1 and 2 with invasion of corporal bodies and/or tunica albuginea?
The current recommendation is to perform a superficial lymph node dissection, followed by total lymphadenectomy if the superficial lymph nodes are positive, with either partial or total penectomy.

13. What is the current recommendation for treatment of Jackson stage 3 carcinoma of the penis?
In patients with lymphadenopathy a 6-week course of antibiotic therapy should be initiated because of the inflammatory inguinal lymphadenopathy frequently associated with ulcerated and/or infected penile lesions. Once therapy is completed, the lymphatic tissue should be reevaluated. Bilateral lymphadenopathy requires bilateral inguinal lymph node dissection, whereas unilateral lymphadenopathy requires a superficial and deep node dissection of the ipsilateral inguinal nodes.

14. What treatment is currently recommended for Jackson stage 4 penile carcinoma?
The usual treatment for such patients is palliative radiotherapy and/or chemotherapy (most commonly a single-agent application of bleomycin, methotrexate, or cysplatin).

BIBLIOGRAPHY

1. DeVita VT, Hellman S, Rosenberg S (eds): Cancer: Principles and Practice of Oncology, vol. 1, 2nd ed. Philadelphia, J. B. Lippincott, 1993.
2. Resnick MI, Kursh ED (eds): Current Therapy in Genitourinary Surgery, 2nd ed. St. Louis, B. C. Decker–Mosby, 1992.
3. Seidman EJ, Hanno PM (eds): Current Urologic Therapy. Philadelphia, W. B. Saunders, 1994.
4. Walsh PC, Retik AB, Stamey AT, Vaughan ED (eds): Campbell's Urology, 6th ed. Philadelphia, W. B. Saunders, 1992.

31. PREMALIGNANT LESIONS OF THE PENIS

Kurt H. Dinchman, M.D.

1. What is the most common malignant lesion of the penis?
Squamous cell carcinoma of the penis.

2. What is the significance of premalignant lesions of the penis?
Approximately 30–40% of patients with squamous cell carcinoma of the penis have a history of a preexisting penile lesion.

3. What precancerous lesions may be found on the penis?
- Cutaneous horns
- Balanitis xerotica obliterans
- Leukoplakia
- Condyloma acuminatum
- Bowenoid papulosis
- Kaposi's sarcoma
- Buschke-Löwenstein tumor

4. Which of the above are related to viral etiology?
Condyloma acuminatum, bowenoid papulosis, and Buschke-Loewenstein tumors are related to infections with the human papilloma virus (HPV), whereas Kaposi's sarcoma is seen in patients infected with the human immunodeficiency virus (HIV).

5. What is a cutaneous horn?
A cutaneous horn is a hyperkeratotic lesion and may be related to preexisting lesions, such as a wart or traumatic injury. Because of their malignant potential, such lesions should be excised, and the area of excision should be watched carefully.

6. What is balanitis xerotica obliterans?
Balantis xerotica obliterans is a patchy white lesion involving the glans and prepuce. Such lesions predispose patients to painful erosions and fissures, along with obstructive symptoms due to meatal stenosis. Treatment consists of a biopsy followed by local application of steroids to the lesions. Meatotomy may be needed to alleviate outlet obstruction. Close observation is required to look for changes of malignant transformation.

7. What is leukoplakia of the penis?
Leukoplakia is a hyperkeratotic lesion of the prepuce or glans that is associated with chronic irritation. Although the malignant potential of such lesions is low, circumcision for lesions involving the prepuce or removing the source of irritation on the glans is the therapeutic regimen of choice, along with close observation.

8. What is condyloma acuminatum?
Also called venereal or genital warts, condyloma acuminatum is a common form of sexually transmitted disease caused by a family of related viruses grouped under the name human papilloma viruses (HPV). Recent reports from the Centers for Disease Control show new cases at approximately 1 million per year. HPV is also considered the main etiologic agent in cervical cancer and dysplasia.

9. How is condyloma acuminatum detected?
Most cases of condyloma acuminatum are detected by the patient as clusterlike lesions on a narrow stalk or sessile base. Frequently patients are evaluated after HPV is discovered on a

cervical smear of a partner on a routine Papanicoloau test. In addition to appearing on the foreskin, glans, and shaft, such lesions may be found on the wall of the scrotum, perineum, and anus. Careful inspections of the distal urethra is warranted to rule out urethral condyloma.

10. How is condyloma acuminatum treated?
Treatment depends on the extent of the disease. Isolated lesions on the shaft may be treated with podophyllin or trichloroacetic acid solution. Surgical excision and electrocautery are also acceptable methods for isolated lesions. More extensive disease may be treated with laser ablation. Nd:YAG and CO_2 lasers have been used successfully with good control of lesions and satisfactory cosmetic results. Intraurethral and meatal condyloma have been treated successfully with 5-fluorouracil cream.

11. Define Buschke-Löwenstein tumor.
Buschke-Löwenstein tumor, also known as giant condyloma, is similar to condyloma acuminatum in appearance but may cause invasive erosion into surrounding tissue. Surgical excision is the treatment of choice.

12. Define bowenoid papulosis.
Bowenoid papulosis is a papulelike lesion of genitalia with pathologic features similar to carcinoma in situ; a connection to HPV has been made in multiple studies. All modalities outlined for the treatment of condyloma acuminatum may be used. To date, no invasive form of the disease has been documented.

13. Why is recognition of Kaposi's sarcoma important?
Kaposi's sarcoma (KS) consists of dark-colored, bleeding, tender papules of the penile skin. In patients with acquired immunodeficiency syndrome (AIDS), KS may be the initial presenting manifestation. Treatment is palliative, including laser treatment and surgical excision.

BIBLIOGRAPHY

1. Gillenwater JY, Grayhack JT, Howards SS, Duckett JW (eds): Adult and Pediatric Urology, 2nd ed. St. Louis, Mosby, 1991.
2. Resnick MI, Elder JS: Office Urology (entire issue). Urol Clin North Am 15(4):1988.
3. Resnick MI, Kursh ED (eds): Current Therapy in Genitourinary Surgery, 2nd ed. St. Louis, B. C. Decker–Mosby, 1992.
4. Walsh PC, Retik AB, Stamey AT, Vaughan ED (eds): Campbell's Urology, 6th ed. Philadelphia, W. B. Saunders, 1992.

32. URETHRAL CANCER

Mark A. Wainstein, M.D., and Elroy D. Kursh, M.D.

1. What is the incidence of urethral cancer?

Urethral cancer is relatively rare, representing < 1% of all genitourinary cancers in men and < 0.02% in women. This malignancy generally occurs during the sixth to seventh decades of life. It is the only genitourinary malignancy that is more common in women than men by a ratio of 4:1.

2. Describe the anatomic differences between the male and female urethra.

The **female urethra** is 2–4 cm long and approximately one-fifth the length of the male urethra. The distal two-thirds is lined with stratified squamous epithelium, and the proximal one-third is lined with transitional epithelium. The anterior urethra is defined as the distal one-third and drains into the superficial and deep inguinal nodes. The posterior urethra, or proximal two-thirds, drains into the pelvic lymph nodes. The anterior female urethra can be excised without destroying the urinary continence mechanism.

The **male urethra** is approximately 21 cm long and divided into three regional segments: penile, membranous, and prostatic. The urethra can also be divided into an anterior portion, composed of the penile urethra with its bulbar and pendulous segments, and the posterior urethra, consisting of the membranous and prostatic segments. Most authors, however, classify lesions of the bulbar urethra as being posterior because of their similarity in presentation, management, and prognosis to other posterior lesions. The epithelial lining varies along its length—transitional epithelium in the prostatic urethra, pseudostratified columnar epithelium in the membranous, bulbar, and penile segments, and stratified squamous epithelium in the fossa navicularis and meatus. The lymphatic drainage of the anterior urethra parallels the glans and corpus spongiosum and drains the deep inguinal nodes. The posterior urethra drains into the pelvic lymph nodes.

3. What etiologic factors are associated with the development of urethral cancer?

Like many genitourinary malignancies, urethral cancer has no known etiology. In women, factors such as chronic irritative voiding symptoms and recurrent urinary tract infections have been implicated, though no direct etiology has been proven. In males, approximately 25–75% of men with urethral cancer have a history of stricture disease, most commonly in the bulbomembranous urethra, which is the most common site of urethral cancers, and up to 50% have a history of venereal disease.

4. List the pathologic types of urethral cancer and their frequencies.

Pathologic Types of Urethral Cancers

TYPE OF CARCINOMA	FREQUENCY	NOTES
Women		
Squamous cell	>50%	Arises in distal two-thirds of urethra. Cell type reflects normal histology of this segment.
Transitional cell	15%	Must be differentiated from primary bladder cancer.
Adenocarcinoma	10–15%	May arise from neoplastic differentiation of transitional cell epithelium or glandular epithelium of paraurethral glands. Presents at later stage and carries worse prognosis than squamous carcinomas.
Men		
Squamous cell carcinoma	75%	Occurs most commonly in penile and bulbomembranous urethra.
Transitional cell	15%	Occurs most commonly in prostatic urethra.
Adenocarcinoma	5%	Must be differentiated from adenocarcinoma arising from prostate.
Undifferentiated	1%	—

5. What are the presenting signs and symptoms?

Females: Bleeding (60–75%), irritative voiding symptoms (dysuria, urinary urgency, frequency) (20–65%), obstructive voiding symptoms (25–50%), and perineal pain (25–40%). Urinary incontinence does not occur until advanced stages of disease. The most common clinical sign is a palpable indurated mass along the urethra.

    Males: Bleeding (40%), obstructive voiding symptoms (40%), and irritative voiding symptoms (28%). Physical findings include a palpable periurethral mass (40%) and, less commonly, perineal abscess or urethrocutaneous fistula (a communication between the urethra and perineum resulting in the leakage of urine). The average delay between the onset of symptoms and the time of diagnosis is considerable, usually 5–6 months.

6. What is the differential diagnosis of urethral cancer?

Women	*Men*
Urethral caruncle	Urethral strictures
Cyst	Perineal abscess
Diverticulum	Urethrocutaneous fistula
Condylomata acuminata	Metastatic disease involving the corpora caver-
Urethral prolapse	nosa (i.e., prostate cancer)
Periurethral abscess	

7. Compare the staging systems for males and females.

Staging of Urethral Carcinomas

STAGE	FEMALES	MALES
0	Carcinoma-in-situ, tumor limited to mucosa.	Tumor limited to mucosa (in situ).
A	Tumor involving and limited to submucosa.	Tumor into but not beyond lamina propria.
B	Tumor involving periurethral musculature.	Tumor into but not beyond corpus spongiosum or prostate.
C	Periurethral involvement	Direct extension into tissue beyond corpus spongiosum (corpora cavernosa, muscle, fat, fascial, skin, direct skeletal involvement) or beyond prostatic capsule.
C1	Infiltration of vaginal wall musculature.	—
C2	Infiltration of vaginal wall with invasion of vaginal mucosa.	—
C3	Infiltration of adjacent organs (e.g., bladder, labia, clitoris)	—
D	Metastatic disease	Metastatic disease
D1	—	Regional metastasis including inguinal and/ or pelvic lymph nodes (with any primary lesion).
D2	—	Distant metastasis (with any primary lesion).

8. Describe the various methods of diagnosis.

If urethral cancer is suspected, a careful **physical examination** should be performed, checking for the presence of a periurethral mass, fistula, or abscess. In women, a careful bimanual examination is necessary to assess the extent of the mass. In both men and women, the inguinal lymph nodes must be palpated since metastasis to this site occurs in approximately 15–30% of patients.

    Cystoscopy should be performed under anesthesia so that an adequate biopsy can be obtained to establish the diagnosis and help stage the cancer. Cystoscopy also allows assessment of tumor size, extent, and bladder involvement. In men, **retrograde urethrography** (injection of contrast media into the urethra) serves as a primary imaging technique for estimating the extent of local disease.

    Other imaging modalities include computed tomography (CT) and, at times, magnetic resonance imaging (MRI), both of which allow better estimation of regional disease involvement.

Chest radiography and bone scanning complete the staging of most patients. The most common sites of metastatic disease are the liver, lung, and bone.

9. How is urethral cancer treated?

The treatment is surgical extirpation of the lesion and depends on the location and extent of the cancer. Although various therapeutic options are available, the rarity of this lesion has made prospective studies impossible, and there is no routine approach. In general, distal lesions are more easily treated and have a more favorable prognosis. Because of the substantial anatomic differences between the male and female urethra, management of each sex varies considerably.

10. What is the surgical treatment of female urethral carcinoma?

Treatment of female urethral carcinoma, as in males, is based on the stage of the disease.

Lower-stage urethral tumors that are restricted to the mucosa can be effectively treated with laser resection, radiotherapy, or local excision. Because the goal of these therapeutic modalities is to preserve normal voiding, the best results have been obtained with cancers of the anterior urethra. Partial urethrectomy should be reserved for stage 0, A, and B lesions arising from and localized to the anterior urethra. The distal one-half of the urethra can be resected with limited risk of postoperative incontinence.

Higher-stage tumors (stage B, C) require more aggressive surgery. At times, adjuvant preoperative radiation with or without chemotherapy is employed. Therapeutic options for these tumors include total urethrectomy with bladder preservation (which is only possible with anterior tumors) or an anterior exenteration, which involves removal of the pelvic lymph nodes, entire urethra, uterus with ovaries and fallopian tubes, bladder, and anterior and lateral vaginal walls, and en bloc resection of the pubic symphysis and inferior pubic rami. Radiation therapy alone has not been very effective for advanced disease, with a mean 5-year survival of 34%. Combined radiation and surgical therapy for advanced urethral cancer provides the best 5-year survival (mean 55%).

11. What is the treatment of male urethral cancer?

In general, anterior urethral carcinoma is more amenable to surgical control than posterior urethral lesions. Superficial or local lesions can be treated with transurethral resection, although this carries a high risk of local recurrence. Carcinoma of the distal urethra in males should be treated with partial penectomy, and a 2-cm tumor-free margin should be resected proximal to the cancer. When there is not enough urethra to allow for an adequate urinary stream, a radical penectomy and perineal urethrostomy (repositioning of the proximal urethra to the perineum) should be performed. The 5-year survival in the absence of positive nodes is approximately 50%.

For stage C tumors, a radical surgical approach including en bloc resection of the penis, pubis, prostate, and bladder have provided the best long-term survival. Despite radical surgical resection, the experience with higher stage carcinomas has been disappointing, with 5-year survival rates of approximately 20%.

Unlike carcinoma of the penis, groin adenopathy usually represents metastasis and does not result from inflammation. In advanced disease, the lymph nodes are involved in > 50% of patients. Inguinal nodes are excised if they are palpable, since 80% contain metastasis. If the nodes are not palpable, the groin should be followed expectantly since there does not appear to be a therapeutic advantage of prophylactic node dissection.

Radiation therapy has been attempted in treating urethral cancer, but the results have been disappointing and even worse than surgical intervention.

12. Do any factors affect the prognosis in patients with urethral cancer?

The prognosis in carcinomas involving the anterior and posterior urethra varies considerably. In general, there is a better prognosis associated with anterior compared to posterior urethral cancers, because they tend to present at a lower stage at the time of clinical diagnosis. The earlier presentation of anterior urethral cancers results from their becoming symptomatic at an earlier stage than more proximal lesions.

The prognosis for urethral cancer is related to the stage at diagnosis and seems to be independent of the histologic type or grade. Patients with tumors of the anterior urethra have a better 5-year survival rate of approximately 50%, compared to 10–15% for posterior urethral cancers.

BIBLIOGRAPHY

1. Carroll PR: Surgical management of urethral carcinoma. In Crawford ED, Das S (eds): Current Genitourinary Cancer Surgery. Malvern, Lea & Febiger, 1990.
2. Droller MJ: Urethral carcinoma in females. In Resnick MI, Kursh ED (eds): Current Therapy in Genitourinary Surgery, 2nd ed. St. Louis, Mosby-Year Book Inc., 1992.
3. Fair WR, Yang C: Urethral carcinoma in males. In Resnick MI, Kursh ED (eds): Current Therapy in Genitourinary Surgery, 2nd ed. St. Louis, Mosby-Year Book Inc., 1992.
4. Grabstald H, Hilaris B, Heuschke U, et al. Cancer of the female urethra. JAMA 197:835–842, 1966.
5. Narayan P, Konety B: Surgical treatment of female urethral carcinoma. Urol Clin North Am 19(2):373–380, 1992.
6. Zeidman EJ, Desmond P, Thompson IM: Surgical treatment of carcinoma of the male urethra. Urol Clin North Am 19(2):359–371, 1992.

33. TESTICULAR TUMORS IN ADULTS

Eric A. Klein, M.D.

1. What is the most common type of tumor affecting the testis?
More than 90% of testis cancers are germ-cell tumors derived from the germinal epithelium of the mature testis (see table below). The tumors occur in both pure and mixed forms, slightly more commonly on the right; they are bilateral in 1–2% of patients. Approximately 5% of testis cancers are gonadal stromal tumors, derived from cells that support the generation and maturation of sperm. About 1% of testis tumors are metastatic from another site.

Histologic Classification of Testicular Neoplasms

Germ-cell tumors	Other tumors
Seminoma	Epidermoid cyst
Embryonal carcinoma	Adenomatoid tumor
Choriocarcinoma	Adrenal rest
Yolk sac tumor	Adenocarcinoma of the rete testis
Teratoma	Carcinoid
Mixed tumors	
Gonadal stromal tumors	
Leydig-cell tumors	
Sertoli-cell tumors	
Gonadoblastoma	
Mixed tumors	

2. What non–germ-cell cancers affect the testis?
Primary tumors of the other cellular elements of the testis include tumors of specialized stroma such as Leydig-cell tumors, Sertoli-cell tumors, and mixed forms; other stromal tumors include gonadoblastoma, adenocarcinoma of the rete testis, carcinoid, and mesenchymal tumors (see table). Secondary tumors include leukemia, lymphoma, and metastases from solid tumors at other sites.

3. Name the histologic subtypes of germ-cell tumors.
Seminoma, embryonal carcinoma, teratoma, choriocarcioma, and yolk sac tumor.

4. What is the most common histologic form of germ-cell tumors?
The most common histologically pure form is seminoma, but mixed tumors occur more frequently than pure ones.

5. What is the most common solid tumor in men between the ages of 15 and 40 years?
Germ-cell tumors of the testis.

6. What are risk factors for germ-cell tumors?
Age, race, and cryptorchidism (with a 3- to 14-fold increase in risk) are the only known risk factors. Although testis cancer can occur at any age, there are three peaks of incidence: men aged 20–40 years, men older than 60 years, and boys from birth to age 10. Caucasians are four times more likely to develop testis cancer than blacks. Approximately 10% of all testis tumors occur in undescended testes. A cryptorchid testis has 3–5% chance of developing cancer, with the risk proportional to the degree of maldescent. Intraabdominal testes and dysgenetic testes associated with a chromosomal syndrome (intersex) have the highest risk of malignancy.

7. Does family history increase the risk of testis cancer?
Testis cancer has been reported in fathers and sons, twins, and in two or more male siblings. However, except for the known forms of intersex, a defined familial inheritance pattern has not been established.

8. How does age influence the histology of testis tumors?
The histology of the primary tumor is closely correlated with age. Seminoma and mixed germ-cell tumors are most common in postpubertal men up to age 40 years; yolk sac tumors and pure teratoma predominate in infants; and men over 50 years of age are most commonly affected by spermatocytic seminoma, lymphoma, or other secondary tumors.

9. Does testicular trauma cause testis cancer?
Although cancer is often diagnosed after an episode of testicular trauma, no evidence suggests that trauma is an etiologic agent. It is more likely that the traumatic episode brings an underlying tumor to attention.

10. What are the primary lymphatic drainage areas of the testes?
Testicular lymphatics exist via the mediastinum testis and coalesce into larger channels in the spermatic cord. These channels travel through the inguinal canal, follow the testicular artery into the retroperitoneum, and fan out medially over the great vessels. Primary drainage of the right testis occurs in the interaortocaval area at the level of the L2 vertebral body. The left testis drains to the paraaortic area lateral to the aorta and medial to the ureter.

11. How do germ-cell tumors metastasize to the inguinal nodes?
The scrotal skin and underlying layers are drained by the inguinal and perianal lymph nodes; tumors that invade the scrotum therefore may drain to inguinal nodes. Prior inguinal or scrotal surgery (such as orchidopexy) also may put the inguinal nodes at risk. In addition, massive retroperitoneal adenopathy may lead to retrograde lymphatic deposits in the inguinal region.

12. What is the most common presenting complaint in patients with testis tumors?
The most common presenting complaint is painless unilateral swelling or nodule, usually as an incidental finding by the patient or his sexual partner. Scrotal or lower abdominal pain occurs in about one-third of patients. In 10% the presenting symptoms are due to systemic metastasis and may include a neck mass due to supraclavicular nodal disease; cough or dyspnea due to lung metastases; gastrointestinal symptoms or back pain due to retroperitoneal metastases; bone pain; central nervous system symptoms; or gynecomastia.

13. How common is a delay in diagnosis of testis tumors?
Delayed diagnosis is common. Ample evidence suggests that a delay in diagnosis leads to more advanced clinical stage, higher morbidity, and excessive mortality. Both patients and physicians may be the source of delay. Reasons for patient delay include misunderstanding the significance of testicular symptoms, attribution of symptoms to minor testicular trauma, transience of symptoms, and fear of cancer. Reasons for physician delay include attribution of symptoms to a benign condition, such as infection, epididymitis, or hydrocele, and neglect of testicular examination.

14. Outline the clinical evaluation of patient with a testis tumor.
Physical examination should include palpation of the testis with particular attention to possible involvement of the spermatic cord, scrotum, or skin by the primary tumor. Examination of the abdomen, chest, and cervical regions may disclose obvious metastases. A scrotal ultrasound may confirm the presence of an intratesticular mass. Serum tumor markers, including alpha fetoprotein (AFP), the beta subunit of human chorionic gonadotropin (βHCG), and lactic acid dehydrogenase (LDH), should be measured. A chest radiographic and computed tomographic (CT) scan of the abdomen and pelvis are performed routinely. A chest CT scan may be performed if the radiograph discloses metastatic disease.

15. What is the *sine qua non* for diagnosis of germ-cell tumor?
Inguinal orchiectomy with pathologic examination of the testis.

16. Describe the clinical and pathologic staging system for germ-cell tumors.

Two systems are in common use. The primary tumor, regional nodes, metastasis (TNM) system has gained popularity recently, because it better describes the local extent of the primary tumor.

Clinical Pathologic Staging of Germ-Cell Tumors

TUMOR EXTENT	CLINICAL STAGE	TNM STAGE	
Tumor confined to testis	I or A	Tx	Unknown status
		T0	No evidence of primary tumor
		T1	Confined to testis
		T2	Beyond tunica
		T3	Invasion of rete testis or epididymis
		T4a	Invasion of cord
		T4b	Invasion of scrotum
Spread to regional nodes	II or B	Nx	Not assessed
	IIA OR B1 <2 cm	N0	Confined to testis
	IIB OR B2 >2, <5 cm	N1	Microscopic tumor
	IIC OR B3 >5 cm	N2a	< 6 positive nodes, all < 2 cm
		N2b	> 6 nodes or any node > 2cm
		N3	Extranodal extension
		N4	Incomplete resection
Spread beyond regional nodes	III or C	M0	No metastases
		M1	Systemic metastases

17. What serum tumor markers are important in germ-cell tumors?

AFP, HCG, LDH, and placental alkaline phosphatase (PLAP) are useful for diagnosis, staging, monitoring response to therapy, predicting prognosis, and monitoring for tumor recurrence.

18. What is AFP? By which histologic types is it secreted?

AFP, a 70-kD, single-peptide-chain glycoprotein, is present in the developing fetus, but only minute amounts remain in adults. Serum AFP elevations (above 10 ng/dl) are detectable in 50–70% of patients with germ-cell tumors, including embryonal carcinoma, yolk sac tumor, and mixed tumors containing these elements.

19. What is HCG? By which histologic types is it secreted?

HCG is a 38-kD glycoprotein composed of alpha and beta subunits. The alpha subunit is homologous to the alpha peptides of several other hormones, including luteinizing hormone (LH), thyroid-stimulating hormone (TSH), and follicle-stimulating hormone (FSH). The beta subunit, which is antigenically distinct, is the clinically relevant marker for germ-cell cancer. Elevated βHCG levels (above 5 mIU/ml) are found in 40–60% of patients with testis cancer, including choriocarcinoma, embryonal carcinoma, and some cases of pure seminoma.

20. What other diseases may cause elevations in serum AFP and βHCG?

Hepatocellular, pancreatic, gastric, and lung cancers and benign liver conditions, including hepatitis and cirrhosis, may cause elevations in serum AFP levels. Multiple myeloma and hepatocellular, pancreatic, gastric, lung, and bladder tumors may cause elevated levels of serum βHCG.

21. What are the serum half-lives of AFP and βHCG?

The half-life of AFP is 5–7 days; of βHCG, 24–36 hours.

22. What is the significance of LDH and PLAP?

Elevations in serum LDH usually indicate advanced or bulky metastatic disease. PLAP, a fetal isoenzyme of alkaline phosphatase, is secreted by some seminomas.

23. What cytogenetic abnormalities are characteristic of germ-cell tumors?
Duplication of the short arm of chromosome 12, known as isochromosome 12p or i(12p).

24. Does an elevated level of serum βHCG after orchiectomy always indicate the presence of residual tumor?
No. Some assays for βHCG cross-react with LH and may lead to a false-positive interpretation. The typical scenario is in patients who are clinically free of disease but who have physiologically elevated concentrations of LH after unilateral orchiectomy and slightly elevated levels of βHCG. This cross-reactivity is distinguished from a true elevation of βHCG by repeating the assay 48 hours after the injection of 200 mg of testosterone, which suppresses the secretion of LH. Any elevations in βHCG attributable to cross-reactivity should return to normal after testosterone injection.

25. What is the significance of an elevated level of serum βHCG in patients with a histologically pure seminoma?
An elevated level of βHCG implies the presence of syncytiotrophoblasts that secrete HCG, but these tumors behave identically to non–HCG-secreting pure seminomas and are treated as such. The syncytiotrophoblastic elements may not be apparent by light microscopy, but usually are demonstrated by immunohistochemistry.

26. What is the significance of an elevated level of serum AFP in patients with a germ-cell tumor?
An elevated level of serum AFP always implies the presence of nonseminomatous elements; such tumors should be treated as mixed or nonseminomatous tumors.

27. Do normal serum markers after inguinal orchiectomy preclude the presence of residual active cancer?
No. Small-volume metastases may produce insufficient amounts of markers to be detectable in the blood, and even massive amounts of teratoma are usually marker-negative.

28. What pathologic factors in the primary tumor are associated with a high risk of metastases?
- Advanced local stage (T3 or T4)
- Presence of lymphatic or vascular invasion
- Percentage of embryonal carcinoma.

29. What is meant by nonseminomatous tumor?
Nonseminomatous tumors are composed histologically of embryonal carcinoma, teratoma, choriocarcinoma, and yolk sac elements alone or in combination. Tumors with both seminomatous and nonseminomatous elements behave and are treated as nonseminomatous tumors. Tumors with more than one element of any type are called mixed germ-cell tumors.

30. Define teratoma. Distinguish between its mature and immature forms.
Teratoma is a tumor that contains elements derived from more than one germ-cell layer (mesoderm, ectoderm and endoderm). Mature teratoma contains benign-appearing, differentiated structures, such as glands, cartilage, bone, muscle, or neural tissue. Immature teratoma consists of undifferentiated tissue from the three layers. Occasionally malignant changes are seen in otherwise mature tissue, leading to teratoma with malignant differentiation.

31. What is the treatment for pure seminoma at clinical stage I?
Inguinal orchiectomy and radiation therapy to the retroperitoneal and ipsilateral iliac lymph nodes yield a 5-year NED (no evidence of disease) survival rate of 95%. Recently, surveillance for stage I seminomas has been advocated as a way of avoiding the cost and toxicity of radiotherapy. However, the toxicity of radiotherapy in this setting is usually minor and self-limited. Surveil-

lance requires more intensive follow-up, and the potential for a much greater burden of therapy if relapse occurs.

32. Describe treatment for low-volume seminoma at clinical stage II (retroperitoneal lymph nodes of 5 cm or less).

Inguinal orchiectomy and radiation therapy to the retroperitoneal and ipsilateral iliac lymph nodes yield a 5-year NED survival rate of 90%.

33. Describe the treatment for advanced seminoma (bulky stage II or stage III).

More than 90% of patients have a complete response to inguinal orchiectomy followed by platinum-based combination chemotherapy; most remain disease-free at 5 years.

34. Describe the management of a residual mass in the retroperitoneum after chemotherapy for seminoma.

Treatment is controversial. Approaches include retroperitoneal lymphadenectomy, radiation therapy, and observation. Surgery in this setting is difficult because of severe fibrosis, and a clean retroperitoneal dissection is usually not attainable. Most residual masses less than 3 cm do not contain viable tumor and probably do not require surgical excision.

35. Describe the treatment for a nonseminomatous tumor at clinical stage I.

The recommended treatment is inguinal orchiectomy with careful pathologic analysis to determine the presence of adverse factors that increase the likelihood of retroperitoneal metastases (see question 28). In patients with no adverse histologic factors, either surveillance or nerve-sparing retroperitoneal lymphadenectomy (RPLND) may be offered. In patients with one or more adverse histologic factors, RPLND should be performed.

36. What are the advantages and disadvantages of surveillance vs. RPLND for clinical stage I nonseminomatous tumors?

The main advantage of surveillance is avoidance of major surgery in the 70% of patients who are cured by orchiectomy alone. The disadvantages of surveillance are the more intensive follow-up regimen required and the uncertainty about cure. The main advantage of RPLND is complete pathologic staging in all patients, early identification of the 30% who harbor occult retroperitoneal metastases, and identification of a small subset who require adjuvant chemotherapy. In the past the main disadvantage of RPLND was loss of seminal emission, but recently described nerve-sparing techniques result in preservation of emission and ejaculation in virtually 100% of patients with stage I disease.

37. Describe nerve-sparing RPLND.

The key element in nerve-sparing RPLND is the prospective identification and preservation of postganglionic sympathetic nerves that arise from the lumbar sympathetic chains and form an anastomosing network (the hypogastric plexus) anterior to the abdominal aorta and surrounding the origin of the inferior mesenteric artery. Nerves from the hypogastric plexus travel anteriorly along the aorta across the aortic bifurcation; descend into the pelvis to innervate the bladder neck; enter the seminal vesicles, vas deferens, prostate, and external urinary sphincter; and subserve emission and ejaculation. Older techniques of RPLND routinely disrupted these nerves and often resulted in failure of seminal emission, leading to dry ejaculation.

38. Describe the treatment for a clinical stage I nonseminomatous tumor found to have metastatic cancer at the time of RPLND.

Treatment of such a tumor, described as pathologic stage IIA or IIB, depends on the number, size, and histology of the involved nodes. For patients with N1 or N2a disease (see table in question 16), the risk of relapse is about 25–30%, and most patients are observed. For N2b or greater disease, the risk of relapse is 50%, and two cycles of adjuvant chemotherapy are recommended. If the nodes contain mature teratoma only, observation is usually recommended regardless of the number or size of nodes involved.

39. Describe the treatment for small-volume (< 5 cm retroperitoneal mass) nonseminomatous tumors at clinical stage II.
Treatment depends on the level of postorchiectomy tumor markers. If the markers are normal, RPLND is performed; if metastatic disease is confirmed, patients generally are treated with adjuvant chemotherapy, although observation may be advised if the volume of metastases is small or only mature teratoma is found. Stage II nonseminomatous and mixed tumors with elevated serum markers after orchiectomy are treated with systemic chemotherapy, followed by surgical resection of residual metastases.

40. What is the treatment of advanced (clinical stage IIC or III) nonseminomatous tumors?
The recommended treatment is systemic platinum-based multiagent chemotherapy, followed by surgical excision of residual pulmonary or retroperitoneal masses. If the initial diagnosis was made by lymph node or retroperitoneal biopsy, the ipsilateral testis also should be removed.

41. Describe the clinical presentation of gonadal stromal tumors.
Gonadal stromal tumors, like germ-cell tumors, usually present with a painless mass or swelling. Except for Leydig-cell tumors, which may present with feminization or other endocrinologic manifestations, gonadal stromal tumors usually are not suspected before orchiectomy.

42. Do gonadal stromal tumors produce clinically useful tumor markers?
Gonadal stromal tumors do not secrete AFP or HCG, but some (especially Leydig-cell tumors) produce estrogens and estrogen metabolites, which may be useful in monitoring for tumor recurrence.

43. How are gonadal stromal tumors treated?
About 90% of gonadal stromal tumors are benign and are cured by inguinal orchiectomy. RPLND may be considered if the histologic appearance suggests malignancy.

44. What other mesenchymal tumors may occur in the testis?
The most common mesenchymal tumors are fibromas, angiomas, leiomyomas, and neurofibromas, although any other stromal element may give rise to a tumor. They are important chiefly because they must be distinguished from germ-cell tumors.

45. Describe epidermoid cysts and their treatment.
Epidermoid cysts are round, sharply circumscribed lesions composed of fibrous tissue and keratinized squamous epithelium. They are uniformly benign and treated by inguinal orchiectomy, although some authors advocate partial excision, especially in children. This lesion may be suspected on testicular ultrasound because of its well-defined edge and associated calcification.

46. Name the most common secondary tumor of the testis.
The most common secondary tumor is lymphoma, which typically causes diffuse enlargement of the involved testis and may be the initial presenting sign of disease.

47. What are the most common metastatic tumors to the testis?
Adenocarcinomas of the prostate, lung, gastrointestinal tract, and kidney, and melanoma.

BIBLIOGRAPHY

1. Donohue JP, Zachary JM, Maynard BR: Distribution of nodal metastases in nonseminomatous testis cancer. J Urol 128:315, 1981.
2. Donohue JP, Foster RS, Rowland RG, et al: Nerve-sparing retroperitoneal lymphadenectomy with preservation of ejaculation. J Urol 144:287, 1990.

3. Jewett MA, Kong YS, Goldberg SD, et al: Retroperitoneal lymphadenectomy for testis tumor with nerve sparing for ejaculation. J Urol 139:1220, 1987.
4. Klein EA, Kay R: Testis cancer in adults and children. Urol Clin North Am 20(1), 1993.
5. Klein EA: Tumor markers in testis cancer. Uro Clin North Am 20:67–74, 1993.
6. Lange PH, Neurin P, Fraley EE: Fertility issues following therapy for testicular cancer. Semin Urol 2:264, 1984.
7. Lowe BA: Surveillance vs nerve sparing RPLND in stage I nonseminomatous germ cell tumors. Urol Clin North Am 20:75, 1993.
8. McLeod DG, Weiss RB, Stablein DM, et al: Staging relationships and outcome in early stage testicular cancer: A report from the testicular cancer intergroup study. J Urol 145:1178, 1990.
9. Marshall FF, Elder J: Cryptorchidism and Related Anomalies. New York, Praeger, 1982.
10. Motzer RJ, Bosl GJ: Role of adjuvant chemotherapy in patients with stage II nonseminomatous germ-cell tumors. Urol Clin North Am 20:11, 1993.
11. Recker F, Tscholl R: Monitoring of emission as direct intraoperative control for nerve sparing retroperitoneal lymphadenectomy. J Urol 150:1360, 1993.
12. Sheinfeld J, Bajorin D: Management of the postchemotherapy residual mass. Urol Clin North Am 20:133, 1993.
13. Vugrin D, Whitmore WF, Golbey RR: VAB-6 Combination chemotherapy without maintenance in treatment of disseminated cancer of the testis. Cancer 51:211, 1983.
14. Wishnow KW et al: Prompt orchiectomy reduces morbidity and mortality from testis cancer. Br J Urol 65:629, 1990.

34. TESTICULAR TUMORS IN CHILDREN

Robert Kay, M.D.

1. What is the most common type of testicular tumor in children?
Yolk sac tumor. It represents 63% of all testicular tumors in children.

2. Is a yolk sac tumor the same as embryonal cell tumor in an adult?
No. Yolk sac tumors differ histologically and biologically from embryonal cell tumors, and the treatment is different.

3. How do children with a testicular tumor usually present?
Most children with testicular tumors present with an asymptomatic mass. It may be misdiagnosed as a hydrocele, delaying diagnosis for up to 6 months because of the confusion.

4. What are the best diagnostic tests for a testicular tumor?
Ultrasound may be definitive with testicular tumors. If a child has a scrotal mass in which the testis cannot be felt or if the diagnosis is unclear, an ultrasound should be obtained. It can clearly delineate the testis and determine if there is an intratesticular mass.

Serum alpha-fetoprotein levels should also be analyzed. Alpha-fetoprotein is a protein that occurs in the fetus but disappears after birth. It is also produced by yolk sac tumors. Although elevated levels may be seen in a newborn and in the first six months of life, it is an excellent tumor marker that can be used both preoperatively and postoperatively to follow the tumor.

5. What tests should be ordered after a diagnosis of yolk sac tumor is made?
Assuming the alpha-fetoprotein was ordered preoperatively or immediately postoperatively, one should obtain a chest x-ray and an ultrasound or computed tomographic (CT) scan of the retroperitoneum to assess for retroperitoneal metastasis. This will allow the physician to stage the patient clinically.

6. What is the half-life of alpha-fetoprotein? How long before elevated levels return to normal?
The half-life of alpha-fetoprotein is 5 days. Thus, five half-lives or approximately 25–30 days should elapse before normal values are seen.

7. What are the survival statistics for children with yolk sac tumors?
Greater than 90% of children with yolk sac tumors will survive.

8. Besides yolk sac tumors, are other testicular tumors malignant?
Most other testicular tumors are benign. The second most common tumor in children, the teratoma, is always benign in infants and children. Although most gonadal stromal tumors are benign, there has been the very rare case of a malignant gonadal stromal tumor.

9. Does radiation therapy have a role in the treatment of prepubertal testicular tumors?
No. Surgery is curative in almost all cases, and only in the unusual metastatic yolk sac tumor is chemotherapy needed. Chemotherapy is effective, so radiotherapy does not play a role except in the palliative care of the child or in metastatic disease that is resistant to chemotherapy.

10. Can tumors be seen in the newborn?
Almost all types of testicular tumors can be seen in the newborn. However, juvenile granulosa cell tumor and yolk sac tumor are the most common tumors in the neonatal period. The tumors present as a hard mass and must not be misdiagnosed as in utero torsion of the testis.

11. What other testicular tumors occur in children?

Classification of Prepubertal Testicular Tumors

Germ cell tumors
  Yolk sac
  Teratoma
  Mixed germ cell
  Seminoma
Gonadal stromal tumors
  Leydig cell
  Sertoli cell
  Juvenile granulosa cell
  Mixed
Gonadoblastoma
Tumors of supporting tissues
  Fibroma
  Leiomyoma
  Hemangioma
Lymphomas and leukemias
Tumor-like lesions
  Epidermoid cysts
  Hyperplastic nodule secondary to congenital adrenal hyperplasia
Secondary tumors
Tumors of the adenexa

12. Which testicular tumor leads to precocious puberty in children?

Leydig cell tumor.

13. Is a retroperitoneal node dissection routinely indicated in yolk sac tumor?

No. The tumor metastasizes via both the hematogenous and lymphogenous system. A retroperitoneal node dissection should be done only if there is radiologic evidence of metastatic disease.

14. What is occult testicular leukemia?

Occult testicular leukemia refers to children with acute lymphogenous leukemia in remission but in whom routine biopsy of testis reveals disease confined to the testis. This occurs in 11% of patients with acute lymphogenous leukemia.

15. Why would leukemia present in the testis but not be detected anywhere else?

Although there are different theories, most believe there is a blood testis barrier. This allows the testis to be a protected haven from chemotherapy, and thus, isolated cells are not destroyed by the systemic treatment.

BIBLIOGRAPHY

1. Connolly JA, Gearhart JB: Management of yolk sac tumors in children. Urol Clin North Am 20:7–14, 1993.
2. Kay R: Genital tumors in children. In Kelalis PP, King LR, Belman AB (eds): Clinical Pediatric Urology, 3rd ed. Philadelphia, W. B. Saunders Co., 1992, pp 1457–1467.
3. Kay R: Prepubertal Testicular Tumor Registry. Urol Clin North Am 20(1):1–5, 1993.
4. Kay R, Kaplan GW: Testicular tumors in infants and children. Am Urol Assoc Update Ser 9(15):114–118, 1992.
5. Lange PH, Vogelzang NJ, Goldman A, et al: Marker half-life analysis as a prognostic tool in testicular cancer. J Urol 128:708, 1982.
6. Levy D, Kay R, Elder J: Neonatal testis tumors: A review of the Prepubertal Testis Tumor Registry. J Urol 151:715, 1994.

III. Congenital and Acquired Disease

35. Congenital Renal Cystic Disease

Jonathan H. Ross, M.D.

1. Explain the difference between polycystic kidney disease and a multicystic kidney.
The polycystic kidney diseases are congenital cystic diseases of the kidneys in which otherwise normal renal elements become cystically dilated. In contrast, the cysts of a multicystic kidney are not due to dilatation of specific renal elements, but rather, the entire kidney is dysplastic and composed of immature dysplastic stroma and cysts of various size.

2. What is the prognosis for an infant with bilateral multicystic kidneys?
Dismal. Multicystic kidneys do not function. As in renal agenesis, this results in anhydramnios and fatal pulmonary hypoplasia.

3. What is the most common cause of an abdominal mass in a newborn?
A multicystic dysplastic kidney. A hydronephrotic kidney, usually due to ureteropelvic junction obstruction, is a close second.

4. How are most multicystic kidneys currently diagnosed?
By prenatal ultrasound. Historically, only palpable multicystic kidneys were detected. Most went undetected and probably regressed. Many adults with an incidentally noted solitary kidney probably had a multicystic kidney originally.

5. What entities may be confused with a multicystic kidney?
Any of the other congenital cystic kidney diseases may be confused with a multicystic kidney, but these are quite rare. The most important distinction is between a multicystic kidney and a severe ureteropelvic junction obstruction.

6. How do you distinguish a multicystic kidney from a ureteropelvic junction obstruction?
A diethylenetriamine pentaacetic acid (DTPA) or mercaptoacetyltriglycine (MAG-3) renal flow scan is used to make the distinction. Multicystic kidneys appear photopenic, while even severe ureteropelvic junction obstructions generally demonstrate some function on a renal scan. In rare equivocal cases, a percutaneous nephrostomy tube can be placed and an antegrade pyelogram obtained. The cysts of a multicystic dysplastic kidney do not communicate, whereas the dilated portions of an obstructed collecting system will all fill on an antegrade study.

7. Are there any other urologic anomalies associated with multicystic dysplastic kidneys?
Yes. Contralateral ureteropelvic junction obstruction and vesicoureteral reflux are the most common.

8. Are there any absolute indications for surgical removal of a multicystic kidney?
Hypertension or massive size.

9. What features distinguish autosomal-recessive polycystic kidney disease (ARPKD) from autosomal-dominant polycystic kidney disease (ADPKD)?

ARPKD Versus ADPKD

	ARPKD	ADPKD
Gross appearance	Massively enlarged but still reniform	Renal contour distorted by cysts of varying size
Portion of nephron that is cystically dilated	Collecting ducts and tubules only	All portions of the nephron including the glomeruli
Lesions in other organs	Proliferation and dilatation of biliary ducts with periportal fibrosis	Hepatic, pancreatic and splenic cysts and cerebral berry aneurysms
Age of onset	Infancy/childhood	Usually adulthood

10. Which polycystic kidney disease occurs in children?
A trick question. ARPKD is typically a disease of infancy and childhood, and ADPKD usually presents in adulthood. However, a few patients with ADPKD become symptomatic in childhood.

11. Do infants and older children with ARPKD generally present with the same problems?
No. All children with ARPKD have renal and hepatic involvement, but the renal involvement tends to be more prominent in infants. In the most severe cases, there is extensive renal involvement and death occurs due to pulmonary hypoplasia. Older children tend to present with complications of hepatic fibrosis, such as bleeding esophageal varices or hepatosplenomegaly due to portal hypertension.

12. What is the outlook for patients with ARPKD?
Not as grim as it used to be. Because of improvements in neonatal intensive care, the 2-year survival rate for those presenting in the neonatal period is roughly 50%. However, nearly all patients develop end-stage renal disease by adulthood (50% by adolescence). Hepatic involvement is variable. Some patients require treatment for portal hypertension, whereas others have subclinical disease detectable only by ultrasound or biopsy. Hepatic failure does not occur.

13. Can ARPKD be detected by prenatal ultrasound?
Yes, in about 50% of cases.

14. How may ADPKD present in childhood?
It presents rarely in infancy with nephromegaly or pulmonary hypoplasia. Older children may develop the same spectrum of problems seen more commonly in adults: hematuria, urinary tract infection, flank pain, hypertension, proteinuria, palpable kidneys, or intracerebral hemorrhage.

15. Although most affected children with ADPKD are asymptomatic, can they be detected by ultrasound?
Ultrasound can detect 22% of affected individuals in the first decade of life, and 66% during the second decade.

16. Can ADPKD be detected prenatally?
Prenatal ultrasound is abnormal in a minority of affected fetuses. DNA probes have been used for prenatal diagnosis, but this technique is expensive and not readily available.

17. What is the prognosis for ADPKD presenting in childhood?
Approximately half of patients with clinical manifestations in infancy die of respiratory failure or sepsis. Cases which become evident later in childhood rarely progress to renal failure before adulthood.

18. How is ADPKD in childhood treated?

The same as in adulthood—aggressive management of complications such as hypertension and urinary tract infection.

19. Can simple renal cysts be diagnosed in childhood?

Yes, but they are rare. Any young child with a renal cyst requires careful evaluation of family members (including renal ultrasonography of both parents) and periodic follow-up to rule out polycystic kidney disease.

CONTROVERSY

20. What is the appropriate management of multicystic dysplastic kidneys detected by prenatal ultrasonography?

The options for managing a multicystic dysplastic kidney are to remove it, follow it, or ignore it. Surgical excision is supported by the reports of hypertension and malignancy (both Wilms' tumor and renal cell carcinoma) occurring in patients with multicystic kidneys. However, the number of reported cases is small, and the total number of multicystic kidneys, while unknown, is undoubtedly large. Therefore, the risk for any given patient is probably extremely small and may not justify the surgical risk of excision.

Most pediatric urologists therefore recommend following patients with multicystic kidneys with periodic ultrasound and blood pressure monitoring. Obviously, any patient developing hypertension or a renal mass would undergo nephrectomy. Some surgeons also remove multicystic kidneys that fail to regress. Conversely, once a multicystic kidney has regressed on ultrasound, monitoring is discontinued.

However, this approach is not entirely logical. It bases management on the progression (or regression) of the cystic component of these lesions (the part discernible on ultrasound). Yet, the hypertension and tumors reported undoubtedly arise from the stromal component. Must patients therefore undergo periodic flank ultrasounds for life? Would it be simpler just to remove the multicystic kidney in infancy—an operation which can be done as an outpatient procedure through a relatively small incision? Or, given the anecdotal nature of reports of hypertension and tumors, and the difficulties of ultrasonographic follow-up, perhaps we should just ignore them? After all, that is how nearly all of them were successfully managed before the era of prenatal ultrasound (because we did not know they were there). Perhaps this is a case "Where ignorance is bliss, 'tis folly to be wise." To address these issues, a multicystic kidney registry has been instituted by the Section of Urology of the American Academy of Pediatrics.

BIBLIOGRAPHY

1. Elder JS, Duckett JW: Perinatal urology. In Gillenwater JY, Grayhack JT, Howards SS, Duckett JW (eds): Adult and Pediatric Urology, 2nd ed. St. Louis, Mosby, 1991, pp 1755–1757.
2. Elder JS, Klacsmann PG, Sanders RC, Jeffs RD: Flank mass in a neonate. J Urol 126:94–98, 1981.
3. Gagnadoux AF, Habib R, Levy M, et al: Cystic renal diseases in children. Adv Nephrol 18:33–58, 1989.
4. Glassberg KI, Stephens FD, Lebowitz RL, et al: Renal dysgenesis and cystic disease of the kidney: A report of the Committee on Terminology, Nomenclature and Classification, Section on Urology, American Academy of Pediatrics. J Urol 138:1085–1092, 1987.
5. Kaplan BS, Kaplan P, Rosenberg HK, et al: Polycstic kidney disease in childhood. J Pediatr 115:867–880, 1989.
6. Lippert MC: Renal cystic disease. In Gillenwater JY, Grayhack JT, Howards SS, Duckett JW (eds): Adult and Pediatric Urology, 2nd ed. St. Louis, Mosby, 1991, pp 711–743.
7. Ross JH, Elder JS: Renal dysplasia, hypoplasia, multicystic kidney, and polycystic kidney disease in childhood. In Resnick MI, Kursh ED (eds): Current Therapy in Genitourinary Surgery. St. Louis, Mosby, 1992, pp 198–202.
8. Susskind MR, Kim KS, King LR: Hypertension and multicystic kidney. Urology 34:362–366, 1989.
9. Wacksman J, Phipps L: Report of the Multicystic Kidney Registry: Preliminary findings. J Urol 150:1870–1872, 1993.

36. CUSHING'S SYNDROME

David A. Goldfarb, M.D.

1. What is Cushing's syndrome?
Cushing's syndrome is an endocrine disorder characterized by the excessive secretion of glucocorticoids (cortisol).

2. How does it differ from Cushing's disease?
Cushing's disease refers to a type of Cushing's syndrome produced by pituitary adenomas or hyperplasia. It is a subset of patients with Cushing's syndrome.

3. What are the causes of Cushing's syndrome?

ACTH-Dependent
Pituitary (70%)
Ectopic ACTH (10%)
Excessive corticotropin releasing factor production (2%)

ACTH-Independent
Adrenal adenoma (10%)
Adrenal carcinoma (5%)
Adrenal hyperplasia (3%)

4. What are the clinical findings?
Patients with Cushing's syndrome have a characteristic appearance with a round face, truncal obesity, and increased scapular fat pad (buffalo hump). Other features include thin skin, easy bruisability, and proximal muscle weakness. Many patients have hypertension, diabetes mellitus, or psychiatric symptoms.

5. How is the diagnosis made?
When the diagnosis is suspected clinically, the following biochemical tests can be performed:
   1. **AM and PM plasma cortisol.** Normal serum cortisol is highest in the early morning and lowest in the evening. This normal diurnal variation is lost in Cushing's syndrome, with high levels of cortisol remaining unchanged through the day.
   2. **24-Hour urinary cortisol.** This is the best and most widely available test to measure the integrated cortisol secretion over a 24-hour period. It is elevated in Cushing's syndrome.
   3. **Overnight dexamethasone suppression test (DST).** Serum cortisol is measured at 8 AM following 1 mg of dexamethasone given at 11 PM the evening before. Failure to suppress AM cortisol is consistent with Cushing's syndrome.
   4. **Low-dose DST.** Plasma and 24-hour urinary cortisol are measured at baseline and after 2 days of dexamethasone (0.5 mg every 6 hrs). Failure to suppress cortisol secretion is diagnostic for Cushing's syndrome.

6. Can the different pathologies be differentiated biochemically?
A **low plasma ACTH** value suggests primary adrenal cortical disease. When this value is elevated, it suggests pituitary disease or ectopic ACTH syndrome.
   Suppression of cortisol secretion after **high-dose DST** (2.0 mg every 6 hrs for 2 days) suggests pituitary disease, whereas failure to suppress cortisol occurs with primary adrenal disease and ectopic ACTH syndrome. The false-positive and false-negative rates are 20%.

7. How are patients evaluated radiographically?
   1. When the plasma ACTH is low and the high-dose DST does not suppress cortisol, computed tomography (CT) or magnetic resonance imaging (MRI) of the adrenals should be performed. In most cases, a mass will be identified, although in a few cases hyperplasia may be found.

2. When the plasma ACTH is elevated and the high-dose DST suppresses cortisol, an MRI of the pituitary should be obtained. This examination is only 70–80% sensitive in identifying an adenoma.

3. When the plasma ACTH is elevated and the high-dose DST fails to suppress cortisol, ectopic ACTH is likely. Because of the relatively high false-negative rate with a high-dose DST, an MRI of the pituitary should be obtained.

4. When the MRI fails to disclose a pituitary tumor in ACTH-dependent Cushing's syndrome, petrosal venous sinus sampling can be performed. This is a highly sensitive and specific test to differentiate the causes of Cushing's syndrome, but it is invasive.

5. When ectopic ACTH is suspected, a CT of the abdomen and chest should be obtained to identify the responsible tumor.

8. What is the treatment of Cushing's syndrome?
Pituitary disease is responsible for Cushing's syndrome and is treated by transsphenoidal pituitary surgery. Eighty percent of cases respond. Radiation therapy can be used for surgical failures.

9. How are adrenal tumors treated?
If the mass is small, an extra-peritoneal approach, such as a flank or posterior incision, can be used. If the tumor is large and suspicious for cancer, an anterior transperitoneal approach (subcostal incision) or thoracoabdominal approach may be used.

10. Is any preoperative treatment required?
For adrenal tumors, a steroid preparation should be administered. The contralateral adrenal is suppressed, and until it recovers, supplemental steroid will be required.

11. Who are candidates for medical treatment?
- Patients who are not surgical candidates due to concomitant medical illness.
- Patients in whom thranssphenoidal surgery and radiation have failed.
- Patients with ectopic ACTH and no identifiable tumor.

12. What are available adrenolytic agents?
Mitotane (o, p'-DDD) (patients may require supplemental steroids), aminoglutethimide (patients may require supplemental steroids), ketoconazole, and metyrapone.

13. When is bilateral adrenalectomy indicated?
- Macronodular adrenal hyperplasia, which is bilateral.
- Medical treatment failures in a patient who is otherwise a surgical candidate.

BIBLIOGRAPHY

1. Atkinson AB: The treatment of Cushing's syndrome. Clin Endocrinol 34:507–513, 1991.
2. Orth DN: Differential diagnosis of Cushing's syndrome. N Engl J Med 325:957–959, 1991.
3. Sheeler LR: Cushing's syndrome. Urol Clin North Am 16:447–456, 1989.
4. Straffon RA: Cushing's syndrome and Cushing's disease. In Resnick MI, Kursh ED (eds): Current Therapy in Genitourinary Surgery. 2nd ed. St. Louis, Mosby, 1992, pp 1–3.
5. Trainer PJ, Grossman A: The diagnosis and differential diagnosis of Cushing's syndrome. Clin Endocrinol 34:317–330, 1991.
6. Vaughan ED, Blumenfeld JD: The adrenals. In Walsh PC, Retik AB, Stamey TA, Vaughan ED Jr (eds): Campbell's Urology, 6th ed. Philadelphia, W. B. Saunders, 1992, pp 2360–2412.

37. ADULT POLYCYSTIC KIDNEY DISEASE

Ernest E. Hodge, M.D.

1. Explain the genetic aspects of adult polycystic kidney disease.

Adult polycystic kidney disease is a hereditary disorder with autosomal-dominant transmission. There is virtually 100% penetrance by age 80, with perhaps a slightly less penetrance before that age. However, a positive family history is not always obtainable, possibly because other family members with the disease die of other causes prior to the disease being diagnosed or because the patient lacks knowledge of the family history. Although the actual gene responsible for transmission is unknown, it has been located to the short arm of chromosome 16. Spontaneous mutations occur infrequently (< 10% of the time) and may also contribute to the lack of a family history.

2. How many individuals are affected?

The incidence is approximately 1 in every 1000–1250 live births, and currently 500,000–600,000 Americans have the disease. Patients with adult polycystic kidney disease account for 5–10% of all patients with end-stage renal disease.

3. What are the other cystic diseases of the kidney?

Hereditary	**Nonhereditary**
1. Infantile (autosomal-recessive) polycystic kidney disease	1. Medullary sponge kidney
2. Juvenile nephronophthisis/medullary cystic disease complex	2. Multicystic kidney disease
3. Congenital nephrosis	3. Multiocular cysts of the kidney
4. von Hippel–Lindau disease	4. Glomerulocystic kidneys
5. Tuberous sclerosis	5. Acquired cystic disease of the kidneys
6. Other multiple malformation syndromes	

4. Does adult polycystic kidney disease occur only in adults?

No. Although the highest incidences occur between ages 45 and 65 and most patients exhibit manifestations of the disease after age 30, the disease can occur at all ages and has even been diagnosed in utero.

5. Does adult polycystic kidney disease affect organs other than the kidney?

Yes. Once again, the term "adult polycystic kidney disease" underemphasizes the true magnitude of the systemic nature of the disease. Cysts have been found in many other organs, including the liver (most commonly), pancreas, spleen, arachnoid, thyroid, testes, seminal vesicles, and ovaries. Other manifestations include intracranial (berry) aneurysms, mitral valve prolapse and other cardiac valvular abnormalities, and colonic diverticula.

6. What causes adult polycystic kidney disease?

While the exact cause remains unknown, several theories are favored:

- An abnormality in the renal tubular basement membrane with altered compliance of the tubular wall allowing cyst formation
- Epithelial hyperplasia with resultant tubular obstruction and cyst formation
- Abnormal synthesis or metabolism of tubular basement membranes with an alteration in the protein composition of the extracellular connective tissue matrix

The latter theory appears to best describe the extrarenal manifestations seen in patients with adult polycystic kidney disease. However, identification of the gene responsible for adult polycystic kidney disease and its function may be necessary before the pathogenesis of the disease is fully understood.

7. How is adult polycystic kidney disease diagnosed?

Although the diagnosis may be suspected due to a strong family history, characteristic symptoms, physical findings, or radiographic imaging is used to confirm the diagnosis. The radiographic hallmark of adult polycystic kidney disease is bilateral renal enlargement with multiple cysts of varying sizes.

8. Which radiographic tests are best for making the diagnosis?

Renal ultrasonography provides an excellent, inexpensive screening tool for diagnosing adult polycystic kidney disease. It has the advantage of avoiding radiation and the need for contrast, but it may be slightly less sensitive in the younger patient.

Computed tomography (CT) demonstrates excellent sensitivity and may provide better imaging of other organs, including the liver, pancreas, and spleen.

Although **intravenous urography** will show the characteristic features of bilateral renal masses with distortion of the collecting system, the results are often equivocal and further study is required with either ultrasound or CT. The addition of nephrotomograms to the intravenous urogram increases the sensitivity.

9. Describe the associated physical findings.

Flank mass represents the most common physical finding in patients with adult polycystic kidney disease. However, patients with severe hydronephrosis (especially from ureteropelvic junction obstruction) as well as other large renal masses (angiomyolipomas, renal cell carcinoma, etc.) may also have detectable flank masses. Some patients with significant extrarenal involvement of adult polycystic kidney disease may have **hepatomegaly** or **splenomegaly** detected on physical examination.

10. Are there any abnormal laboratory values seen in these patients?

Most of the abnormal laboratory values are related to complications of the disease, especially uremia:

- Anemia (related to uremia or recurrent bleeding episodes)
- Mild proteinuria (< 1g/24 hrs)
- Loss of renal concentrating ability (first indicator of renal impairment)
- Azotemia with elevated serum creatinine and blood urea nitrogen
  (in advanced renal failure)

The urinalysis typically shows microscopic hematuria, pyuria, and bacteriuria.

11. Which are the most common signs, symptoms, and related complications of adult polycystic kidney disease?

1. **Pain** (60% of patients) usually presents as lateral abdominal or flank pain and is commonly related to distention of the renal capsule due to enlarging cysts.

2. **Hematuria** (50–70% of patients), either gross or microscopic, is the presenting symptom in approximately one-third of patients and is most commonly associated with bleeding into a cyst.

3. **Nephrolithiasis** (15–20% of patients) may be related to either structural (i.e., obstruction) or metabolic abnormalities.

4. **Hypertension** (40–80% of patients) is more common in patients with renal function impairment, and probably relates to a renin-mediated cause due to a compression of normal renal tissue by enlarged cysts resulting in relative ischemia.

5. **Urinary tract infections** (50–60% of patients) tend to be recurrent and affect women predominantly (90% of infections occur in females).

6. **End-stage renal disease** (50% of patients by age 60) appears to be less aggressive in women but develops approximately 10 years earlier in blacks than whites.

12. How is adult polycystic kidney disease treated?

Treatment is largely directed at the individual complications. Most episodes of bleeding resolve spontaneously, although an occasional life-threatening episode will require intervention such as angiographic embolization or surgery. The hypertension should be aggressively treated, and the angiotensin-converting enzyme (ACE) inhibitors may be of particular benefit. Analgesics usually provide pain relief, and appropriate antimicrobials are employed for urinary tract infections. As renal insufficiency progresses, conservative measures such as low protein diet and phosphate binders are instituted. Many patients ultimately require dialysis or transplantation.

13. Can surgery prevent the progression of renal failure?

Except in the rare case in which ureteral obstruction is caused by an enlarged cyst, surgical decompression of the cyst does not appear to affect renal function. Surgical decompression of the cyst can be dramatic in relieving intractable pain and is more effective than percutaneous aspiration of the cyst for this purpose. Also, surgical cyst decompression only rarely appears to improve blood pressure substantially.

14. Are dialysis and transplantation effective for patients with adult polycystic kidney disease?

Yes. Despite these patients being slightly older at the time of development of end-stage renal disease, the results of dialysis and transplantation are at least as good as in other nondiabetic patients.

15. If adult polycystic kidney disease is hereditary, can family members safely donate kidneys?

Yes. With appropriate genetic studies and ultrasound screening, family members, especially those beyond age 25–35, can be accurately assessed for the presence of adult polycystic kidney disease. In the absence of any evidence for this disease, such family members may safely donate a kidney for transplantation.

BIBLIOGRAPHY

1. Delaney VB, Adler S, Bruns JF, et al: Autosomal dominant polycystic kidney disease: Presentations, complications, and prognosis. Am J Kidney Dis 5:104, 1985.
2. Elzinga LW, Barry JM, Torres VE, et al: Cyst decompression surgery for autosomal dominant polycystic kidney disease. J Am Soc Nephrol 2:1219–1226, 1992.
3. Gabow PA: Autosomal dominant polycystic kidney disease. N Engl J Med 329:332–342, 1993.
4. Glassberg KI: Renal dysplasia and cystic diseases of the kidney. In Walsh PC, Retick AB, Stamey TA, Vaughan ED Jr (eds): Cambell's Urology, 6th ed. Philadelphia, W.B. Saunders, 1992, pp 1443–1495.
5. Ho-Hsieh H, Novick AC, Steinmuller D, et al: Renal transplantation for end-stage polycystic kidney disease. Urology 4:322–326, 1987.
6. Lippert MC: Renal cystic disease. In Gillenwater JY, Grayhack JT, Howards SS, Duckett JW (eds): Adult and Pediatric Urology, 2nd ed. St. Louis, Mosby, 1991, pp 711–743.

38. ACQUIRED CYSTIC DISEASE OF THE KIDNEY

Stuart M. Flechner, M.D.

1. What is acquired renal cystic disease (ARCD)?

ARCD is the term used to describe the development of cystic degeneration of the kidneys in patients without a congenital predisposition to form renal cysts. Usually, 25% or more of the mass of one or both kidneys is involved when the diagnosis is made, predominantly in patients with chronic renal failure. The association of ARCD with renal failure, especially in patients treated with hemodialysis, was first described by Dunnill in 1977, although reports of cysts in the kidneys of autopsied patients with renal failure date to the 19th century.

2. Where do the cysts form?

Multiple cysts are usually found in both kidneys, predominantly in the renal cortex, although cysts can be found in the medulla or corticomedullary junction. Because end-stage renal disease kidneys are usually small and contracted, the cysts cause an increased renal mass. The cysts have also been associated with multiple small renal adenomas and frank renal cell carcinomas.

3. How is ARCD different from other forms of renal cystic disease?

The aging kidney has a propensity to form benign simple cysts. They may develop in either kidney and be single or multiple. However, in ARCD many tens or hundreds of cysts develop.

There are two main types of congenital polycystic renal diseases: one is genetically transmitted in an autosomal dominant fashion and the other in autosomal recessive. There is usually a family history of these forms of cystic kidney disease, and they are also usually associated with cyst formation in other organs, such as the liver and gastrointestinal tract. In contrast, ARCD occurs in renal failure patients, absent a family history of cystic disease, and is isolated to the kidney. In addition, microdissection studies show that ARCD cysts lack the arboral-like proliferation found in congenital cystic disease of the kidney.

4. How often are cysts found in renal failure patients?

This depends on when patients undergo evaluation for cystic disease. The prevalence of ARCD in dialysis patients undergoing autopsy is 28–47%. ARCD is reported to exist in 14–65% of dialysis patients undergoing random radiologic screening studies. It appears that about one-third of patients develop ARCD within the first 3 years of dialysis, with the number approaching 80–90% in those who survive on dialysis for 5–10 years. Males appear to have a two-fold increased risk for the development of ARCD.

5. Does the type of renal replacement therapy affect the risk for ARCD?

The early reports of ARCD were confined to patients undergoing chronic hemodialysis, and indeed the artificial kidney and/or dialysis tubing were once suggested to be linked to the pathogenesis of cyst formation. However, cysts have been found in patients who were treated only by peritoneal dialysis, as well as in patients with slowly progressive renal insufficiency prior to the initiation of dialysis. Therefore, the length of time an individual suffers from chronic renal insufficiency may be the most important risk factor for ARCD. For this reason, younger patients may harbor the greatest risk for ARCD during their lifetime.

6. Are some patients more likely to form cysts?

Yes. ARCD develops more commonly in patients with tubulointerstitial diseases. It is less likely in those with membranoproliferative glomerulonephritis and in type I diabetics with renal failure.

7. Do the cysts ever go away?
There is some evidence that successful renal transplantation, with the return of near-normal renal function, can cause a regression of established ARCD in native kidneys. In addition, new cases of ARCD are uncommon in successfully transplanted patients. However, a few new cases of ARCD have been identified in patients with acceptable renal transplant function and can be associated with polycythemia post-transplant.

8. Why do cysts form in end-stage renal disease (ESRD) kidneys?
The pathogenesis is currently not known. Animal experiments and clinical observations have led to a number of theories:

1. **Occlusive theory.** Obstruction of renal tubules by a combination of interstitial fibrosis, epithelial proliferation, and/or intratubular oxalate crystal leads to cyst formation.

2. **Chemical theory.** Toxic endogenous substances or metabolites accumulated in renal failure, such as polyamines or exogenous substances from dialysis tubing or the artificial kidney, could be responsible.

3. **Ischemic theory.** Experimentally, ischemia and obstruction to a renal segment can induce cyst formation. Both are present in ESRD kidneys.

4. **Growth factor theory.** As-yet-unidentified polypeptides with renotrophic activity could be locally released and induce cystic degeneration.

5. **Immune theory.** Uremia is known to be immunosuppressive. ESRD kidneys may be susceptible to escape mechanisms predisposing to cellular proliferation.

6. **Hormonal theory.** The increased incidence of ARCD in males suggest that alterations of sex steroid production and metabolism induced by uremia may predispose to cyst formation. An up-regulation of epidermal growth factor receptors in renal tissue has been shown to result from altered androgen/estrogen ratios in uremic males.

9. How do the cysts form?
Cysts are generally 1–25 mL in size and contain clear fluid in which oxalate crystals are often found. They have regular cuboidal or columnar epithelium, but papillary hyperplasia and thickened basement membranes are generally observed. Microdissection studies have confirmed that cysts are always in continuity with renal tubules and may represent fusiform tubular dilations or saccular outpouchings. The lumens of over 80% of the proximal and distal tubules are patent. These data suggest that cyst formation results from dilation and hyperplasia of remaining nephrons rather than obstruction and fibrosis.

10. Do cysts cause any clinical symptoms?
Yes. Depending upon their relative size and position in the kidney, they may result in hematuria, stone formation, infection, hypertension, pain, etc. Although these symptoms tend to be reported infrequently, they can be significant and may require nephrectomy for resolution.

11. Are there any other reasons to worry about cysts in ESRD kidneys?
Yes. Several studies have confirmed an association between ARCD and renal tumors, and there have been case reports of patients with ARCD who developed metastatic renal cell carcinomas. Tumors can be found in areas of the kidney where cystic degeneration is prominent, as well as in areas without cystic involvement. It is possible that some tumors arise from the hyperplastic multilayered epithelium, often with papillary projections, found in many cysts. Conversely, about 80% of reported patients on dialysis with renal adenocarcinomas have had ARCD.

Estimated Occurrence of Renal Adenocarcinoma

GROUP	CASES/1000 POPULATION
General population	1.3
Renal insufficiency	1.5
ESRD population	6.0
Kidneys with cysts	22.8
ESRD patients with ARCD	45.5

12. Are all renal tumors found in ARCD patients malignant?

No. About 20–40% of patients with ARCD have small solid renal tumors, compared with a 10–20% incidence in an age-matched general autopsy population. Only about 1–2% of patients with ARCD develop a frank renal adenocarcinoma, and about 15% of those with cancer develop metastases. Males also exhibit a seven-fold increased risk for developing renal adenocarcinoma when ARCD is present. The risk for neoplastic transformation appears to correlate more with length of time renal failure is present rather than age of the patient. Therefore, younger patients with ESRD harbor the greatest risk and require close monitoring.

13. How does one tell if a small renal tumor is malignant?

This remains a highly controversial issue in urology. Some believe the size of the lesion is an accurate discriminator, as lesions under 3 cm in diameter rarely if ever metastasize, and consider these to be adenomas. Others believe that renal adenomas are small renal adenocarcinomas and will demonstrate malignant behavior in time. The association of clinical symptoms at the time of presentation has also been suggested as a marker for more rapid growth—e.g., gross hematuria would be most unlikely to result from a small slow-growing adenoma. Currently, the presence of tissue invasion and/or metastases continues to be the only truly diagnostic feature separating these two entities.

14. What is the best way to determine if an ARCD kidney contains a renal tumor?

The **renal ultrasound** evaluation is uniformly considered the most accurate and efficient way to screen ESRD kidneys for cystic disease. In most cases, cysts can be confidently identified. The computed tomographic (CT) scan is more accurate (but more costly and delivers contrast and radiation) if a complex cyst or solid mass is identified by ultrasound. On very rare occasions, other modalities such as angiography, isotopic renal scans, and magnetic resonance imaging may supply additional information. The altered architecture of the kidney caused by ARCD makes delineation of renal masses more difficult than in otherwise normally functioning kidneys.

15. Because renal adenocarcinoma can develop in ARCD kidneys, how often should a patient be evaluated?

This is also a controversial question which involves the true incidence of kidney cancer in ESRD patients, the costs of large-scale screening programs, and the ultimate benefit to patients. Important facts that apply to this consideration are the average life expectancy of new patients beginning dialysis in the United States (under 5 years for patients over age 50) and the infrequent finding of kidney cancer (< 2%) as a cause of death in dialyzed patients.

A reasonable approach would be to perform an ultrasound examination when the diagnosis of ESRD is made, and then repeat the study after about 3 years. Higher risk groups, such as young males in good health on hemodialysis, should undergo closer scrutiny than elderly females on continuous ambulatory peritoneal dialysis with cardiac disease, for example.

16. What is the best treatment for a solid renal mass in an ARCD kidney?

If a solid renal mass > 3 cm in diameter is found or a smaller mass associated with symptoms is uncovered, the patient should undergo **radical nephrectomy.** This approach should be modified only by coexisting medical conditions that would significantly limit life expectancy or preclude the safe administration of anesthesia and surgery. Smaller asymptomatic masses can either be removed or followed with CT scans. Elective nephrectomy can be done if progression is demonstrated.

BIBLIOGRAPHY

1. Boileau M, Flechner SM, Foley R, Weinman E: Renal adenocarcinoma and end-stage kidney disease. J Urol 138:603–606, 1987.
2. Concolino G, Lubrano C, Ombres M, et al: Acquired cystic kidney disease: The hormonal hypothesis. Urology 41:170–175, 1993.

3. Dunnill MS, Millard PR, Oliver D: Acquired cystic disease of the kidneys: A hazard of long-term intermittent dialysis. J Clin Pathol 30:868–877, 1977.
4. Ishikawa I, Yasuhito S, Naoto S, et al: Ten-year prospective study on the development of renal cell cancer in dialysis patients. Am J Kidney Dis 26:452–458, 1990.
5. Levine E: Renal cell cancer in uremic acquired renal cystic disease: Incidence, detection, and management. Urol Radiol 13:203–210, 1992.
6. Levine E, Slusher S, Grantham J, Wetzel L: Natural history of ARCD in dialysis patients: A prospective CT study. AJR 156:501–506, 1991.
7. Lien Y, Kam I, Shanley P, Schroter G. Metastatic renal cell carcinoma associated with ARCD 15 years after transplantation. Am J Kidney Dis 28:711–715, 1991.
8. Mallofre C, Almirall J, Campistol JM, et al: Acquired renal cystic disease in HD: A study of 82 nephrectomies in young patients. Nephrology 50:297–302, 1992.
9. Mindell HJ: Imaging studies for screening native kidneys in long-term dialysis patients [commentary]. AJR 153:768–769, 1989.
10. Vandeursen H, Van Damme B, Baert J: Acquired cystic disease of the kidney analyzed by microdissection. J Urol 146:1168–1169, 1991.

39. URETEROPELVIC JUNCTION OBSTRUCTION

Allen D. Seftel, M.D.

1. What is ureteropelvic junction obstruction?
It is a blockage of the ureter at the level of the renal pelvis–proximal ureteral junction.

2. What are the causes?
The causes can be divided into congenital or acquired. Congenital ureteropelvic junction obstruction is an entity that is often now found prenatally. Inasmuch as prenatal ultrasonography is routinely performed, it will present as one of the differential diagnoses of prenatal or postnatal hydronephrosis or abdominal mass. Acquired ureteropelvic obstruction may be the result of ureteral manipulation, urinary calculi, or retroperitoneal disease.

3. What are the physical findings and symptoms?
One might be able to appreciate an abdominal mass. In the older child, there might be flank or abdominal pain.

4. How is the diagnosis of ureteropelvic junction obstruction made?
Renal ultrasonography, intravenous pyelography, or radionuclide renogram.

5. What are the causes of congenital anomaly?
It is believed that there is a disorganization of the renal pelvis–upper ureteral junction during the recanalization process in utero. This disorganization of the smooth muscle leads to a lack of motility or perhaps collagen deposition, and thus there is a lack of peristalsis, with narrowing at this site.

6. How does one treat this entity?
A pyeloplasty is usually performed in the neonate. There are several types of pyeloplasy procedures, the most common being the dismembered pyeloplasy.

7. Are there any other causes for pediatric ureteropelvic junction obstruction?
It may be that vesicoureteral reflux may cause a secondary ureteropelvic junction obstruction. This is most commonly found in children.

8. How does one make a diagnosis of ureteropelvic junction obstruction in children?
Diuretic renal nuclide scanning is usually performed either to make the diagnosis of ureteropelvic junction obstruction or to confirm the diagnosis.

9. Is ureteropelvic junction obstruction more common in male or female children?
Boys more than girls by a 5:2 ratio.

10. Is ureteropelvic junction obstruction more common on the right, left, or both (bilateral)?
It is more common on the left than the right, again with a 5:2 ratio. Bilateral obstruction occurs in 15% of cases.

11. How does ureteropelvic junction obstruction usually present in the adult?
Flank pain, flank mass, or a urinary tract infection.

12. How is ureteropelvic junction obstruction diagnosed in the adult?

This diagnosis usually is made by intravenous pyelography, renal ultrasonography, or diuretic renal scanning.

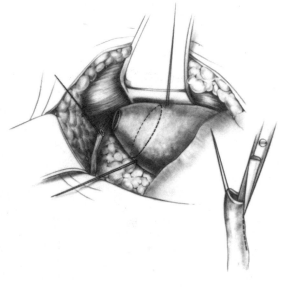

On the pelvis. 4-0 chromic sutures are placed at the margins where excess pelvis will be excised. A small tacking suture is placed in the proximal end of the ureter to minimize handling and traumatic injury. The ureter is then incised for approximately 1–2 cm on the lateral portion of the ureter. (From Novick AC (ed): Stewart's Operative Urology, 2nd ed. Baltimore Williams & Wilkins, 1989, with permission.)

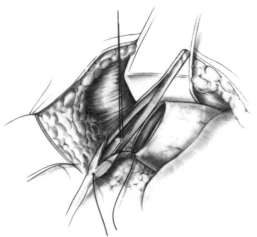

A 4-0 or 5-0 chromic suture is then placed at the apex of the incised ureter to the inferior portion of the pelvis. A pair of forceps is used to spread the internal diameter of the ureter to facilite the placement of this suture. (From Novick AC (ed): Stewart's Operative Urology, 2nd ed. Baltimore Williams & Wilkins, 1989, with permission.)

13. What are the causes of this obstruction in the adult?

1. A crossing renal vessel at the ureteropelvic junction
2. Previous passage of a urinary calculus
3. Manipulation of the urinary system either with a ureteroscope or nephroscope.
4. A retroperineal process impinging on the ureter externally (e.g., inflammation or enlarged lymph nodes)
5. Nonurologic malignancies such as gynecologic cancers or colonic cancers can causing obstruction either through enlarged lymph nodes or actual compression of that area by the tumor burden
6. Abdominal and aortic aneurysm leakage may produce an inflammatory response in the

retroperineal area near the upper ureteropelvic junction, causing uretopelvic junction obstruction as well

   7. Infection, either hematogenous or ascending

14. How is the obstruction treated in the adult?
Most commonly, a dismembered pyeloplasty is performed in the adult. Other types of pyeloplasties also may be performed. Minimally invasive techniques such as endopyelotomy, a procedure performed via a percutaneous opening through the skin to the kidney, allowing access to the ureteropelvic junction area from below, or through the ureter in a retrograde fashion (a retrograde ureteral endopyelotomy) can be performed as well.

40. VESICOURETERAL REFLUX

Jack S. Elder, M.D.

1. What is vesicoureteral reflux?
Vesicoureteral reflux refers to the regurgitation of urine from the bladder into the ureter and usually into the kidney.

2. What is low-pressure reflux?
Low pressure reflux is vesicoureteral reflux that occurs during bladder filling.

3. What is high-pressure reflux?
High pressure reflux is vesicoureteral reflux that occurs during micturition. Reflux may occur during bladder filling, voiding, or both.

4. Describe the anatomy of the normal ureterovesical junction.
The smooth muscle of the renal calyces, pelvis, and extravesical ureter is composed of helically-oriented fibers that allow peristaltic activity. The ureter passes obliquely through the bladder wall for 1 to 2 cm, and the fibers are reoriented into a longitudinal plane, making the ureter incapable of peristalsis in that location.

5. What is the trigone?
The trigone is the triangle formed by the two ureteral orifices and the bladder neck.

6. What is Waldeyer's sheath?
It is the external layer of longitudinal smooth muscle surrounding the ureter. This sheath passes through the bladder wall. As this layer enters the bladder lumen, the fibers diverge to join with the contralateral ureter, forming the deep trigonal layer.

7. How does vesicoureteral reflux occur?
Reflux occurs when the intravesical (intramural) ureteral length is too short. Usually the ureter is positioned superolateral to the normal position.

8. Discuss the causes of vesicoureteral reflux.
There are numerous causes of vesicoureteral reflux. The most common is termed primary reflux and is thought to be a congenital condition. If the ureteral bud is too close to the urogenital sinus on the wolffian (mesonephric) duct, then it may not acquire sufficient mesenchymal tissue around it to have sufficient support to prevent reflux.

Reflux also may occur in association with high-pressure voiding states, including posterior urethral valves, certain cases of neuropathic bladder, and detrusor sphincter dyssynergia. Furthermore, reflux may occur in association with a duplex collecting system, in which the kidney is drained by two ureters. In children with an ectopic ureterocele, the insertion of the lower pole ureter into the bladder may be altered, allowing reflux. In children with an ectopic ureter draining into the bladder neck, there may be reflux into the upper pole ureter. Reflux also may occur following bladder surgery. For example, if one divides the trigone during a bladder operation, the ureteral orifice(s) may retract, allowing reflux to occur.

9. What is the normal ratio of the length of the intramural ureter to the diameter of the ureteral orifice?
Normally the ratio of the length of the intramural ureter to the diameter of the ureteral orifice is 2.5:1. If this ratio is less, then reflux occurs.

10. What is the prevalence of primary vesicoureteral reflux?
The prevalence has been estimated to be as high as 1 in 100.

11. What is the ratio of girls to boys with reflux?
The female to male ratio is approximately 10:1.

12. Define secondary reflux. Give examples.
Secondary reflux is an anatomic or clinical abnormality in which reflux occurs. Examples include ureterocele, in which reflux may occur from distortion of the base of the bladder from a ureterocele, posterior urethral valves, and neuropathic bladder.

13. What is the significance of vesicoureteral reflux?
Vesicoureteral reflux directly or in association with urinary tract infection may result in renal injury, termed reflux nephropathy.

14. How does a urinary tract infection cause renal injury?
If bacteria from the bladder ascend to the renal pelvis and renal parenchyma, a process that is facilitated by reflux, renal injury may occur by several mechanisms.
    1. The bacteria may produce an endotoxin that has a direct effect on the renal tubule.
    2. By chemotaxis, there is granulocyte aggregation in the area of the bacteria, resulting in capillary obstruction, which causes focal renal ischemia. During ischemia the purine pool is consumed due to anaerobic metabolism. During reperfusion the remaining hypoxanthine pool is metabolized to xanthine, which, in the presence of xanthine oxidase, is converted to uric acid and superoxide. Superoxide can be converted to peroxide and hydroxyl radicals, both of which may cause cell damage. Experimentally this ischemic damage has been prevented by treatment with allopurinol, which blocks xanthine oxidase and thus prevents toxic oxygen radical formation during reperfusion.
    3. During the inflammatory response endotoxin causes complement activation, which by chemotaxis leads to phagocytosis. The respiratory burst of phagocytosis results in the release of superoxide with formation of peroxide and hydroxyl radicals. All tissues in the body contain superoxide dismutase, which rapidly degrades superoxide, which naturally occurs in the presence of oxygen. However, urine contains no superoxide dismutase, allowing these radicals to act on the renal tubules unopposed. In addition, lysosomal enzymes are released during phagocytosis, which also may damage renal tubules.

15. How common is primary reflux in children with a urinary tract infection?
Approximately 50% of children with a urinary tract infection have reflux. The incidence of reflux in children with urinary tract infections is similar in boys and girls. Primary reflux is much less common in black children than in white children.

16. Who should be evaluated for reflux?
Any child with pyelonephritis (i.e., febrile UTI), all boys with a UTI, all girls < 5 years old with a UTI, and girls > 5 years with two or more episodes of cystitis.

17. How is reflux detected?
Reflux is usually detected by performing a voiding cystourethrogram (VCUG). This study is performed by inserting a catheter into the bladder, distending the bladder with contrast material, and observing the bladder and kidneys during bladder filling and voiding. In boys the study is performed using fluoroscopy, because it is important to assess the urethra for an abnormality (e.g., posterior urethral valves). In girls, the VCUG may be performed either with serial x-rays performed during bladder filling and voiding, or with fluoroscopy.
    An alternative method of assessing reflux is to perform the nuclear (also termed radionuclide) cystogram. In this study a solution containing radionuclide is instilled into the bladder and the

bladder and kidneys are monitored with a gamma camera during bladder filling and voiding. There is much less radiologic detail with this study, but also much less radiation exposure to the gonads.

18. Describe the grading system for vesicoureteral reflux.
Numerous grading systems have been used over the years. The current system is that adopted by the International Reflux Study in Children and is termed the International System. There are five grades.

Grade I: The contrast material enters the ureter but does not enter the renal pelvis.

Grade II: The contrast material reaches the renal pelvis but does not distend the collecting system.

Grade III: The collecting system is filled and either the ureter or pelvis is distended but the calyceal demarcations are not distorted.

Grade IV: The dilated ureter is slightly tortuous and the calyces are blunted significantly.

Grade V: The entire collecting system is tremendously dilated without a visible papillary impression, and there is significant ureteral tortuosity.

19. What is the typical distribution of grades of vesicoureteral reflux?
Approximately 5–8% have grade I, 35% grade II, 25–35% grade III, 15–25% grade IV, and 5% grade V. Approximately half of children have bilateral reflux.

20. Name the relative advantages and disadvantages of performing a VCUG compared to a nuclear cystogram in the initial evaluation of a child for reflux.
The International System for grading reflux is based on the VCUG. The grading system has important prognostic features that allow one to predict the likelihood of spontaneous reflux resolution. In addition, the radiographic VCUG allows one to see certain features in the bladder that may predispose to reflux, such as a duplication of the upper urinary tract, periureteral diverticulum, and ectopic insertion of the ureter. During a VCUG in girls, signs of voiding dysfunction, as well as intrarenal reflux, may be seen. The main disadvantage of the VCUG (radiographic) is the higher radiation exposure. The nuclear cystogram causes only 1–2% of the radiation exposure to the gonads compared to a standard radiographic VCUG. Currently most obtain a VCUG as the initial study and utilize the nuclear cystogram for follow-up studies.

21. Can ultrasound be used to detect vesicoureteral reflux?
Only 25% of children with primary reflux have hydronephrosis, which is the most common sonographic finding in children with reflux. Consequently, a VCUG must be done to determine whether a child has reflux.

22. What is intrarenal reflux?
Intrarenal reflux is the reflux of urine into the renal parenchyma during voiding. If intrarenal reflux exists in conjunction with infection, renal inflammation occurs. In general, intrarenal reflux occurs in compound papillae, which are located in the polar regions of the kidney. Most papillae are convex, with slit-like openings of the collecting ducts opening obliquely onto the papilla. In concave or flat papilla, however, collecting ducts open at right angles and allow reflux.

23. When is vesicoureteral reflux most likely to cause renal injury?
Reflux is most likely to cause renal injury during the first year of life, although it may occur at any age.

24. Does sterile reflux cause renal injury?
In general, sterile reflux is not thought to cause renal injury. However, if a high-pressure voiding situation exists, as in a boy with posterior urethral valves, a neuropathic bladder, or detrusor-sphincter dyssynergia, renal injury may occur in the absence of infection.

25. What is the likelihood of renal scarring in patients with reflux?

Approximately 85% with grade V reflux, 50% of children with grade IV, 30% of those with grade III, 15% of those with grade II, and 5–10% of those with grade I reflux have renal scarring. Thus, renal scarring is more common in those with higher grades of reflux.

26. What is the long-term significance of renal scarring?

The main complications of renal scarring are hypertension, which occurs in approximately 10% of children with renal scarring, and renal insufficiency or end-stage renal disease.

27. Describe the "big bang" theory of vesicoureteral reflux.

The big bang theory of Ransley and Risdon postulates that during a child's first urinary tract infection with vesicoureteral reflux, infected urine is carried into areas of the kidney subject to intrarenal reflux, which leads to a fixed scar that prevents further renal growth in that area. It is now recognized that scarring in one area of the kidney may distort adjacent papillae sufficiently to allow intra-renal reflux in areas not previously subject to this phenomenon, resulting in progressive renal scarring.

28. Of children with reflux, what proportion of their siblings also have reflux?

Approximately 30–35% of siblings have reflux. In most series, 75% of siblings with reflux are asymptomatic, i.e., they have not had urinary tract infections. The incidence of sibling reflux is unrelated to the index patient's reflux grade, sex, or renal scarring.

29. Should all siblings of index patients with reflux undergo a VCUG?

Most recommend that if a sibling is < 2–3 years old, then a nuclear cystogram should be obtained. In children > 3 years, a renal ultrasound should be done, and if an abnormality is discovered, then a VCUG should be performed.

30. What are the signs of reflux on an IVP?

Renal scarring (blunted calyx, thin parenchyma, or global atrophy), hydronephrosis, caliectasis, and vertical striations of the upper ureter.

31. Which imaging studies are commonly used to detect renal scarring? What are the characteristic findings?

A dimercaptosuccinic acid (DMSA) renal scan may show areas of diminished uptake in the cortex. Single photon emission computed tomography (SPECT) increases the sensitivity of DMSA slightly in detecting scarring. On an intravenous pyelogram (IVP), renal scarring is evident as a blunted calyx, renal cortical thinning, or cortical atrophy if a segment of the entire kidney. Ultrasound also may demonstrate global atrophy or atrophy of a part of the kidney, but calyceal morphology usually is indistinct.

32. Which study is most sensitive in detecting renal scarring?

The DMSA renal scan is the most sensitive study. Renal scarring also might be apparent on a MAG-3 or glucoheptonate renal scan, but these studies are not thought to be as sensitive as the DMSA scan. Ultrasound is one of the least sensitive methods of detecting renal scarring.

33. What is the Weigert-Meyer rule?

This rule applies to children with complete duplication of the urinary tract, which results from two ureteral buds leading to the formation of two separate ureters and separate renal pelves within one kidney. The ureter to the upper segment arises from a cephalad position on the mesonephric duct, remains attached to the mesonephric duct longer during embryogenesis, and thus migrates farther, ending inferomedial to the ureter draining the lower segment. Thus, the ureter draining the lower pole is more cephalolateral, and the ureter draining the upper pole is more inferomedial in the bladder, and is prone to becoming ectopic.

34. What is the significance of the Weigert-Meyer law in reflux?
Because the ureter draining the lower pole of the kidney drains in a more lateral position in the bladder, its intramural tunnel is shorter, predisposing to reflux.

35. How common is upper urinary tract duplication?
Approximately 1 of 125 individuals have duplication of the upper urinary tract.

36. In a child with complete duplication of the urinary tract and reflux, into which segment(s) does the reflux occur typically?
Approximately 85% have reflux only into the lower pole, whereas 15% have reflux into both the upper and lower pole systems.

37. Describe the natural history of vesicoureteral reflux.
With growth and maturation of bladder function, reflux often resolves spontaneously. The likelihood of spontaneous resolution is related directly to reflux grade. Approximately 90% of children with grade I reflux, 75% with grade II, 50% with grade III, 40% with grade IV, and 5% or fewer of those with grade V reflux show spontaneous resolution.

38. How is a patient's age related to the likelihood of spontaneous resolution of reflux?
The younger the child, the greater the likelihood that reflux will resolve.

39. Are children with upper urinary tract duplication as likely to show spontaneous resolution as those with single systems?
Comparing identical reflux grades, the likelihood of spontaneous reflux resolution in children with complete duplication is significantly lower than in those with a single system.

40. What is the likelihood of spontaneous resolution of reflux in a child with bilateral grade III or IV reflux?
Approximately 10% will have spontaneous resolution.

41. What is the mean age at diagnosis of reflux?
The mean age is 2 to 3 years.

42. What is the mean age at spontaneous resolution of reflux?
Approximately 5 to 6 years.

43. At what age is reflux no longer likely to resolve?
In most children with reflux, reflux is unlikely to resolve beyond 10 or 11 years. However, in children with grade II reflux, spontaneous resolution has been shown to occur at 14 to 15 years.

44. How are children with reflux managed medically?
Medical management involves assessment of a child's voiding habits and patterns of infection. In children who are toilet trained, regular frequent voiding is encouraged. In children with bladder instability (urge incontinence), often anticholinergic therapy (e.g., oxybutynin chloride, propantheline bromide) is administered.

Antimicrobial prophylaxis is administered in an attempt to prevent urinary tract infection. In general, trimethoprim/sulfamethoxazole, trimethoprim, or nitrofurantoin are used, because these drugs have the least effect on the bacterial flora in the stool, which is the source of urinary tract infections. The dosage used for prophylaxis is approximately 1/4 to 1/3 the dosage commonly used to treat a UTI.

The child should have a urinalysis and/or culture performed every 3–4 months. Every 12–18 months, a follow-up cystogram is done to monitor the reflux, usually with a nuclear cystogram. In addition, an upper tract study such as an ultrasound, an IVP, or a DMSA scan is performed to assess renal growth. Children with reflux who are not placed on prophylaxis have a much higher incidence of renal scarring than those receiving prophylaxis.

45. What is a breakthrough UTI?
This term refers to a urinary tract infection that occurs while the patient is receiving prophylaxis.

46. What is the incidence of breakthrough UTI in children with VUR?
Approximately 25–35% with reflux have a breakthrough UTI.

47. Of children with grade I to III reflux managed medically, what is the likelihood of reappearance of reflux after one normal cystogram?
Approximately 20% will show reflux on a follow-up study.

48. Of children with no reflux on one side and contralateral grade I–III reflux, what is the likelihood of reflux on the nonrefluxing side on a follow-up cystogram?
Approximately 20% of those with no reflux on one side will show reflux into that ureter on a subsequent study.

49. What constitutes a failure of medical management?
A child who develops a breakthrough UTI, is allergic to antimicrobial medication, is poorly compliant, or has persistent reflux until the age of 10 or 11 years would be considered to have failed medical management.

50. Define bladder instability.
It is uninhibited detrusor (bladder) contractions that persist beyond 2–4 years, the usual age at which toilet training occurs. In a neurologically normal child, typical symptoms include urgency with urge incontinence and frequency.

51. What is the significance of bladder instability in children with reflux?
Bladder instability is common in children with reflux and seems to worsen their reflux grade. Children with bladder instability are managed with anticholinergic medication (e.g., oxybutynin chloride, propantheline bromide) and regular timed voiding. Children with bladder instability managed with anticholinergic therapy and antimicrobial prophylaxis are more likely to show spontaneous resolution than those who are treated with prophylaxis alone.

52. What are the indications for surgical management of children with reflux?
In general, ureteroneocystostomy is recommended for all children with grade V reflux. In children with lesser grades of reflux, failure of medical management constitutes a strong indication. Thus breakthrough UTI, noncompliance with medical management, allergies to prophylactic medications, and persistent reflux, particularly in 10-year-old children, are indications. Currently, most pediatric urologists recommend antireflux surgery for primary grade IV reflux because of its low likelihood of spontaneous resolution and the high risk of renal scarring.

53. What are the principles of surgical management for vesicoureteral reflux?
The principles of antireflux surgery include creation of an intramural ureter that is 4–5 times as long as wide. The ureter is placed in the submucosal layer between the mucosa and detrusor (muscle).

54. What types of open surgical techniques are used to correct reflux?
The term for this operation is ureteroneocystostomy. The most common method of correcting reflux consists of opening the bladder, mobilizing the ureter, and advancing it across the trigone (Cohen or transtrigonal repair). Alternatively, the ureter may be reinserted in a higher more medial position in the bladder and brought down to its normal position (Leadbetter-Politano).

There are also extravesical repairs, in which the ureter is anchored in the bladder base and the bladder muscle is sutured around the ureter (Lich-Gregoir; detrusorrhaphy).

55. In a child with duplication of the urinary tract and reflux into the lower pole, how is the reflux managed surgically?
In these children the ureters are in a single sheath near the bladder and share a common blood supply. Even though only the lower pole ureter may reflux, it is necessary to perform a "common sheath" ureteroneocystostomy, in which both ureters are mobilized together and reimplanted as one unit. Alternatively, the refluxing lower pole ureter may be detached from the bladder and anastomosed to the upper pole ureter near the bladder (ureteroureterostomy).

56. What is the success rate of ureteroneocystostomy?
Approximately 95–98% of children undergoing ureteroneocystostomy have a successful surgical result.

57. What are the complications of ureteroneocystostomy?
Obstruction of the ureterovesical junction and reflux each occurs in approximately 1–2% of cases.

58. In children with primary reflux, which patients are most likely to experience a complication?
Children who have untreated voiding dysfunction are most likely to have a surgical complication.

59. What is J-hooking of the ureter?
In children undergoing a Leadbetter-Politano repair, if the ureter is anastomosed to a mobile portion of the bladder, kinking of the ureter may occur where it inserts into the bladder. In most of these patients, when the bladder is empty there is normal urinary drainage, but with bladder filling, the lower ureter becomes kinked and progressive hydroureteronephrosis occurs. This condition also is termed the **high reimplant syndrome.**

60. If the ureter is extremely wide, what modifications of surgical technique are necessary?
If the ureter is wide, a tunnel of satisfactory length may be difficult to achieve. In these patients the ureter must be tailored, i.e., narrowed, to achieve a sufficient width to allow a successful ureteroneocystostomy. This is done in one of two ways. Excisional tapering may be performed, in which the lateral aspect of the ureter is excised to a point 2–3 cm above the level of implantation. Alternatively, the ureter may be plicated, or folded, to narrow its width.

61. Describe the typical cystoscopic appearances of the ureteral orifice in children with reflux.
Normally the ureteral orifice has a cone shape. Refluxing ureters may have a stadium orifice, a horseshoe orifice, a golf-hole orifice, or patulous ureteral orifice. These terms refer to a progressively abnormal appearances of the ureter in the bladder.

62. What is the endoscopic form of antireflux surgery?
Reflux may be corrected by injecting a substance deep into the ureter to create an intramural tunnel. This procedure has been called the "STING," which stands for subtrigonal injection. In the past polytef paste was used. This substance consists of pyrolyzed Teflon particles suspended in glycerin. Migration of these Teflon particles to the pelvic lymph nodes, liver, lung, and brain has been demonstrated in laboratory models, and currently few procedures are performed using Teflon. Other substances such as collagen or autologous fat may be used in the future.

63. What are the results of the STING?
The results of the STING are inferior to open surgical management. Approximately 70% of patients have reflux resolution with one procedure. With repeat STING procedures, however, the cure rate is as high as 90–95%.

64. What is the likelihood of new renal scarring in children with grade III or IV reflux?
New renal scarring will develop in approximately 20% managed medically.

65. Can reflux be diagnosed prenatally?
Reflux may be detected prenatally by detecting hydronephrosis. However, reflux is not the most common cause of hydronephrosis in the fetus.

66. In children with prenatally diagnosed reflux, what proportion are boys?
Approximately 80% are boys, because boys have higher grades of reflux than girls.

BIBLIOGRAPHY

1. Arant BS: Vesicoureteric reflux and renal injury: In-depth review. Am J Kidney Dis 17: 491–511, 1991.
2. Arant BS: Medical management of mild and moderate vesicoureteral reflux: Follow-up studies of infants and young children. A preliminary report of the Southwest Pediatric Nephrology Study Group. J Urol 148: 1683–1687, 1992.
3. Arant BS Jr, Sotelo-Avila C, Bernstein J: Segmental "hypoplasia" of the kidney (Ask-Upmark). J Pediatr 95: 931–939, 1979.
4. Bellinger MF, Duckett JW: Vesicoureteral reflux: A comparison of nonsurgical and surgical management. Contrib Nephrol 39: 81–93, 1984.
5. Elder JS: Importance of antenatal diagnosis of vesicoureteral reflux [Commentary]. J Urol 148: 1750–1754, 1992.
6. Goldraich NP, Goldraich IH: Followup of conservatively treated children with high and low grade vesicoureteral reflux: A prospective study. J Urol 148: 1688–1692, 1992.
7. Goldraich NP, Ramos OL, Goldraich IH: Urography versus DMSA scan in children with vesicoureteric reflux. Pediatr Nephrol 3: 1–5, 1989.
8. Koff SA, Lapides J, Piazza DH: Association of urinary tract infection and reflux with uninhibited bladder contractions and voluntary sphincteric obstruction. J Urol 122: 373–376, 1979.
9. Koff SA, Murtagh DS: The inhibited bladder in children: Effect of treatment on recurrence of urinary infection and vesicoureteral reflux. J Urol 130: 1138, 1983.
10. Noe HN: The long-term results of prospective sibling reflux screening. J Urol 148: 1739–1742, 1992.
11. Obling H, Claesson K, Ebel D, et al: Renal scars and parenchymal thinning in children with vesicoureteral reflux: A 5-year report of the international reflux study in children (European Branch). J Urol 148: 1653–1656, 1992.
12. Ransley PG, Risdon: Reflux and renal scarring. Br J Radiol Suppl 14: 1–34, 1978.
13. Roberts JA: Vesicoureteral reflux and pyelonephritis in the monkey: A review. J Urol 148: 1721–1725, 1992.
14. Rushton HG and Massoud M: Dimercaptosuccinic acid renal scintigraphy for the evaluation of pyelonephritis and scarring: A review of experimental and clinical studies. J Urol 148: 1726–1732, 1992.
15. Tamminen-Mobius I, Brunier E, Ebel KD, et al: Cessation of vesicoureteral reflux for 5 years in infant and children allocated to medical treatment. J Urol 148: 1662–1666, 1992.
16. Weiss R, Duckett J, et al: Results of a randomized clinical trial of medical versus surgical management of infants and children with grades III and IV primary vesicoureteral reflux (United States). J Urol 148: 1667–1673, 1992.

41. URETEROCELE

Robert Kay, M.D.

1. What is a ureterocele?
A ureterocele is the cystic dilatation of the distal end of the ureter in the intravesical segment.

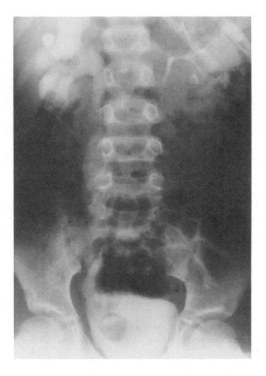

Intravenous pyelogram demonstrating a simple orthotopic ureterocele.

2. In what settings does a ureterocele occur?
Although ureteroceles may occur in single systems (orthotopic ureteroceles), they are most commonly seen in duplicated ureters (ectopic ureteroceles) and come from the ureter draining the upper segment.

3. Why do ureteroceles occur?
There are three current theories to explain the development of ureteroceles:
- Ureteral meatal obstruction
- Inadequate muscularization of the distal ureter
- Excessive dilatation of the distal ureter during development

4. Do ureteroceles occur equally in both sexes?
No. Single-system ureteroceles occur mostly in boys and rarely are seen in girls. Conversely, ectopic ureteroceles, as seen in duplicated systems, occur more frequently in girls than boys.

5. How do ureteroceles present?

Ureteroceles are most commonly diagnosed today by in-utero ultrasound. During fetal ultrasound, a diagnosis of hydronephrosis is made, which is corrected to ureterocele during evaluation in the postpartum period.

Ureteroceles also may be seen during physical examination. An ectopic ureterocele may prolapse through the urethra and present as an intralabial mass, or it may extend underneath the urethra and present between the labia as a cystic mass. Before the advent of ultrasound, urinary tract infection was the most common presentation, and many children still present with this complaint.

6. What is the best way to diagnose a ureterocele on ultrasound?

1. **Ultrasonography** is the best initial step to diagnose a ureterocele. The ultrasound will be ordered as follow-up to the in-utero diagnosis or as evaluation of a urinary tract infection. The technique can evaluate the upper tract and define hydronephrosis. It also may see the cystic mass at the end of the distal ureter and into the bladder.

2. The suspicion of ureterocele on ultrasound may be confirmed by a **voiding cystoure-thrography.**

3. Finally, a **renal scan** is needed to assess the function of the upper tracts.

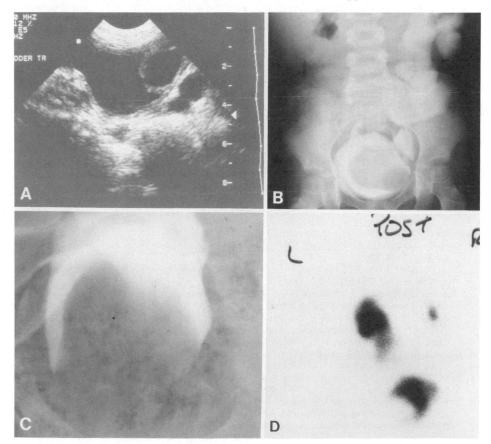

A, Ultrasound demonstrating large ureterocele in bladder. **B,** Intravenous pyelogram revealing large ureterocele in bladder with function of lower pole and dilated ureter. **C,** Cystogram demonstrating large ureterocele. **D,** Renal scan demonstrating hydronephrotic lower pole with nonfunctioning upper pole draining into ectopic ureterocele in bladder.

7. What is the preferred treatment for a single-system (orthotopic) ureterocele?
Although there is a risk of a vesicoureteric reflux, the initial step in treatment is a simple, endoscopic incision of the ureterocele. If reflux occurs and the kidney is salvageable, surgical reimplantation may be performed.

8. List the possible management modalities for ectopic ureteroceles.
   1. Endoscopic incision of the ureterocele
   2. Upper pole nephrectomy with possible ureterectomy
   3. Upper pole pyelo-pyelostomy for functioning kidneys
   4. Upper pole nephrectomy with total ureterectomy and repair of the bladder

9. What is the functional status of the upper pole associated with an ectopic ureterocele?
The upper pole associated with a ureterocele usually has poor or no function. In many cases, the segment might be dysplastic. In some cases, however, there is functioning tissue that should be salvaged.

10. Does reflux occur in ureteroceles?
Reflux can occur in up to 50% of ipsilateral ureters that are associated with ureteroceles. This may be due to poor musculature backing and distortion of the bladder wall from the ectopic ureter. It may also be seen in the contralateral ureter, probably due to distortion of the trigone.

11. Can the reflux disappear spontaneously?
Mild reflux in the ipsilateral ureter and contralateral ureter may spontaneously resolve. Significant degrees of reflux, however, do not usually resolve and require surgical reimplantation.

12. Can ureteroceles be bilateral?
Yes. Bilateral ureteroceles may be seen in up to 10% of all cases of ectopic ureteroceles.

13. What is a cecoureterocele?
A cecoureterocele is an ectopic ureterocele that extends suburethrally into the proximal or even distal urethra.

BIBLIOGRAPHY

   1. Balchick RJ, Nasrallah PF: Cecoureterocele. J Urol 137:100, 1987.
   2. Blyth B, Passerini-Glazel G, Camuffo C, et al: Endoscopic incision of ureteroceles: Intravesical versus ectopic. J Urol 149:556, 1993.
   3. Caldamone AA, Snyder HM, Duckett JW: Ureteroceles in children: Follow-up of management with upper tract approach. J Urol 131:1130, 1984.
   4. Churchill BM, Sheldon CA, McLorie GA: The ectopic ureterocele: A proposed practical classification based on renal unit jeopardy. J Pediatr Surg 27:497, 1992.
   5. Decter RM, Roth DR, Gonzales ET: Individualized treatment of ureterocele. J Urol 142:535, 1989.
   6. Gonzales ET: Anomalies of the renal pelvis and ureter. In Kelalis PP, King LR, and Belman AB (eds): Clinical Pediatric Urology, 3rd ed. Philadelphia, W.B. Saunders, 1992.
   7. King LR, Koglowski JM, Schacht MJ: Ureteroceles in children: A simplified and successful approach to management. JAMA 249:1461, 1983.
   8. Retik AB: Ectopic ureter and ureterocele. In Walsh PC, Gittes RE, Perlmutter AD, Stamey TA (eds): Campbell's Urology. Philadelphia, W.B. Saunders, 1986.
   9. Rich MA, Keating MA, Snyder HM, Duckett JW: Low transurethral incision of single system intravesical ureteroceles in children. J Urol 144:120, 1990.
  10. Stephens FD: Congenital Malformations of the Urinary Tract. New York, Praeger, 1983, pp 320–322, 329.
  11. Tank ES: Experience with endoscopic incision and open unroofing of ureteroceles. J Urol 136:241, 1986.

42. STRESS URINARY INCONTINENCE

Rodney A. Appell, M.D.

1. What is urinary incontinence?

Urinary incontinence is not a single disorder. Rather, it is a symptom of some underlying disorder. It is defined as the involuntary loss of urine and is a major clinical problem and a significant cause of disability and dependency.

2. Is urinary incontinence a consequence of aging?

While normal aging is not a cause of urinary incontinence, age-related changes in lower urinary tract function do predispose older individuals to urinary incontinence. These include anatomic or physiologic insults to the lower urinary tract and systemic disturbances common in the older population.

3. What are the types of urinary incontinence?

These can be defined by function or symptoms.

Types of Incontinence

FUNCTIONAL	SYMPTOMATIC
Detrusor overactivity	Total
Detrusor underactivity	Urge
Outlet incompetence	Stress
Outlet obstruction	Overflow
	Transient
	Functional

The essential organs involved relate to the lower urinary tract and consist of the bladder and urethra, and one can distinguish urinary incontinence that is caused by problems at the level of the bladder as compared to urinary incontinence caused by problems at the level of the urethra. More commonly, the symptomatic definition is used. The six symptomatic types are as follows.

1. **Total incontinence.** Urinary loss which is not associated with any particular event.

2. **Urge incontinence.** The inability to delay voiding after perceiving that the bladder is full—i.e., the bladder contracts without its owner's permission.

3. **Stress urinary incontinence.** Urine loss due to increases in intra-abdominal pressure (Valsalva maneuver).

4. **Overflow incontinence.** Urinary loss due to obstruction or a poorly contracting bladder which allows for a continuous drip of urine.

5. **Transient urinary incontinence.** Acute urinary loss which is precipitated by a nonurinary tract factor, such as change in medications.

6. **Functional incontinence.** Incontinence occurs despite a normal-functioning lower urinary tract, but the patient has a cognitive disorder.

4. Explain the problem causing stress incontinence.

Stress incontinence is a poor term since *stress* is usually associated with such abnormalities as coronary artery disease and peptic ulcer disease. Here, *stress* is meant as the effect of increased abdominal pressure on the lower urinary tract which occurs during times of coughing, laughing, bending, lifting, and defecating.

Normally, the bladder and functional portion of the urethra are located above the pelvic floor so that both are within the true pelvis as intra-abdominal organs. At rest, the urethral pressure is higher than the bladder pressure, preventing urinary leakage. When a Valsalva maneuver increases abdominal pressure, this pressure is transmitted equally onto the bladder and urethra, since both organs are confined within the true pelvis. In stress incontinence, there is hypermobility of the urinary outlet consisting of the bladder neck and proximal functional urethra. The weakening of supportive muscular tissues of the pelvic floor allows the urethra to move out of the true pelvis during a Valsalva maneuver, which results in unequal transmission of the intra-abdominal pressure onto the bladder only and not the urethra. This results in the bladder pressure rising significantly above urethral pressure for that moment and urinary loss.

5. What can cause pelvic floor weakness?
- Anatomic: congenital or traumatic (pelvic floor fracture, pelvic surgery, labor)
- Hormonal
- Neurologic: Congenital or traumatic

6. Is the underlying problem in stress incontinence what is meant by urethral incompetence?
No! Genuine stress urinary incontinence involves the hypermobility of a normally functioning urethral sphincteric mechanism. The problem is anatomic in that the urethra has moved out of the true pelvis and pressures are transmitted unequally. In **urethral incompetence,** the sphincteric mechanisms do not function properly. This results in an open bladder outlet at rest in the absence of a bladder contraction and produces total urinary incontinence usually in any position.

7. What causes urethral incompetence?
It is caused by damage to the sympathetic neural input to the bladder neck and proximal urethra. This area is innervated by the hypogastric nerve, which branches from the thoracolumbar sympathetic outflow tract. Trauma, such as fracture of the pelvis or pelvic surgery, may damage these nerves. Congenital problems such as myelodysplasia (spina bifida) also result in a decrease in innervation to this area of the lower urinary tract, resulting in a nonfunctioning sphincteric mechanism.

8. In that case, are there two types of stress incontinence?
Yes! These are caused by two different mechanisms:
- Hypermobility due to changes in anatomic support
- Urethral dysfunction due to sympathetic neural injury

It is extremely important to differentiate between hypermobility of the urethra and the poor or nonfunctioning urethra because their treatments are very different. The treatment for hypermobility primarily relates to replacing the urethra into its proper position such that pressures will once again be equally transmitted onto the bladder and urethra. In sphincteric nonfunction, elevating and stabilizing the urethra will not result in a return of continence since the urethra itself is dysfunctional; compression and coaptation of the proximale urethra are required.

9. How does one evaluate a patient complaining of urinary incontinence?

Evaluation of Incontinence

History
   Medical
   Obstetrical
Urinary diary
Physical examination
   Observe urinary loss
   Stress test
   Q-tip test
   Bonney/Marshall test
   Vaginal speculum exam
Urinalysis
Urodynamic testing
Cystourethroscopy

---

10. What is the point of the history?

Because the history is not helpful in arriving at a precise diagnosis, its primary value is to direct further investigative efforts to define the cause of the patient's urinary incontinence. During the history, one attempts to define the type of urinary incontinence while recognizing that there is a significant overlap in many of the "types" of urinary incontinence. In general, pathology in five major areas causes lower urinary tract symptoms:

1. Urinary tract pathology
2. Extrinsic local anatomic changes
3. Neurologic disorders
4. Psychiatric disorders
5. Local effects of systemic disease and/or its treatment

Therefore, specific questions will suggest a category for the patient's problem, placing it into one of the above general areas rather than trying to focus on a specific diagnosis.

11. How is the incontinence documented?

The patient should keep a diary of intake of fluid and output of urine, recording the time and volume of each voiding and incontinent episode. Also, during the physical examination, the physician must be able to reproduce the urinary incontinence and observe it.

12. Are there special aspects of the physical examination in female patients?

The proximity of the lower urinary tract to the female reproductive tract makes simultaneous assessment of both a necessity in the proper evaluation of female incontinence problems. For example, estrogen deprivation not only manifests itself with atrophic changes in the vulva and vagina, but also produces a variety of lower urinary tract symptoms due to atrophic urethritis. In addition, both a vesicovaginal fistula or urethral diverticulum may produce incontinence, and a thorough examination may help to detect this particular defect.

13. Explain the specific tests used during the physical examination.

1. **Q-tip test.** This helps determine the amount of urethral hypermobility on straining. With the patient in the lithotomy position, the physician inserts a lubricated Q-tip into the urethra to the level of the urethrovesical junction and then measures the angle between the Q-tip and horizontal when the patient strains maximally. Normally, the angle is $10°-15°$ above horizontal at rest with minimal changes on straining. In the patient with genuine stress urinary incontinence, this angle usually increases by $> 20°$, suggesting that the descent of the urethra and bladder neck is due to weakness of the anatomical support.

2. **Stress test.** The patient with a full bladder stands with one leg up on a stool, and while the physician closely observes the urethral meatus, the patient bears down or coughs. If a short spurt of urine escapes simultaneously with the cough, this suggests genuine urinary incontinence. A slight delay in the leakage after the cough suggests an unstable bladder, as contractions in the bladder may have been provoked by the Valsalva maneuver.

3. **Bonney test.** The physician places two fingers in the vagina to elevate the neck of the bladder up toward the pubic bone, taking care not to compress the urethra. Unfortunately, this is extremely difficult to do without compressing the urethra. In a patient who has demonstrated a positive stress test, the Bonney test usually stops the urinary loss by elevating and compressing the urethra.

4. **Marshall test.** In this variation on the Bonney test, the vagina is anesthetized locally to allow a section of the vagina to be grasped with a clamp and elevated in a fashion that does not compress the urethra. Neither the Bonney or Marshall test is diagnostic, as occlusion of the urethra prevents leakage regardless of the pathophysiology of the urinary incontinence. Therefore, these tests are of limited value.

5. **Speculum evaluation.** A full pelvic examination often reveals evidence for pelvic relaxation with herniation of the bladder (cystocele) or rectum (rectocele) into the vagina. Of course, other disease such as a pelvic mass may also be found.

14. Are any laboratory tests necessary?
A urinalysis should be performed. Evidence of hematuria requires further evaluation with urinary cytology, intravenous urography, and cystourethroscopy. Any and all urinary tract infections should be treated appropriately.

15. What is the purpose of urodynamic testing?
Urodynamic studies are the most important set of examinations because they evaluate the motor function of the three specific muscle groups making up the lower urinary tract: the bladder, smooth muscle of the urethra, and external striated muscle sphincter. When urodynamic testing is combined with contrast placed into the urinary tract, the lower urinary tract may be visualized, and an anatomic and physiologic evaluation can be performed simultaneously; this is called **videourodynamics.** Although this is not necessary for every patient, in those with confusing symptoms it helps elucidate the actual dysfunction that is occurring.

Urodynamic tests are done with small catheters which measure the pressure within the bladder and urethra. It is important to do these studies while the patient is in an upright position, especially if the patient denies having any leakage while lying down. The most important of these tests is the cystometrogram, which evaluates the stability of the bladder while it is filling with urine. Unstable bladder contractions are usually interpreted by the patient as the urge to void and, if the pressure is high enough, can result in urge incontinence. The presence of unstable bladder contractions in a patient who has stress incontinence may alter the recommended therapy.

16. When is urodynamic testing indicated?
- Failed previous incontinence surgery
- Previous radical pelvic surgery
- Symptoms of mixed incontinence
- No objective evidence of urinary leakage
- Abnormal neurologic examination
- History of neurologic disorder

17. When is cystoscopy indicated?
1. In patients shown to have an unstable bladder either by history or cystometrogram, it is important to exclude bladder pathology, which could cause the symptoms. Bladder tumors, bladder stones, urinary infections, and even carcinoma-in-situ may result in unstable bladder contractions.

2. If a patient has stress incontinence or another form of incontinence requiring surgical repair, then preoperative cystourethroscopy can prevent errors in patient management. Coexisting disease, if detected before the scheduled incontinence surgery, then can be appropriately handled at the same time. For example, patients who have mixed incontinence may be cured by removal of permanent suture material which has perforated the bladder from previous pelvic surgery.

18. How do you identify patients with a nonfunctioning urethra?
In these patients, urodynamic evaluation is mandatory to evaluate the sphincteric function. Specific tests designed to do this include the **urethral closure profile.** Pressure in the urethra below 20 cm H_2O indicates a poorly functioning urethra (the normal urethral closure pressure is > 40 cm H_2O). **Leak point pressures** can be determined during cystometrography. If the bladder pressure resulting in urinary leakage is < 60 cm H_2O, this indicates severe urethral dysfunction.

19. Once the diagnosis of genuine stress incontinence is made, what medical treatments are available?
The only medical treatment that has been helpful is the use of estrogen in postmenopausal women who have demonstrated estrogen deprivation. No other medications have been effective because this is an anatomic disorder.

Treatment of Stress Incontinence

HYPERMOBILITY	URETHRAL INCOMPETENCE
Medical	Slings
Estrogen	Artificial urinary sphincter
Behavioral	Injectables
Pelvic floor exercise	
Bladder drill	
Timed voidings	
Biofeedback	
Surgery	
Abdominal	
Vaginal	

20. Are any other nonsurgical methods helpful?

Most definitely, noninvasive methods may be helpful in controlling patient symptoms if they are not too severe. These include Kegel pelvic muscle exercises, behavior modification and retraining, and biofeedback. In addition, pelvic floor electrical stimulation with a vaginal probe is effective in approximately 50% of patients with mild stress urinary incontinence. This stimulation acts directly on the pudendal nerve to cause contraction of the levator muscles and periurethral skeletal muscle and appears to strengthen the sphincter and pelvic floor muscles without actually correcting the underlying anatomic defect.

21. What role does surgery play in the management of stress urinary incontinence?

Some have suggested that the name *stress incontinence* be replaced by the phrase *surgically curable urinary incontinence.* Surgery clearly has been successful in managing patients with genuine stress urinary incontinence, curing about 75% of patients and improving continence in 85% no matter which technique of surgical repair is used.

A multitude of surgical repairs has been developed in attempts to reduce the amount of surgical trauma and hospitalization time and to return patients to work quicker. However, none of the procedures works 100% of the time, and these new procedures are also attempts to improve surgical success. No one method can be recommended over another, as it relates to the surgeon's experience with a particular procedure and patient selection for that procedure. Some procedures are done via an abdominal surgical approach and others through the vagina.

22. What about patients with intrinsic sphincteric deficiency with urethral incompetence?

Here, standard urethral resuspension procedures will not be effective if the continence mechanism is defective. Rather, compression and coaptation of the urethral mucosa are necessary. There are three approaches to this:

1. **Pubovaginal sling.** An autologous, heterologous, or synthetic material is used as a broad base of support under the urethra and then brought up through the abdominal wall and anchored to either the abdomen or pelvic bones in order to provide compression of the urethra.

2. **Artificial urinary sphincter.** A small cuff is placed around the neck of the bladder, and a hydraulic pump mechanism is placed inside the labia of the patient. When she has the urge to void, she merely pushes the pump once or twice, and this drives the fluid out of the cuff and opens up the neck of the bladder to allow unobstructed voiding.

3. **Injectable treatment.** The use of bovine collagen injected under local anesthesia into the submucosa of the urethra at the level of the bladder neck is extremely effective in controlling urethral incompetence.

BIBLIOGRAPHY

1. Appell RA: Injectables for urethral incontinence. World J Urol 8:208–211, 1990.
2. Appell RA: Techniques and results in the implantation of the artificial urinary sphincter in type III stress urinary incontinence by a vaginal approach. Neurourol Urodyn 7:613–619, 1988.

3. Blaivas JG, Fisher DM: Combined radiographic and urodynamic monitoring: Advances in technique. J Urol 125:541–544, 1981.
4. Burgio KL: Behavioral training for stress and urge incontinence in the community. Gerontology 38(suppl 2):27–34, 1990.
5. Cardozo L: Role of estrogens in the treatment of female urinary incontinence. J Am Geriatr Soc 38:326–328, 1990.
6. Henalla SM, Kirwan P, Castleden CM, et al: The effect of pelvic floor exercise in the treatment of genuine stress urinary incontinence in women at two hospitals. Br J Obstet Gynaecol 95:602–606, 1988.
7. Kelley MJ, Leach GE: Long term results of bladder neck suspension procedures. Probl Urol 5:94–105, 1991.
8. McGuire EJ: Bladder instability and stress incontinence. Neurourol Urodyn 7:563–567, 1988.
9. McIntosh LJ, Richardson DA: Thirty-minute evaluation of incontinence in the older woman. Geriatrics 49:35–44, 1994.
10. Staskin DR: Sling surgery for the treatment of female stress incontinence. Probl Urol 5:106–122, 1991.
11. Staskin DR, Zimmern PE, Hadley HR, et al: The pathophysiology of stress incontinence. Urol Clin North Am 12:271–278, 1985.
12. Wall LL, Norton PA, DeLancey JOL: Practical Urogynecology. Baltimore, Williams & Wilkins, 1993.

43. VESICOVAGINAL FISTULA

Elroy D. Kursh, M.D.

1. What is a vesicovaginal fistula (VVF)?
A VVF is a hole between the bladder and vagina, causing the patient to suffer varying degrees of urinary incontinence.

2. How does a VVF develop?
In undeveloped countries, most VVFs develop following labor and delivery. Prolonged labor and delivery, which may be associated with cephalopelvic disproportion (newborn's head is too large for mother's pelvis), causes excessive pressure on the bladder, leading to bladder necrosis and the development of a VVF. Advances in obstetrics in developed nations have greatly reduced the incidence of obstetric VVFs.

Far and away the most common cause of VVF in developed areas is iatrogenic damage to the bladder during surgery. Gynecologic surgery accounts for approximately 70–80%, with most occurring after abdominal hysterectomy and, less commonly, vaginal hysterectomy. Radiation injury to the bladder may also be responsible for the development of a VVF, which usually occurs 6–12 months after cessation of therapy but may occur years later.

3. What is the etiology of a VVF following gynecologic or pelvic surgery?
Various theories have been proposed to explain how a VVF develops after hysterectomy. The most commonly stated explanations have been that the fistula results from avascular necrosis of the base of the bladder or erosion from sutures placed between the bladder and vaginal cuff.

Recent data suggest that most VVFs following gynecologic surgery result from an unsuspected bladder perforation. The urine that drains from the perforation site forms a collection in the pelvis behind the bladder known as a **urinoma.** The undrained urinoma may be responsible for abdominal pain, distention, or a paralytic ileus after abdominal hysterectomy, which are relatively common findings in patients who later develop a VVF. The logical site of urine leakage from the injured bladder is the vaginal cuff, which is dependent and usually left open. A VVF develops when the tract between the bladder and vagina becomes epithelialized.

4. What are the symptoms of a VVF?
Patients usually note the onset of a painless, watery discharge of varying amounts from the vagina, most often occurring 7–14 days after surgery. The volume of leakage can vary substantially, depending on the size and location of the fistula. Most VVFs are located in the dependent portion of the base of the bladder and are large enough to result in leakage of most, if not all, of the urine from the vagina. On the other hand, a very small fistula may result in vaginal leakage of a small amount of urine intermittently.

5. How can you prove that the fluid draining from the vagina is urine?
If it is unclear that the drainage represents urine, an aliquot of the fluid should be analyzed for blood urea nitrogen (BUN) and creatinine. If the BUN and creatinine values exceed those of serum (usually 20 times), urinary leakage is proven.

6. What is the differential diagnosis of a VVF?
Small amounts of vaginal drainage following a hysterectomy may result from drainage of serous fluid from the vaginal cuff. Gynecologists may often attribute vaginal drainage to such a vaginal cuff seroma, which may delay establishing a correct diagnosis. Otherwise, leakage of urine from the vagina following pelvic surgery may occur from other urinary fistulas, with a ureterovaginal fistula being far and away the most common. Other possible urinary fistulas include urethrovaginal fistula, vesicouterine fistula, and various fistulas from the bowel to the bladder that may

include the vagina. Patients with very small VVFs, which may result in a small amount of intermittent vaginal leakage, may be misdiagnosed as having stress urinary incontinence.

7. How is a diagnosis of a VVF established?

The most reliable means of establishing a diagnosis of VVF is by a **bladder filling test.** The bladder is filled with fluid through a catheter or cystoscope, while the vagina is observed with use of a vaginal speculum; fluid can usually be readily observed exiting the fistula site in the vagina. Inspection of the vagina almost always reveals considerable inflammation of the vaginal cuff, which is the inevitable site of most VVFs.

If the diagnosis is still in doubt, various **dye studies** can be performed. Methylene blue or indigo carmine solution is instilled into the bladder from a catheter, with care taken to avoid leakage from the urethra. The suspected fistula site in the vagina is observed for leakage of the blue dye solution. Another technique is to insert a tampon into the vagina after the bladder is filled with the dye solution. Staining of the uppermost part of the tampon indicates a VVF, while staining of the outermost part may represent urinary incontinence or a urethrovaginal fistula.

A cystogram (x-ray of the bladder) may be helpful in establishing a diagnosis but is not generally required.

8. Are any other diagnostic studies indicated?

Even if a diagnosis is readily established by other studies, a cystoscopic examination must be done to identify the number, size, and location of the fistulas and to assess the degree of associated inflammation in the bladder in order to plan appropriate treatment.

Because it is not uncommon for an ureterovaginal fistula to be associated with a VVF and because ureterovaginal fistula represents the next most common cause of urinary leakage following pelvic surgery, it is important to rule out this diagnosis before planning therapy. Ureterovaginal fistulas are usually associated with normal spontaneous voiding from the bladder and continuous urinary leakage from the vagina. An intravenous pyelogram (IVP) can demonstrate not only the fistula site with varying degrees of leakage into the vagina, but also the associated ureteral obstruction and accompanying hydronephrosis. Retrograde urography may also be helpful in establishing a diagnosis of ureterovaginal fistula.

9. What is the treatment of a VVF?

Almost all VVFs require surgical closure. A very small VVF can be successfully managed by electrocoagulation of the epithelialized tract and placement of an indwelling Foley catheter in the bladder for several weeks; adequate bladder drainage may allow the tract to scar and the respective mucosal surfaces of the bladder and vagina to heal.

Both vaginal and suprapubic approaches to surgical correction have been employed. The choice of surgery depends on the experience of the surgeon and is determined by the location of single or multiple fistulas and the complexity of the fistula. Overall cure rates using the abdominal approach are slightly lower than for vaginal repairs, but this is because abdominal techniques are generally employed for more complicated fistulas. For complex fistulas, such as recurrent VVFs or VVFs that develop following radiation therapy, various pedicle materials (e.g., omentum, labial fat pad, rectus abominis muscle, gracilis muscle) can be interposed between the bladder and vagina during repair.

10. Can anything be done to reduce the amount of incontinence while the patient awaits surgery?

The continual wetness, odor, and discomfort present difficult social problems while the patient awaits surgical repair. Unfortunately, most fistulas are in the dependent portion of the bladder base and tend to cause considerable leakage. In general, incontinence underpants with various urine collection pads are necessary. Today there are a number of well-constructed silica-impregnated pads that are preferable since they trap urine and help prevent extensive contact with the perineum. Another alternative is to use a well-fitted contraceptive diaphragm to attempt to trap urine to reduce urinary leakage. Although some patients may require an indwelling Foley catheter for hygenic and psychological reasons, they are best avoided because of risk of associated infection and inflammation.

BIBLIOGRAPHY

1. Badenoch DF, Tiptaft RC, Thakar DR, et al: Early repair of accidental injury to the ureter or bladder following gynaecological surgery. Br J Urol 59:516, 1987.
2. Lee RA, Symmonds RE, Williams TJ. Current status of genital-urinary fistula. Obstet Gynecol 72:313, 1988.
3. Kursh ED, Morse RM, Resnick MI, Persky L: Prevention of the development of a vesicovaginal fistula. Surg Gynecol Obstet 166:409, 1988.
4. O'Conor VJ Jr: Review of experience with vesicovaginal fistula repair. J Urol 123:367, 1980.
5. Wang W, Hadley HR. Non-delayed transvaginal repair of high lying vesicovaginal fistula. J Urol 144:34, 1990.
6. Wein AJ, Malloy TR, Carpincello VC, et al: Repair of a vesicovaginal fistula by a suprapubic transvesical approach. Surg Gynecol Obstet 150:57, 1980.

44. EXSTROPHY OF THE BLADDER

Jonathan H. Ross, M.D.

1. Define bladder exstrophy.

Bladder exstrophy is a congenital anomaly in which the bladder is exposed and everted on the lower abdominal wall.

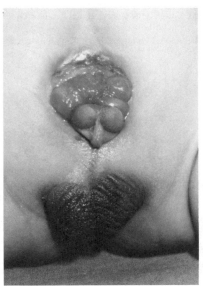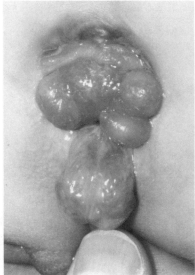

A newborn with bladder exstrophy.

2. Is it common?

No. It occurs in approximately 1 in 35,000 live births. It is three to four times more common in boys than in girls.

3. What causes it?

It is probably caused by a failure of the cloacal membrane to retract. The cloacal membrane covers the mid-lower abdomen in the first weeks of gestation. In the fourth week of gestation, the membrane retracts caudally, allowing the medial migration of mesoderm on the lateral borders of the membrane to produce the abdominal wall and roll the bladder into a spherical structure. If the membrane persists inappropriately, then this portion of the abdominal wall fails to develop, and when the cloacal membrane ruptures, the bladder is left exposed and everted.

4. What are the usual associated anomalies?

Vesicoureteral reflux is present in most patients. Inguinal hernias are common, particularly in boys. Epispadias (both male and female) and a widely separated pubic symphysis are always present.

5. Are upper urinary tract changes common at birth in patients with bladder exstrophy?
No. But anomalies such as horseshoe kidney and dysplasia have been described. Therefore, newborns should undergo a renal ultrasound.

6. What problems does the exposed bladder mucosa present?
Actually, very few. The main concern is protecting the mucosa from injury and preventing mucosal edema, which will make bladder closure more difficult. To that end, the mucosa is covered with a piece of Silastic or plastic wrap, and care is taken to prevent irritation from diapers and the umbilical cord clamp.

7. List the three operations which most boys with bladder exstrophy undergo.
    1. **Primary bladder closure.** This is usually accomplished in the first days of life. The bladder is closed, but no attempt is made to tighten the bladder neck. Thus, the infants are totally incontinent following the procedure. Iliac osteotomies are performed in most patients at the same time so that the pubic rami can be brought together in the midline, allowing for a more secure bladder closure.
    2. **Epispadias repair.** This is usually performed at 6–18 months of age. It is hoped that the added passive resistance created contributes to increasing bladder size, which facilitates the third operation.
    3. **Bladder neck reconstruction.** Bilateral ureteral reimplantation is performed simultaneously to correct vesicoureteral reflux and to move the ureteral orifices away from the caudal portion of the bladder, which is tubularized in reconstructing the bladder neck.

8. How successful is this approach?
Approximately 70% of patients gain an acceptable level of continence (a dry interval of at least 3.5–4 hours).

9. If patients remain incontinent, what other procedures are available?
The most common reason for failure is a persistently small bladder. This can be corrected with a **bladder augmentation.** Indeed, if the bladder is < 70–80 ml at the time of bladder neck reconstruction, a preemptive augmentation is considered. If persistent incontinence is due to low outflow resistance, then **collagen injection,** a **bladder neck revision,** or placement of an **artificial sphincter** may be undertaken. An ultimate solution, which a minority of patients require, is a **continent urinary diversion.**

10. Name two obstetric/gynecologic complications that occur in women with a history of bladder exstrophy.
Uterine prolapse and fetal malpresentation.

11. What happens if you do not operate on newborns with exstrophy?
Actually, they may live long and healthy lives, but intervention is always undertaken. The continuous incontinence is intolerable, and they are at risk for adenocarcinoma in the chronically exposed bladder mucosa. Irritation of mucosa at the ureteral orifices may also lead to hydroureteronephrosis.

12. What is cloacal exstrophy?
Cloacal exstrophy is a rare, complex disorder occurring in 1 in 200,000 live births. It results from premature rupture of the cloacal membrane before separation of the cloaca into an anterior and posterior portion. This results in two halves of an exstrophied bladder separated by an exstrophied ileocecal segment.

BIBLIOGRAPHY

1. Adams MC, Retik AB: Exstrophy of the bladder. In Resnick MI, Kursh ED (eds): Current Therapy in Genitourinary Surgery. St. Louis, Mosby, 1992, pp 272–275.
2. Caldamone AA: Anomalies of the bladder and cloaca. In Gillenwater JY, Grayhack JT, Howards SS, Duckett JW (eds): Adult and Pediatric Urology, 2nd ed. St. Louis, Mosby, 1991, pp 2023–2053.
3. Connor JP, Lattimer JK, Hensle TW, Burbige KA: Primary closure of bladder exstrophy: Long-term functional results in 137 patients. J Pediatr Surg 23:1102–1106, 1988.
4. Gearhart JP, Canning DA, Peppas DS, Jeffs RD: Techniques to create continence in the failed bladder exstrophy closure patient. J Urol 150:441–443, 1993.
5. Gearhart JP, Jeffs RD: Augmentation cystoplasty in the failed exstrophy reconstruction. J Urol 139:790–793, 1988.
6. Gearhart JP, Jeffs RD: Bladder exstrophy: Increase in capacity following epispadias repair. J Urol 142:525–526, 1989.
7. Gearhart JP, Jeffs RD: State-of-the-art reconstructive surgery for bladder exstrophy at the Johns Hopkins Hospital. Am J Dis Child 143:1475–1478, 1989.
8. Lepor H, Jeffs RD: Primary bladder closure and bladder neck reconstruction in classical bladder exstrophy. J Urol 130:1142–1145, 1983.

45. ACQUIRED URETHRAL STRICTURE

Kenneth W. Angermeier, M.D.

1. What is a urethral stricture?
A urethral stricture is a scar that results from tissue injury. As the scar heals, circumferential contraction may result in narrowing of the urethral lumen.

2. Describe the anatomic divisions of the urethra.
    1. **Glanular urethra**—the portion surrounded by the erectile tissue of the glans penis.

    2. **Pendulous or penile urethra**—the segment extending from the corona of the glans penis to the distal fusion of the ischiocavernosus muscles.

    3. **Bulbous urethra**—the portion covered by the fusion of the ischiocavernosus muscles, extending proximally to the level of the perineal membrane.

    4. **Membranous urethra**—the section of the urethra surrounded by the striated urethral sphincter. Embryologically, the membranous urethra extends from the perineal membrane to the verumontanum.

    5. **Prostatic urethra**—the portion proximal to the verumontanum and surrounded by the prostate gland.

    The prostatic and membranous portions of the urethra are often termed the posterior urethra, whereas the combined bulbous, pendulous, and glanular portions are often termed the anterior urethra.

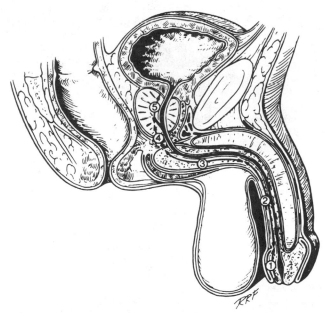

Sagittal section of the penis and perineum demonstrates the divisions of the urethra as enumerated in the text. (From Devine CJ Jr, Angermeier KW: Anatomy of the penis and male perineum. Part 1. American Urological Association Update Series. Vol. 13, Lesson 2, 1994, with permission).

3. Where is the corpus spongiosum in relation to the urethra?
The corpus spongiosum, which consists of erectile tissue, lies in the ventral groove between the two corpora cavernosa. It completely surrounds the anterior urethra throughout its course. The

corpus spongiosum expands distally to form a broad cap of tissue, called the glans penis, that encompasses the glanular urethra and proximally to form the bulb of the penis. Within the bulb the urethra lies closer to the dorsal than the ventral aspect of the corpus spongiosum and exits the dorsal surface of the bulb before its attachment to the perineal body.

4. What are the most common causes of urethral stricture?
In the past inflammatory urethritis, such as that caused by gonococcal infection, was the leading cause of urethral stricture disease. With the development of modern antibiotic therapy, this is no longer the case. Currently urethral strictures result most commonly from urethral trauma or instrumentation.

5. How do patients with urethral stricture usually present?
As the urethral lumen gradually narrows, the onset of obstructive voiding symptoms is often insidious. Symptoms may include decreased urinary stream, prolonged voiding time, and hesitancy and/or straining to void. Some patients present with prostatitis or epididymitis, which may be recurrent.

6. What is spongiofibrosis?
Spongiofibrosis is fibrosis or scarring within the corpus spongiosum adjacent to a urethral stricture. It is important to assess the depth of spongiofibrosis, which helps to delineate the severity of stricture disease and affects the success of subsequent treatment modalities.

7. Describe the evaluation of a patient suspected of having urethral stricture.
A retrograde urethrogram is performed, using contrast suitable for intravenous administration. If enough contrast has entered the bladder, the patient is asked to void, and a voiding urethrogram is also obtained. These studies provide information about the location, length, and caliber of stricture disease. Urethroscopy confirms the findings on urethrography and visually assesses the urethral mucosa and associated scarring. Palpation of the urethra also may reveal evidence of spongiofibrosis or periurethral scarring. With experience one can estimate reliably the depth of spongiofibrosis on the basis of the above information.

8. What is the role of ultrasound in the evaluation of urethral stricture?
Several reports describe the use of ultrasound in the evaluation of patients with urethral stricture, suggesting improved assessment of the depth of spongiofibrosis. In clinical practice, however, it has been our impression that ultrasound adds little information to the evaluation described above.

9. Describe the "reconstructive ladder" approach to the treatment of urethral strictures.
The reconstructive ladder approach is based on the concept of beginning with the simplest procedure available and progressing to more complex procedures as initial efforts fail. Management of urethral stricture is initiated with urethral dilation, followed by internal urethrotomy and then by open urethral reconstruction, as necessary. With progress in modern techniques of tissue transfer, this protocol has become outdated. More recently an anatomic approach has been adopted, which matches a particular treatment modality to the individual patient on the basis of anatomy of the stricture and likelihood of success.

10. How is urethral dilation performed?
In general, urethral dilation should be performed by gradually dilating a stricture over a period of several weeks, increasing the caliber of the dilation by 2–4 French until a maximum of 24–26 French is reached. This approach minimizes further urethral trauma due to dilation. In the past gradual dilation was accomplished by blind passage of a thin filiform catheter through the area of stricture to serve as a guide, with subsequent dilation by the passage of progressively larger "follower" catheters that attach to the filiform. A more recent technique involves manipulation of a soft wire through the stricture under direct vision with a flexible cystoscope, with subsequent passage of a balloon-dilating catheter over the wire. The balloon is then inflated to dilate the

urethra. The radial forces exerted by the balloon catheter may lead to less urethral trauma than the shearing forces generated by filiforms and followers.

11. Can urethral dilation be curative?

Urethral dilation is primarily a management modality in patients with urethral stricture. The interval between dilations often may be progressively increased, eventually to every 6–12 months in optimal circumstances. Discontinuing the dilations almost certainly results in recurrence of the stricture. Infrequently a patient with minimal stricture in the form of a urethral mucosal scar and minimal to no spongiofibrosis may be cured by dilation alone. Dilation is used primarily as a form of management in patients who are not candidates for more aggressive surgical intervention.

12. Where are the incisions made during endoscopic direct-vision internal urethrotomy (DVIU)?

Traditionally a cold-knife urethrotome has been used to incise longitudinally through the urethral stricture at the 12-o'clock position. For the procedure to be successful, the incision must be made completely through the spongiofibrosis into the underlying healthy corpus spongiosum. Because of the anatomic position of the urethra, little corpus spongiosum is located dorsally within the bulbous portion. For this reason, some authors advocate incisions at the 10- and 2-o'clock (± 6 o'clock) positions for DVIU within the bulbous urethra.

13. Which patients are good candidates for DVIU?

DVIU may be curative in patients with urethral stricture that involves minimal spongiofibrosis. If the initial attempt is unsuccessful and the stricture recurs, the patient should be reevaluated both radiographically and endoscopically. If the overall situation is somewhat improved, a second DVIU is reasonable. If the stricture is unchanged or worsened, open urethral reconstruction should be considered.

14. What are the indications for open urethral reconstruction?

In patients who are medically fit for surgery, open urethral reconstruction should be considered for stricture disease associated with moderate-to-severe spongiofibrosis or when more conservative measures have failed. The presence of a fistula or other complicating factors also may necessitate this approach. The length of stricture may vary from 1–2 cm to involvement of nearly the entire anterior urethra (panurethral).

15. What is the optimal form of open urethral reconstruction?

Excision of the stricture with a spatulated primary urethral anastomosis is the optimal reconstruction procedure. Unfortunately, this procedure can be applied only to bulbous urethral strictures of < 3 cm because of limitations in mobilizing the corpus spongiosum to allow a tension-free anastomosis.

16. Describe the genital skin islands that may be useful for "flap" urethral reconstruction.

For strictures not amendable to excision and primary anastomosis, the most useful and reliable form of reconstruction is creation of a longitudinal urethrotomy incision through the entire length of the stricture, followed by inlay of viable tissue into the urethrotomy defect. Genital skin islands dissected and mobilized on a dartos fascia pedicle have been found to be the most reliable form of inlay. Several such flaps are available for use, depending on the availability of well-vascularized local skin. Penile island flaps include the following:

    1. **Ventral longitudinal island flap (Orandi)**—useful for strictures of the pendulous urethra.

    2. **Dorsal transverse island flap**—applicable to strictures of the pendulous and distal bulbous urethra.

    3. **Ventral longitudinal/transverse preputial island flap (Quartey)**—mobilized for use throughout the bulbous urethra.

    In addition to the above, some men have an area of truly hairless skin near the inferior midline of the scrotum. This flap can be mobilized on a lateral dartos fascia pedicle and used for reconstruction of the bulbous urethra.

17. What is the surgical approach to the bulbous urethra?
Surgery in this region is accomplished through a perineal incision with the patient in the exaggerated lithotomy position.

18. Are staged procedures ever necessary for urethral reconstruction?
Yes. Although most urethral reconstructive procedures can be performed in one stage, a staged approach is necessary in certain cases, including urethral stricture with severe spongiofibrosis associated with fistula or abscess formation, or lack of sufficient well-vascularized local skin for one-stage flap reconstruction. The first stage generally involves opening or excising the diseased urethra, with transfer of viable, nonhirsute skin to the penis or perineum in the form of a meshed, split-thickness skin graft. In the second stage, which is undertaken approximately 6–9 months later, the skin graft, with its newly established blood supply, is mobilized and closed to form the neourethra.

19. Describe the management of a membranous urethral stricture after transurethral resection of the prostate (TURP).
Development of a membranous urethral stricture after TURP is not uncommon. In this difficult situation, the bladder neck has been resected, and the patient therefore relies solely on the distal urethral sphincter mechanism for continence. DVIU or open reconstruction in this instance carries a high risk of postoperative urinary incontinence, because the striated urethral sphincter encompasses the membranous urethra and may be compromised. Therefore, urethral dilation is the preferred form of management.

BIBLIOGRAPHY

1. Angermeier KW, Devine CJ Jr: Anatomy of the penis and male perineum. Part 2. American Urological Association Update Series. Vol. 13, Lesson 3, 1994.
2. Devine CJ Jr, Angermeier KW: Anatomy of the penis and male perineum. Part 1. American Urological Association Update Series. Vol. 13, Lesson 2, 1994.
3. Devine CJ Jr, Jordan GH, Schlossberg SM: Surgery of the penis and urethra. In Walsh PC, Retik AB, Stamey TA, Vaughan ED Jr (eds): Campbell's Urology, 6th ed. Philadelphia, W.B. Saunders, 1992, pp 2982–2998.
4. Jordan GH: Management of anterior urethral stricture disease. Prob Urol 1:199–225, 1987.
5. Jordan GH: Treatment of urethral stricture disease. In Stein BS (ed): Practice of Urology. New York, Norton Medical Books, 1993, pp 1–38.
6. McAninch JW, Laing FC, Jeffrey RB. Sonourethrography in the evaluation of urethral strictures: A preliminary report. J Urol 139:294, 1988.
7. Orandi A: One-stage urethroplasty: Four year followup. J Urol 107:977, 1972.
8. Quartey JKM: One-stage penile/preputial cutaneous island flap urethroplasty for urethral stricture: A preliminary report. J Urol 129:284, 1983.
9. Webster GD, Koefoot RB, Sihelnik SA: Urethroplasty management in 200 cases of urethral stricture: A rationale for procedure selection. J Urol 134:892, 1985.

46. POSTERIOR AND ANTERIOR URETHRAL VALVES

Jack S. Elder, M.D.

1. Name the four segments of the male urethra.

1. Prostatic urethra: from the bladder neck to the proximal margin of the urogenital diaphragm

2. Membranous urethra: traverses the urogenital diaphragm (external or striated sphincter)

3. Bulbous urethra: the portion from the distal membranous urethra to the penoscrotal junction

4. Penile urethra: the segment traversing the length of the penile shaft, including the glans penis.

2. What is the posterior urethra?
The posterior urethra consists of the prostatic urethra and membranous urethra.

3. What is the anterior urethra?
The anterior urethra consists of the bulbous urethra and penile urethra.

4. Define verumontanum.
The verumontanum, located on the dorsal aspect of the prostatic urethra, is a small mound of tissue into which drains the two ejaculatory ducts and the prostatic utricle. It is an important landmark during cystoscopy, as it is just proximal to the external sphincter.

5. What are posterior urethral valves?
Posterior urethral valves refers to abnormal congenital mucosal folds in the prostatic urethra that look like a thin membrane that impairs bladder drainage.

6. Do girls get posterior urethral valves?
No.

7. What is the incidence of posterior urethral valves?
Approximately 1 in 8000 males.

8. How are posterior urethral valves diagnosed?
A voiding cystourethrogram (VCUG) must be performed. This involves catheterizing the bladder with a pediatric feeding tube or Foley catheter, infusing contrast material into the bladder under gravity, and observing the bladder fill and empty using fluoroscopic monitoring. The posterior urethra is examined very carefully throughout the procedure.

9. What are the radiographic signs of posterior urethral valves?
A VCUG shows a distended prostatic urethra, the valve leaflets, detrusor (bladder) hypertrophy, possibly with cellules and/or diverticula, bladder neck hypertrophy, and a narrow stream in the penile urethra. In addition, there may be incomplete emptying of the bladder.

10. What other studies should be performed?
Usually a renal ultrasound shows bilateral hydronephrosis. Another upper tract study such as a renal scan (MAG-3, DTPA, or DMSA) should be performed to ascertain how well the kidneys are functioning.

11. Discuss the three types of congenital posterior urethral valves.
Hugh Young described three distinct types of congenital PUV. A type I urethral valve is an obstructing membrane that extends distally from each side of the verumontanum toward the membranous urethra where they fuse anteriorly. This type accounts for 90–95% of all cases. Type II valves were described as folds extending cephalad from the verumontanum to the bladder neck. More recently it has become apparent that type II valves do not exist. A type III valve represents a diaphragm or ring-like membrane with a central aperture just distal to the verumontanum.
    There is evidence that types I and III valves represent the same condition. Antegrade cystography (injecting contrast material into the bladder through a small catheter rather than through the urethra) in babies with suspected posterior urethral valves demonstrated the classic radiologic features. Subsequently, during cystoscopy, all of the patients seemed to have a type III valve, but after the cystoscope was inserted, the appearance of the valve changed to a classic type I appearance. Therefore, urethral catheterization seems to disrupt the urethral valve in the vast majority of patients. The subsequent appearance is that of a type I posterior urethral valve.

12. What proportion of boys with urethral valves have vesicoureteral reflux?
Approximately 50% have reflux, with 25% being unilateral and 25% bilateral.

13. What are the long-term consequences of posterior urethral valves?
Posterior urethral valves are the most common obstructive cause of end-stage renal disease, and approximately one-third of surviving males develop renal insufficiency or chronic renal failure.

14. How do infants with posterior urethral valves present?
Often the condition is discovered prenatally with the finding of bilateral hydronephrosis and a distended bladder. In a newborn there may be a palpable abdominal mass (distended bladder, hydronephrotic kidney), ascites, or respiratory distress from pulmonary hypoplasia. Many children with valves present with a febrile urinary tract infection. These infants may have urosepsis, dehydration, uremia, and electrolyte abnormalities. At times a pneumothorax occurs in these newborns. Often the bladder feels like a small walnut in the suprapubic area. Usually the urinary stream is poor. Older boys whose obstruction is less severe may have daytime incontinence as the only symptom.

15. In a boy who is found to have posterior urethral valves, what is the appropriate initial management?
Initially the bladder should be drained with a urethral catheter, ideally a 5F or 8F pediatric feeding tube. A Foley balloon catheter should not be used, because it may not drain satisfactorily, as the balloon has a tendency to occlude the ureteral orifices or cause bladder spasm, which can result in secondary distal ureteral obstruction. Broad-spectrum antibiotics are given intravenously to minimize the chance of nosocomial bacterial urinary tract infection. The serum creatinine is measured, and electrolyte abnormalities, including acidosis and hyperkalemia, need to be managed before surgical treatment of the lesion is undertaken. The kidneys should be assessed at a minimum with a renal ultrasound.

16. What is the treatment of posterior urethral valves?
The simplest treatment is transurethral valve ablation. If the urethra is sufficient in size then the 10.5F pediatric resectoscope may be used for valve ablation under direct vision. The procedure is performed by incising the valves at the 5 and 7 o'clock positions. Some resect the valves at the 12 o'clock position also. If the urethra is too small to accommodate the pediatric resectoscope, an alternative is to visualize the valves with an 8F cystoscope and ablate the posterior urethral valves under direct vision with a Bugbee electrode passed adjacent to the cystoscope.
    If the urethra is too small to accommodate the small cystoscope and Bugbee electrode, then a small insulated crochet hook ("Whitaker hook") may be used. The technique is to pass the hook

into the urethra and engage the valve leaflets at the 5 and 7 o'clock positions. The entire instrument, except for the crotch of the hook, is insulated, protecting the urethra from thermal injury. This procedure can be performed while the neonate is awake in the fluoroscopy suite or under anesthesia. This technique is applicable primarily in babies born prematurely or who are small for gestational age, in whom the larger resectoscope is too big for the urethra. Other techniques for valve ablation include a valve rupture using a small Fogarty catheter. In addition, antegrade valve ablation may be performed through a suprapubic cystostomy tract or through a cutaneous vesicostomy.

If the serum creatinine remains significantly elevated despite catheter drainage, then temporary cutaneous vesicostomy is recommended. In this procedure the dome of the bladder is brought to a point midway between the umbilicus and pubic symphysis to allow continuous urinary drainage. An alternative is bilateral cutaneous pyelostomies, in which the renal pelvis is exteriorized. This technique provides excellent upper tract drainage. An advantage to this approach is that it allows the surgeon to biopsy the kidneys.

17. Describe the most common complications of valve ablation.
The most common complication of valve ablation through a cystoscope is urethral stricture, which results if the resectoscope or cystoscope is too large for the urethra. Another complication is incomplete valve resection. One might think that injury to the external urinary sphincter also is common, but actually it is quite rare.

18. What are favorable prognostic factors following treatment for posterior urethral valves?
Favorable prognostic factors include the serum creatinine falling below 1.0 mg/dl one month following treatment, absence of vesicoureteral reflux on the VCUG, preservation of the corticomedullary junction of the kidneys by ultrasonography, or evidence of radiographic "pop-off valve."

19. What is a "pop-off valve"? What are the three types that can occur in boys with urethral valves?
The term "pop-off valve" refers to a mechanism in which the high intravesical or intrapelvic pressure is dissipated, allowing for normal development of one or both kidneys. Examples include: (1) urinary ascites, in which urine leaks from the fornices of the kidneys or from a bladder rupture; (2) "VURD" syndrome, a syndrome in which there is massive unilateral reflux into a nonfunctioning kidney; and (3) the presence of a large bladder diverticulum, causing aberrant micturition into the diverticulum, taking pressure off the developing kidneys.

20. How is urinary ascites treated?
In patients with urinary ascites secondary to posterior urethral valves, the leakage may be coming from one or both kidneys. At times, however, it may be secondary to a ruptured bladder. In most cases a temporary cutaneous vesicostomy is necessary to allow decompression. In some neonates, paracentesis (removal of the ascitic fluid) must be done, and occasionally renal exploration and high urinary diversion must be performed.

21. What proportion of patients with posterior urethral valves have a protective radiographic feature ("pop-off valve")?
Approximately 25–30%.

22. What is VURD syndrome?
Approximately 15% of patients have this condition, in which there is massive reflux into a dysplastic nonfunctioning kidney. VURD stands for vesicoureteral reflux associated with renal dysplasia. The term applies only to children with posterior urethral valves.

23. List the adverse prognostic factors in children with posterior urethral valves.
- Presentation under 1 year of age
- Failure of the serum creatinine to be below 1.0 mg/dl 1 month following initial therapy
- Bilateral vesicoureteral reflux
- Diurnal incontinence beyond 5 years of age

24. What is the overall prognosis for boys with urethral valves?
Approximately 30% have poor renal function, 10% die of renal failure, 15% have end-stage renal disease, and 5% have chronic renal failure that probably will require dialysis.

25. In a neonate with severe posterior urethral valves, what is the likely cause of death?
Pulmonary hypoplasia. Lung development is dependent on a normal volume of amniotic fluid. In the first trimester, amniotic fluid is a transudate from the placenta. During the second and third trimesters, however, the amniotic fluid comes from urine voided by the fetus. In the presence of severe obstructive uropathy, urine output is significantly reduced and pulmonary development is significantly impaired, resulting in pulmonary hypoplasia, i.e., underdeveloped lungs.

26. Does prenatal decompression of the urinary tract improve survival in a fetus with posterior urethral valves?
To date there have only been a few reports of survival following in utero bladder decompression for posterior urethral valves. Usually the procedure is performed by inserting a small shunt between the bladder and amniotic space, bypassing the urethral obstruction. The procedure is performed by the perinatologist (obstetrician) using ultrasound monitoring. A few centers have performed cutaneous vesicostomy in utero.

   One of the main problems with performing a vesicoamniotic shunt is making the correct diagnosis of obstructive uropathy in utero, as prune belly syndrome and high-grade vesicoureteral reflux have an appearance similar to that urethral valves on prenatal ultrasonography. The technique is indicated primarily to prevent pulmonary hypoplasia. If there is normal amniotic fluid, then the baby is not at significant risk for respiratory complications. Consequently, therapy is directed primarily at those with oligohydramnios. If oligohydramnios is detected around 20 weeks' gestation, nearly always there is irreversible renal dysplasia, so that even if a technically successful vesicoamniotic shunt is inserted, renal development usually is not improved.

27. What is the "full-valve bladder" syndrome?
In boys born with posterior urethral valves, bladder development is abnormal because of the severe congenital bladder outlet obstruction. In addition, often there is a urinary concentrating defect that results in high urine output. Possible defects in bladder function include (1) reduced bladder compliance, meaning that as the bladder fills with urine, the intravesical pressure increases quickly, and this elevated pressure is transmitted to the kidneys, resulting in continued deterioration in renal function; (2) uninhibited bladder contractions, often associated with a nonrelaxing external sphincter (detrusor-sphincter dyssynergia); (3) persistent secondary bladder neck hypertrophy, causing impaired bladder drainage; and (4) myogenic failure with absent bladder contractions. The full-valve bladder syndrome refers to the persistent filling of the bladder secondary to one of these factors, resulting in transmission of elevated intravesical pressures to the kidneys and thereby causing reduction in renal function.

28. At what intravesical pressure is there impaired upper urinary tract drainage?
35 cm of water pressure.

29. What is the treatment for patients with the full-valve bladder syndrome?
Treatment often includes double-voiding, clean intermittent catheterization to allow more effective emptying of the bladder, and anticholinergic medication.

30. In boys with posterior urethral valves, does ureterovesical junction occur?

Some boys with posterior urethral valves develop secondary ureterovesical obstruction, in which there is impaired ureteral drainage into the bladder during bladder filling because the intravesical pressure is higher than in the ureter, but when the bladder is empty, there is normal drainage of urine.

31. When is bladder augmentation recommended in children with posterior urethral valves?

Augmentation cystoplasty may be necessary if there is a noncompliant bladder, severe detrusor-sphincter dyssynergia, or uninhibited bladder contractions that do not respond to medical therapy.

32. What is the source of tissue for augmentation cystoplasty in boys with valves?

Stomach tissue often is recommended for augmentation cystoplasty in boys with posterior urethral valves because it can reduce the acidosis that results from the valve condition, allowing excretion of the hydrogen ion into the urine. The potential complications with use of stomach can be formidable, however. Another option is ureterocystoplasty, in which a dilated ureter associated with a nonfunctioning kidney is used to enlarge the bladder rather than simply performing a total ureterectomy. Finally, the ileum or large bowel often is used.

33. In boys with posterior urethral valves undergoing renal transplantation, what is the prognosis compared to that of a child with glomerulonephritis?

The graft survival rates are identical, but the serum creatinine level at 5 years is significantly higher in the group with posterior ureteral valves, probably because of the associated noncompliant or unstable bladder.

34. What is an anterior urethral valve?

An anterior urethral valve is not a true valve. Rather, it is a wide-mouth anterior urethral diverticulum, with the distal lip of the diverticulum filling during voiding, compressing the distal urethra.

35. What is the location of anterior urethral valves?

All occur in the bulbous or pendulous urethra.

36. What are the physical findings of an anterior urethral valve?

A cystic mass on the ventral aspect of the penoscrotal junction increases in size during voiding. Prolonged urinary strain often is noted. Compression of the cystic mass may result in urinary dribbling.

37. How is the diagnosis of anterior urethral valves made?

The diagnosis is based on physical findings and voiding cystourethrogram. These patients also should undergo a renal ultrasound and serum creatinine. If there is renal insufficiency, a renal scan should be obtained.

38. How are anterior urethral valves treated?

The treatment is based on the size of the diverticulum and renal function. If the diverticulum is small, the cusp may be ablated by transurethral resection. However, in the majority of neonates with this condition, open surgical resection of the diverticulum and valve cusp is necessary. A small Silastic urethral stent should be left in the bladder postoperatively for 10–14 days.

If renal function is significantly impaired, temporary catheter drainage of the bladder may be necessary to stabilize the infant and correct electrolyte abnormalities. If the serum creatinine fails to decrease to a satisfactory level, resection of the diverticulum and perinatal urethrostomy will provide reliable drainage. Alternatively, cutaneous vesicostomy should be considered.

BIBLIOGRAPHY

1. Diamond DA, Ransley PG: Fogarty balloon catheter ablation of neonatal posterior urethral valves. J Urol 137:1209, 1987.
2. Elder JS, Duckett JW: Perinatal Urology. In Gillenwater JY, Grayhack JT, Howards SS, Duckett JW (eds): Adult and Pediatric Urology, 2nd ed. St. Louis, Mosby, 1991 p 1711.
3. Elder JS, Duckett JW, Snyder HM: Intervention for fetal obstructive uropathy: Has it been effective? Lancet 2:1007, 1987.
4. Firlit CG, King LR: Anterior urethral valves in children. J Urol 108:972, 1972.
5. Gonzales ET, Jr.: Posterior urethral valves and other urethral anomalies. In Walsh PC, Retick AB, Stamey TA, Vaughan ED Jr (eds): Campbell's Urology, 6th ed. Philadelphia, W. B. Saunders, 1992, p 1872.
6. Hulbert WC, Duckett JW: Prognostic factors in infants with posterior urethral valves. J Urol 135:121A, 1986.
7. Krueger RP, Hardy BD, Churchill BM: Growth in boys with posterior urethral valves. Primary valve resection vs upper tract diversion. Urol Clin North Am 7:265, 1980.
8. Nakayama DK, Harrison MR, de Lorimier AA: Prognosis of posterior urethral valves presenting at birth. J Pediatr Surg 21:43, 1986.
9. Parkhouse HF, Barratt TM, Dillon MJ, et al: Long-term outcome of boys with posterior urethral valves. Br J Urol 62:59, 1988.
10. Rittenberg MH, Hulbert WC, Snyder HM, et al: Protective factors in posterior urethral valves. J Urol 140:993, 1988.
11. Rushton HG, Parrott TS, Woodard JR, et al: The role of vesicostomy in the management of anterior urethral valves in neonates and infants. J Urol 138:107, 1987.
12. Whitaker TH: Sherwood T: An improved hook for destroying posterior urethral valves. J Urol 135:531, 1986.
13. Zaontz MR, Firlit CF: Percutaneous antegrade ablation of posterior urethral valves in infants with small-caliber urethras: An alternative to urinary diversion. J Urol 136:247, 1986.
14. Zaontz MR, Gibbons MD: An antegrade technique for ablation of posterior urethral valves. J Urol 132:982, 1984.

47. URETHRAL DIVERTICULUM IN FEMALES

Rodney A. Appell, M.D.

1. What is the reported incidence of female urethral diverticula?
The literature reports a 1%–6% incidence, but this may be a significant underestimate.

2. Is the treatment of a urethral diverticulum a simple problem?
The treatment for urethral diverticula requires surgery, and the complication rate approaches 20%, which should be adequate to remove the word *simple* from the description of the diagnosis and management of a urethral diverticulum.

3. What are the causes of urethral diverticula?
  1. Congenital
  2. Acquired
       Surgery/trauma
       Infection
If histologic sections contain smooth muscle, a congenital origin is inferred. However, most female diverticula are acquired.

4. Where are diverticula located? How do they form?
The diverticula always occur on the vaginal aspect of the urethra (anterior vaginal wall) on the distal two-thirds of the urethra where the periurethral glands are known to open. Infection and obstruction of the periurethral glands result in the formation of retention cysts, which rupture into the lumen and give rise to a diverticulum. These retention cysts progressively enlarge and entrap droplets of urine during voiding, and due to the lack of muscle in the diverticular sac, the contents remain stagnant and inflammation occurs. The most common offending organisms are gonococci, *Escherichia coli,* and *Chlamydia.*

5. What are the symptoms of a urethral diverticulum?
Symptoms may vary from mild occasional discomfort to severe pain and frank urinary retention during acute infections. Most patients, however, present with nonspecific irritative symptoms of the lower urinary tract similar to those of cystitis.

Clinical Symptoms and Signs of Urethral Diverticula

Symptoms
  Classic 3 D triad (dribbling, dysuria, dyspareunia)
  Urinary urgency
  Hematuria
  Recurrent urinary tract infection
  Urinary incontinence
  Urinary retention
Signs
  None
  Suburethral mass
  Palpable stone
  Expression of purulent material

6. Is a diverticulum always solitary?
No. Diverticula may be small or large, single or multiple, or multiloculated.

7. Are any disease processes associated with diverticulum formation?
The stasis of urine and infection within the diverticulum provides an ideal condition for stone formation in some patients. In addition, urethral carcinoma may be discovered within the diverticulum.

8. What are the 3 D's?
It has been claimed that the classic symptom triad of **dribbling, dysuria,** and **dyspareunia** is always found in females with urethral diverticula. However, this triad occurs in a very small number of patients.

9. What signs are found on physical examination?
The classic physical finding is a **palpable suburethral mass** on vaginal examination, occasionally with expression of purulent material from the urethra when the mass is compressed. Often, however, no signs may be present and the diverticulum may go unrecognized on physical examination.

10. How does one make the diagnosis?
Physician awareness and an index of suspicion for the possibility of a urethral diverticulum are essential factors in making the diagnosis. Always consider the possibility of a urethral diverticulum in a female with persistent lower urinary tract symptoms resembling cystitis or with recurrent urinary tract infection. If the diagnosis is suspected, then voiding cystourethrography and/or positive-pressure urethrography should be performed.

Voiding cystourethrography depends on the filling of the diverticulum with contrast material when the patient is voiding. Filling the urethra with contrast while a balloon blocks the external urethral meatus and another at the bladder neck is called **positive-pressure retrograde urethrography** (see figure below). Obviously, a special catheter is needed for this examination, but this is the most definitive way in which to make the diagnosis. Methylene blue or indigo carmine can be added to the contrast so that following the x-ray study, **urethroscopy** may be performed and the blue dye will be seen in the opening of the diverticulum.

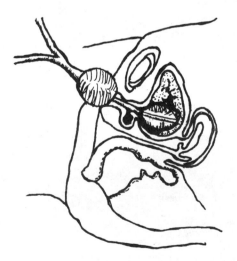

Positive-pressure uretherography allows filling of the diverticulum.

11. How are urethral diverticula treated?
There is no one operative procedure to correct all cases of urethral diverticula. If the diverticulum is very close to the external urethral meatus, it may be incised through the urethra and vagina in a

marsupialization technique (Spence procedure). On rare occasions, they may be managed **endoscopically** through a urethroscope using electrocautery to open the meatus of the diverticulum, which will allow it to drain better.

The classic approach is a **complete urethral diverticulectomy.** There are several approaches, but the essential idea is to expose and mobilize the diverticulum through an incision in the vagina and then excise the complete diverticulum. The small opening in the urethra is closed with fine suture material. This is the procedure of choice because of the possibility of finding carcinoma within the wall of the diverticulum.

BIBLIOGRAPHY

1. Appell RA: Experience with a laterally based vaginal flap approach for urethral diverticulum. J Urol 127:677–678, 1982.
2. Appell RA: Urethral diverticulum and fistula. In Glenn JF (ed): Urological Surgery, 4th ed. Philadelphia, J. B. Lippincott, 1991, p 762.
3. Drutz HP: Urethral diverticula. Obstet Gynecol Clin North Am 16:923–929, 1989.
4. Leech GE, Bavendam TG: Female urethral diverticula. Urology 40:407–415, 1987.
5. Leech GE, Sirls LT, Ganabathi K, Zimmern PE: LNSC3: A proposed classification system for female urethral diverticula. Neurourol Urodyn 12:523–531, 1993.
6. Spence HM, Duckett JW: Diverticulum of the female urethra: Clinical aspects and presentation of a single operative technique for care. J Urol 104:432–437, 1970.
7. Spencer WF, Streem SB: Diverticulum of the female urethral roof managed endoscopically. J Urol 138:147–148, 1987.

48. HYPOSPADIAS

Robert Kay, M.D.

1. What is hypospadias?
Hypospadias refers to any condition in which the meatus, or opening of the urethra, occurs on the undersurface of the penis, rather than the tip. When it occurs on the dorsal side of the penis, it is referred to as epispadias.

2. Is hypospadias an inherited disorder?
There is a genetic factor involved in some cases, although most patients do not give a family history. In one series by Bauer, the father of the affected child had hypospadias in 7% of the cases. The brother was affected in 14% of cases of this series. If a child is born with hypospadias, the risk of the next child having hypospadias is 12% if there is no family history. This increases to 19% if another family member, such as a cousin or uncle, has hypospadias, and to 26% if the father and a sibling have hypospadias.

3. Do all children with hypospadias have a hooded foreskin?
Because of the embryologic development of the penis and urethra and the closure of lateral to medial tissues, the foreskin almost always fails to be complete in boys with hypospadias. Rarely, a variant of hypospadias with a large meatus, the megameatal hypospadias, does have an intact foreskin and usually is detected at the time of circumcision.

4. What is the more common site for hypospadias, in the penoscrotal junction or the distal portion of the penis?
The most common form of hypospadias is distal hypospadias. This is the most mild form of the disease and occurs in the subcoronal or glandular area in approximately 80–85% of all cases. Ten to fifteen percent of cases occur in the penile shaft, with only 5–10% occurring in the severe location of the penoscrotal or perineal location.

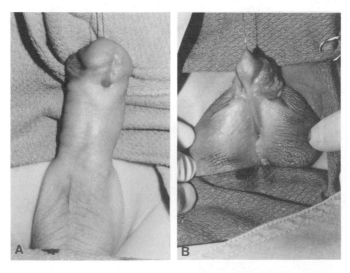

A, Distal hypospadias. **B,** Severe proximal hypospadias in the midscrotal area.

5. Do all children with a hooded foreskin have hypospadias?
No. Some children are born with a normal meatus, yet have a hooded foreskin. The penis should be carefully examined to exclude other penile abnormalities, such as chordee or atretic urethra. Hooded foreskin may also be seen in otherwise normal states and carries no significance other than a cosmetic factor.

6. How often does hypospadias occur?
The incidence of hypospadias ranges from 5.2–8.2/1,000 male births or approximately 1/200 male births.

7. Do boys with hypospadias need urologic evaluation to detect other anomalies?
Only boys with severe hypospadias and sexual ambiguity, which includes testicular abnormalities (e.g., undescended testis), need to be evaluated. Up to 25% of these patients have enlarged utricles or other female structures.

Routine evaluation of other forms of hypospadias is not needed since the incidence of abnormalities approximates the incidence in the general population.

8. What is the optimal age for hypospadias repair?
Emotional issues for both the child and family must be considered when determining the best age for surgical repair. When the factors of genital awareness, separation anxiety, ease of postoperative management, and technical aspects are considered, the ideal age is between 6 and 15 months.

9. How does one repair a severe hypospadias on a small penis?
Testosterone can be used in selective cases to induce growth of the penis. In complex cases, such as a small penis when early repair is desired, parenteral testosterone may be used preoperatively. Also, optical magnification is critical in the surgical repair of these cases.

10. Does the child need to be hospitalized for hypospadias repair?
The overwhelming majority of cases can be done on an outpatient basis. The medical advantage is the avoidance of communicable diseases, such as viral infections which are prevalent in the hospital. Cost savings are also dramatic as an outpatient. However, some of the major advantages are the emotional aspects of the surgery to both the child and family. The child prefers his own environment, the parents' lives are less disrupted, and other siblings are relieved. Postoperative care has become significantly easier with outpatient hypospadias surgery.

11. What is a hypospadias cripple?
A hypospadias cripple is an older term used for the male child or adult who has had numerous operations in attempts to repair the hypospadias defect. Once very common, this problem has been significantly reduced with technical advances and the better understanding of hypospadias.

12. If hypospadias repair has been done several times with no success, what else can be done?
The failed hypospadias repair is a surgical challenge complicated by the presence of severe scar tissue and the lack of skin. Often, skin must be imported to construct the urethra. Although free skin grafts have been used in the past, other tissues such as buccal mucosa are preferred today. These give better results in both the short and long term.

13. List the most important factors for technical success of hypospadias surgery.
1. Use of vascularized tissues
2. Careful tissue handling
3. Tension-free anastomosis
4. Nonoverlapping suture lines
5. Meticulous hemostasis
6. Fine suture material
7. Adequate urinary diversion

14. What complications occur from hypospadias surgery?

Ranging from perfect cosmetics to total dehiscence, a spectrum of complications may. These include fistula formation, urethra strictures, meatal stenosis, urethral diverticulum, excess skin, persistent chordee, and persistent hypospadias.

15. Is urinary diversion required during hypospadias repair?

In most cases, urinary diversion is a preferred tool of management. This allows tissue healing and minimizes the risk of urethra cutaneous fistulas. Although some have advocated no diversions for distal repairs, urinary diversion offers advantages and, theoretically, fewer complications, particularly in complex repairs.

The use of an indwelling urethral stent has replaced a suprapubic cystotomy tube, even in severe cases. Although there may be a limited role for suprapubic diversion, urethral diversion is effective, serves as a stent, has less bladder spasms, and is easier to manage than suprapubic tubes.

16. What is the best operation for hypospadias?

There is no single best operation for hypospadias repair. Over 150 operations have been described. Today, the most common operations are the MAGPI meatal-based flaps and vascularized inner preputial transfer flaps. Free grafts with buccal mucosa are also used in select patients.

BIBLIOGRAPHY

1. Bauer SB, Retick AB, Colodny AH: Genetic aspects of hypospadias. Urol Clin North Am 8:559, 1981.
2. Belman AB: Hypospadias and other urethral abnormalities. In Kelalis PP, King LR, Belman AB (eds): Clinical Pediatric Urology, 3rd ed. Philadelphia, W. B. Saunders, 1992.
3. Belman AB, Kass EJ: Hypospadias repair in children under one year of age. J Urol 128:1273, 1982.
4. Duckett JW: MAGPI (meatoplasty and glanuloplasty): A procedure for subcoronal hypospadias. Urol Clin North Am 8:515, 1981.
5. Duckett JW: The island flap technique for hypospadias repair. Urol Clin North Am 8:503, 1981.
6. Hatch DA, Maizels M, Zaontz MR, et al: Hypospadias hidden by a complete prepuce. Surg Gynecol Obstet 169:233, 1989.
7. Kass EJ, Boling D: Single stage hypospadias reconstruction without fistula. J Urol 144:520, 1990.
8. Manley CB, Epstein ES: Early hypospadias repair. J Urol 125:698, 1981.
9. Rabinowitz R: Outpatient catheterless modified Mattieu hypospadias repair. J Urol 138:1074, 1987.
10. Retik AB, Keating M, Mandell J: Complications of hypospadias repair. Urol Clin North Am 15:223, 1988.
11. Sweet RA, Schrott HG, Kurland R, et al: Study of the incidence of hypospadias in Rochester, Minnesota, 1940–1970, and a case-controlled comparison of possible etiologic factors. Mayo Clin Proc 49:52, 1974.

49. Epispadias

Jonathan H. Ross, M.D.

1. What is epispadias?

Epispadias is a penile anomaly in which the urethra opens on the dorsal aspect of the penis. The penis is generally foreshortened due to separation of the pubic symphysis. Dorsal curvature of the penis and an incomplete foreskin dorsally are also characteristic. The glans generally has a flattened spade-like appearance, and the corporal bodies do not communicate.

2. What is "female epispadias"?

Females with epispadias have a bifid clitoris, patulous urethra, and unformed bladder neck. In addition to genitoplasty, they require bladder neck reconstruction in the same manner as girls with the complete exstrophy–epispadias complex.

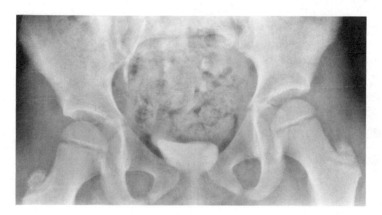

Bladder film of an intravenous urogram in a 6-year-old girl with epispadias demonstrates the typical findings of a small bladder, open bladder neck, and separation of the pubic symphysis.

3. Is epispadias closely related to hypospadias embryologically?

No. It is a form of the exstrophy–epispadias complex (*see* chapter 44). When caudal migration of the cloacal membrane fails, bladder exstrophy (which is always associated with epispadias) results. When partial migration occurs, then epispadias alone occurs. In fact, most patients with epispadias also have bladder exstrophy. The incidence of epispadias alone is approximately 1/100,000 male births, and 1/500,000 female births.

4. What abnormality on KUB examination is universally present in patients with epispadias?

Separation of the pubic symphysis.

5. Are most patients with epispadias incontinent?

Yes. Nearly all females and approximately 70% of males with epispadias are incontinent. Most males have penopubic epispadias, but those with penile shaft or glanular epispadias are usually continent.

6. Describe the bladder abnormalities found in most epispadias patients.

A small bladder capacity and vesicoureteral reflux (the latter being present in 90% of patients).

7. What are the three principles of epispadias repair?

- Penile lengthening
- Correction of chordee
- Urethroplasty

BIBLIOGRAPHY

1. Arap S, Nahas WC, Giron AM, et al: Incontinent epispadias: Surgical treatment of 38 cases. J Urol 140:577–581, 1988.
2. Borzi PA, Thomas DFM: Cantwell-Ransley epispadias repair in male epispadias and bladder exstrophy. J Urol 151:457–459, 1994.
3. Caldamone AA: Anomalies of the bladder and cloaca. In Gillenwater JY, Grayhack JT, Howards SS, Duckett JW (eds). Adult and Pediatric Urology, 2nd ed. St. Louis, Mosby, 1991, pp 2043–2053.
4. Gearhart JP, Peppas DS, Jeffs RD: Complete genitourinary reconstruction in female epispadias. J Urol 149:1110–1113, 1993.
5. Kramer SA, Kelalis PP: Assessment of urinary continence in epispadias: Review of 94 patients. J Urol 128:290–293, 1982.
5. Kramer SA, Mesrobian HGJ, Kelalis PP: Long-term followup of cosmetic appearance and genital function in male epispadias: Review of 70 patients. J Urol 135:543–547, 1986.
7. Lemmers MJ, Tank ES: Epispadias. In Resnick MI, Kursh ED (eds): Current Therapy in Genitourinary Surgery. St. Louis, Mosby, 1992, pp 322–325.
8. Peters CA, Gearhart JP, Jeffs RD: Epispadias and incontinence: The challenge of the small bladder. J Urol 140:1199–1201, 1988.

50. INTERLABIAL MASSES

Jack S. Elder, M.D.

1. What is the differential diagnosis of interlabial masses in young girls?

Urethral prolapse

Paraurethral cysts

Prolapsed ectopic ureterocele

Sarcoma botryoides

Imperforate hymen

Uterovaginal prolapse

2. What is urethral prolapse?

This condition refers to eversion of the urethral mucosa. It has the appearance of erythematous, inflamed mucosa protruding from and surrounding the urethral meatus. One theory of its pathogenesis is that urethral prolapse results from poor attachment between the smooth muscle layers of the urethra in association with episodic increases in intraabdominal pressure.

3. What is the typical presentation of a girl with urethral prolapse?

The disorder occurs predominantly in black girls between 1 and 9 years of age, with an average age of 4 years. The most common signs are bloody spotting on the underwear or diaper, dysuria, and perineal discomfort. Sexual abuse is suspected in many cases of urethral prolapse before the correct diagnosis is made.

4. What is the treatment of urethral prolapse?

Initial management includes topical application of estrogen cream 2 or 3 times daily to the prolapsed urethra for 1–2 weeks as well as sitz baths. If intermittent bleeding persists, however, formal surgical excision is necessary. In general, surgical excision is recommended if the child is under anesthesia for examination because of suspected sexual abuse.

5. What is a paraurethral cyst?

Paraurethral cyst results from retained secretion in Skene's glands, secondary to ductal obstruction. Typically the cyst displaces the meatus in an eccentric manner.

6. How is a paraurethral cyst treated?

Most paraurethral cysts regress is size during the first 4–8 weeks of life, although occasionally it is necessary to remove them.

7. What is a prolapsed ectopic ureterocele?

A ureterocele is a cystic dilatation of the distal ureter within the wall of the bladder. In girls it almost always drains the upper pole of a completely duplicated urinary tract and usually is ectopic, that is, it extends beyond the bladder neck. In approximately 10% of girls with a ureterocele, the lesion may prolapse and appear as a cystic mass arising from the urethra. It may be erythematous or, if ischemic, purplish or even black.

8. What is the typical age of girls with an ectopic ureterocele? Are there other presenting symptoms or signs?

The typical age at presentation is 1 month to 3 years. Most girls with a ureterocele have a history of febrile urinary tract infection, unless the lesion was diagnosed by prenatal ultrasonography. Occasionally the prolapsed ureterocele can cause bladder outlet obstruction.

9. How does the prolapsed ectopic ureterocele differ on examination from a paraurethral cyst?

A prolapsed ectopic ureterocele appears to arise from the urethra. It may be pale, erythematous, and purplish or even black, whereas the paraurethral cyst seems to arise from the wall of the urethra and usually is pale.

10. How is a ureterocele diagnosed?
The initial study in diagnosing a ureterocele is ultrasonography of the kidneys and bladder. Typically a full bladder demonstrates the ureterocele in the bladder base. More than 90% of girls with a ureterocele have a complete duplication of the urinary tract, with the ureterocele draining the upper pole. A voiding cystourethrogram usually shows a filling defect in the base of the bladder. A intravenous urogram or renal scan usually shows a duplication anomaly on the affected side with nonfunction or diminished function in the hydronephrotic upper pole.

11. What is sarcoma botryoides?
This term refers to rhabdomyosarcoma of the vagina.

12. What is the appearance of this lesion? How is it diagnosed?
This lesion has the appearance of a firm grape-like mass protruding from the introitus, and often results in vaginal bleeding and sloughed tissue fragments from the vagina. The diagnosis is usually established by biopsy.

13. What is imperforate hymen?
Imperforate hymen refers to stenosis of the hymen, resulting in retained vaginal secretions that originate from stimulation by maternal estrogens.

14. How does imperforate hymen present?
It presents as a white bulging interlabial mass in the newborn.

15. How is an imperforate hymen treated?
Imperforate hymen is managed by hymenotomy, in which the hymen is incised, allowing release of retained vaginal secretions. Usually signs of upper urinary tract obstruction resolve following decompression of the hydrocolpos.

16. Which type of patient is most likely to develop uterovaginal prolapse?
This condition usually occurs in the newborn and is most common in those with myelodysplasia. It was thought that this anomaly results from partial or complete denervation of the levator ani, which supports the uterus and vagina.

BIBLIOGRAPHY

1. Caldamone AA, Snyder HMcC III, Duckett JW: Ureteroceles in children: Followup of management with upper tract approach. J Urol 131:1130, 1984.
2. Carpenter SE and Rock JA: Procidentia in the newborn. Int J Obstet Gynecol 25:151, 1987.
3. Elder JS: Congenital anomalies of the genitalia. In Walsh PC, Retik AB, Stamey TA, Vaughan ED Jr (eds): Campbell's Urology, 6th ed. Philadelphia, W. B. Saunders, 1992, p 1920.
4. Elder JS: Interlabial masses. In Reece RM (ed): Manual of Emergency Pediatrics, 4th ed. Philadelphia, W. B. Saunders, 1992, p 448.
5. Klein FA, Vick CW III, Broecker BH: Neonatal vaginal cysts: Diagnosis and management. J Urol 135:371, 1986.
6. Lowe FC, Hill GS, Jeffs RD, Brendler CP: Urethral prolapse in children: Insights into etiology and management. J Urol 135:100, 1986.
7. McHenry CR, Reynolds M, Raffensperger JG: Vaginal neoplasms in infancy: The combined role of chemotherapy and conservative surgical resection. J Pediatr Surg 23:842, 1988.
8. Nussbaum AR, Bebowitz RL: Interlabial masses in little girls: Review and imaging considerations. Am J Radiol 141:65, 1983.
9. Richardson DA, Hajj SM, Herbst AJ: Medical treatment of urethral prolapse in children. Obstet Gynecol 59:69, 1982.
10. Rock JA, Azziz R: Genital anomalies in childhood. Clin Obstet Gynecol 30:62, 1987.
11. Wilson DA, Stacy TM, Smith EI: Ultrasound diagnosis of hydrocolpos and hydrometrocolpos. Radiology 128:451, 1978.

51. END-STAGE RENAL DISEASE

Ernest E. Hodge, M.D.

1. What are the causes of end-stage renal disease?

Diabetes has become the most common cause of end-stage renal disease overall, although glomerulonephritis ranks as the number 1 cause in children. The various etiologies and frequency for patients presenting for treatment for end-stage renal disease between 1987 and 1990 are listed in the following table:

Cause and Frequency of End-stage Renal Disease

ADULT		PEDIATRIC	
Diabetes	34.2%	Glomerulonephritis	37.6%
Hypertension	29.4%	Congenital/other hereditary diseases	19.1%
Glomerulonephritis	14.2%	Collagen vascular diseases	9.9%
Cystic kidney diseases	3.4%	Obstructive nephropathy	6 %
Interstitial nephritis	3.4%	Cystic kidney diseases	4.3%
Obstructive nephropathy	2.3%	Interstitial nephritis	4.2%
Collagen vascular diseases	2.2%	Hypertension	4.2%
Malignancies	1.3%	Diabetes	1.4%
		Malignancies	0.4%

2. What is the incidence and prevalence of end-stage renal disease?

The incidence of end-stage renal disease is 180–200 new cases per million population, with 45,153 patients starting therapy during the year 1990. Currently, in excess of 200,000 patients require treatment for end-stage renal disease.

3. Is the incidence of end-stage renal disease uniform for all ages?

No. There is an age-dependent increase in the incidence of end-stage renal disease ranging from 12 cases per million population for the pediatric age group (ages 0–19 years) to 680 cases per million population for patients age 65–74 years.

4. How much does the treatment of end-stage renal disease cost? Who pays?

The cost of treating end-stage renal disease in the United States in 1990 was 7.26 billion dollars and continues to increase significantly each year. In 1973, the End-Stage Renal Disease Medicare Act was passed, and 70–80% of the costs are paid for by the Federal Government (5.22 billion dollars in 1990). The remainder is paid for by patients and insurance, including the state-funded Medicaid programs.

5. Does end-stage renal disease affect life expectancy?

Although the treatment discussed later in this chapter has improved the life expectancy of patients with end-stage renal disease, it is still significantly worse (70–80%) than that of the general population. For the United States population as a whole, life expectancy is 29.8 years for individuals 49 years of age and 21.6 years for those 59 years of age, while it is 7.0 and 4.5 years, respectively, for patients with end-stage renal disease. Approximately 22% of patients die in the first year after developing end-stage renal disease.

6. What is the major cause of mortality in patients with end-stage renal disease?

The primary cause of death in patients with end-stage renal disease is cardiovascular, with infectious complications (sepsis) being the second most common.

7. How do patients with end-stage renal disease present?
Patients developing end-stage renal disease often present with vague symptoms, including general fatigue, anorexia, nausea and vomiting. Itching accompanies more advanced degrees of uremia. Often there are signs of fluid overload, and patients may present with congestive heart failure or pulmonary edema.

8. What degree of renal impairment is usually required before symptoms develop?
Unfortunately, progressive renal insufficiency usually follows an insidious course, and most patients have lost greater than 90% of renal function before significant symptoms ensue.

9. Is it possible to "screen" patients for the development of end-stage renal disease?
Screening for the development of end-stage renal disease is difficult, save for the obvious cases of familial disorders (cystic diseases of the kidney) or known systemic diseases (diabetes) which lead to renal failure. However, a urinalysis performed as part of a routine physical exam can be important, as proteinuria or microscopic hematuria should arouse concern about potential intrinsic renal disease.

10. Which electrolyte disturbances are associated with end-stage renal disease?
Hyperkalemia is the most common and the most dangerous electrolyte imbalance seen in patients with end-stage renal disease. Patients also have varying degrees of metabolic acidosis with decreased serum bicarbonate levels.

11. What clinical findings are noted in patients with end-stage renal disease?
Anemia, often quite severe, is usually present and most likely accounts for symptoms such as fatigue, etc. Recently, the use of synthetic erythropoietin has markedly diminished problems associated with anemia. **Hypertension** occurs frequently and is more common (possibly related to hypervolemia) as renal failure progresses and the patient nears end-stage renal disease. **Peripheral neuropathy** accompanies more advanced stages of uremia, whereas uremic pericarditis is a less common but potentially life-threatening complication. **Renal osteodystrophy,** and in severe cases renal "rickets," result from altered calcium and phosphorus metabolism (secondary and tertiary hyperparathyroidism). Young children with end-stage renal disease exhibit a marked retardation in growth.

12. Are sexual and fertility problems associated with end-stage renal disease?
Yes. Many patients suffer a decreased libido. Women often become anovulatory and are thus unable to conceive. Men commonly have low sperm counts and also experience erectile dysfunction (impotence).

13. Can the development of end-stage renal disease be prevented?
Several measures have been employed that appear to slow or arrest the progression of renal failure, especially in high-risk patients such as diabetics. Aggressive control of high blood pressure is essential, and newer classes of medications, including angiotensin-converting enzyme (ACE) inhibitors and calcium channel blockers, have proved to be of benefit. A low-protein diet is instituted and strict adherence to other dietary restrictions, especially salt and water intake, is essential. Despite these interventions, the disease still progresses in most patients and they eventually require renal replacement therapy.

14. What modalities (replacement therapies) are used to treat end-stage renal disease? How often is each utilized?
The therapeutic options for patients with end-stage renal disease include hemodialysis, peritoneal dialysis, and transplantation. In 1990, 60% of patients with end-stage renal disease were on hemodialysis, 30% had a functioning transplanted kidney, and 10% were managed with peritoneal dialysis.

15. How are hemodialysis and peritoneal dialysis achieved?
Hemodialysis requires placement of a vascular access, which is usually achieved by construction of an arteriovenous fistula or graft. Blood is then removed from the arterial tree and filtered through an artificial membrane and returned to the venous circulation. Peritoneal dialysis is accomplished by placement of an intraperitoneal catheter, which is then tunneled through the subcutaneous tissue and externalized from the skin. Dialysate solution is then instilled into the peritoneum and allowed to "dwell" for varying periods of time. This allows for transport of solute materials across gradients from the mesenteric circulation into the dialysate solution, which is then drained.

16. What are the complications of hemodialysis and peritoneal dialysis?
Complications related to hemodialysis are primarily those associated with thrombosis and infection of the vascular access. Depending on a patient's degree of compliance and adequacy of dialysis, other complications discussed above (hyperkalemia, fluid overload, etc.) may ensue or progress between dialysis sessions. Complications of peritoneal dialysis include infection and mechanical failure related to occlusion of the dialysis catheter, especially from the omentum. Previous studies have suggested that within the first year of peritoneal dialysis, 40% of patients experience a "tunnel" infection and 60% have at least one episode of peritonitis. Newer catheters appear to have decreased the incidence of infectious complications. Excellent detailed descriptions of the technology and complications of hemodialysis and peritoneal dialysis can be found in reference 2 of the bibliography.

17. If a patient requires emergency dialysis and does not have a vascular access or a peritoneal catheter, what are the options?
The most effective means of emergency dialysis are placement of a large-bore intravenous catheter in the jugular, subclavian, or femoral vein; venous blood is removed, filtered, and returned to the venous circulation.

18. What are the results with transplantation?
In January of 1994, more than 25,000 individuals were actively awaiting transplantation in the United States. In 1993, 10,912 patients underwent transplantation, with 2,744 receiving kidneys from live donors and 8,168 patients receiving kidneys from cadaveric donors. Current, 1- and 2-year patient and allograft (kidney) survival are demonstrated in the table below:

Patient and Allograft Survival Following Transplantation

	LIVE DONOR	CADAVERIC DONOR
Patient Survival		
One year	97.1%	93.0%
Two years	95.6%	90.0%
Allograft Survival		
One year	90.6%	78.9%
Two years	87.0%	72.8%

19. Is transplantation better than dialysis for patients with end-stage renal disease?
Most studies, even correcting for sex, age and etiology of renal failure, demonstrate improved survival in patients undergoing transplantation compared with those on dialysis. However, there have been valid criticisms related to the potential bias of healthier patients having been selected for transplantation. It is of note that patients with failed transplants who go back on dialysis appear to have worse survival than patients with successful transplants. Many of the complications of chronic renal failure (anemia, metabolic difficulties including bone disease, sexual/ fertility, neuropathy, etc.) discussed will be reversed following transplantation.

Also, most "quality of life" studies suggest that there is significant improvement with transplantation as opposed to dialysis. Most patients are rehabilitatable following transplantation and, in fact, Medicare reimbursement for nondiabetic persons undergoing successful transplantation covers only the first three years following surgery.

20. If so many patients are awaiting transplantation, why are so few transplants performed?

Despite vigorous efforts to educate the general public as well as the medical profession, there remains a tremendous shortage of donor organs for transplantation. The problem is of a greater magnitude for extrarenal (heart, liver, etc.) organs, as many patients die each year awaiting transplantation. Federal, and in many cases, state legislation has been enacted requiring hospitals and other health care providers to inform families of their right to donate, though this has had only minimal impact to date in the number of organ donors.

21. How soon after kidneys are removed do they need to be transplanted? How are they stored?

Most centers prefer to transplant kidneys with ischemic times (time that the kidney is removed from the circulation) of 24–36 hours. In the case of live donors transplants, the donor and the recipient surgery occur simultaneously, and the kidneys rarely have ischemic times of more than a couple of hours. While kidneys have been successfully transplanted with ischemic times of 48–60 hours or longer, the chances of nonfunction of the kidney increase beyond the 24–36 hour time frame.

One method of storing kidneys is **cold slush (static) storage.** The kidney is flushed (in many cases in situ prior to removing the kidney) with a cold intracellular-like solution that rapidly cools the kidney, decreases metabolic requirements, and washes out blood. The kidney is placed into a sterile plastic bag that contains a similar solution, although magnesium is omitted as it will form a precipitant on the kidney surface. The kidney is placed into an ice solution inside a sterile container. Newer preservation solutions, such as the University of Wisconsin's solution, have added high-energy substrates and have significantly improved early function after transplantation.

An alternative method for preservation is **pulsatile perfusion.** After the initial flushing of the kidney, it is placed in an incubator with a pulsatile pump that perfuses the kidney at 4°C with a denatured plasma (lipoproteins and clotting factors removed). Recently, solutions similar to the University of Wisconsin's cold storage solution have been developed for pulsatile perfusion. However, pulsatile perfusion is more expensive and logistically more cumbersome and thus largely has been abandoned as results with newer cold storage solutions have improved.

22. What determines who gets a transplant?

If a patient has a living, related donor who, after evaluation, has been determined to be compatible and medically suitable, then the patient may receive a kidney from that individual. However, in the absence of a suitable living, related donor, patients are placed on a waiting list for cadaveric kidneys. In an attempt to assure fairness, all patients awaiting cadaveric renal transplantation in the United States must be registered on a **national** waiting list that is managed by the United Network for Organ Sharing. With a few mandated exceptions for extremely good matches, kidneys are allocated on a geographic basis to individuals on the list by a point system that takes into consideration a number of factors, including degree of match between the donor and recipient, length of time waiting for a transplant, and so on.

23. Can patients with cancer receive a transplant?

Active malignancy is one of the few absolute contraindications to transplantation. Studies have shown that placing a patient with a malignancy on immunosuppressive medications can enhance progression of the cancer. However, many cancers such as squamous and basal cell of the skin carry much less risk. Patients who have had appropriate treatment of their malignancy and remain cancer free for various periods of time (usually 1–2 years) are candidates for transplantation.

24. What other screening or evaluation must potential transplant candidates undergo?

As new immunosuppressive medications have been introduced and results with transplantation have improved, patient selection has been significantly liberalized, thus allowing patients who would have been excluded in previous years to undergo transplantation. All potential recipients undergo a thorough evaluation, including a complete history, physical examination, and additional studies to investigate possible high-risk factors. Risk factors for transplantation include **age,** with optimal results in patients 15 to 50 years, although very young and older patients can be successfully transplanted. Also, **race** appears to be a significant factor, as African-Americans appear to have decreased survival rates, especially with cadaveric transplants. Patients with **systemic disease,** especially diabetes, have a higher morbidity and mortality following transplantation than their nondiabetic counterparts. Significant disease in other organ systems also adversely affects the results of transplantation, and patients who have evidence of coronary artery disease, peptic ulcer disease, etc. will require correction of these problems prior to transplantation. Patients with **abnormal lower urinary tracts** (e.g., neurogenic bladder, prostatic obstruction, previous urinary diversion) require extensive evaluation and possible intervention before being accepted for transplantation. Patients requiring intermittent catheterization are candidates for transplantation, although they are at higher risk for urinary tract infections.

25. Do a patient's kidneys need to be removed before a transplant?

No, unless specific indications or conditions exist requiring nephrectomy. Indications include refractory hypertension, although this is now rare due to currently available antihypertensive medications. Other potential indications include vesicoureteral reflux and upper urinary tract infections (pyelonephritis), urolithiasis, and the presence of renal masses suspicious for tumors. Many patients, especially diabetics and those with polycystic kidney disease, appear to do better if their native kidneys are preserved.

26. Is the transplanted kidney placed in the same position as the native kidney?

No. Renal transplant surgery has become fairly standardized, with the transplanted kidney usually placed in the iliac fossa in the pelvis. This location allows for easy access to the bladder for reimplantation of the ureter. The renal artery is usually anastomosed either to the external iliac artery or the internal iliac artery, and the renal vein to the external iliac vein. This location allows for easy monitoring (auscultation, palpation, radiologic studies) following transplantation. Small children who receive larger kidneys require intraabdominal placement of the kidney, with the renal artery being anastomosed to the aorta or common iliac artery and the renal vein to the vena cava. The ureter usually still can be reimplanted directly into the bladder.

27. Why do transplants fail?

Technical complications such as renal artery or venous thrombosis or ureteral obstruction can result in failure of a transplant, although this is rare and accounts for less than 1% of allograft loss. Although a small percentage of kidneys are lost due to other problems such as **infectious complications** or **recurrent disease,** the overwhelming majority of kidneys are lost due to **rejection.** Rejection is mediated by both the humoral and cellular arms of the immune system, and the various forms of rejection are defined according to the immunologic component and the time after transplantation.

Hyperacute rejection occurs within the first 24 hours following transplantation and is humorally mediated by preformed cytotoxic antibodies that result from previous antigen exposure via blood transfusion, previous transplant or, in the case of females, pregnancy. It is irreversible and activates the clotting system, resulting in thrombosis of small vessels with infarction of the kidney. **Accelerated rejection** usually occurs within 4–6 days and has both humoral and cellular components. It can occasionally be reversed with antirejection treatment (discussed below), although it is often refractory. **Acute rejection** occurs within the first 2–3 months, but is most common 2–4 weeks after transplantation. It is manifested by a decrease in urine output, low-grade fever, weight gain, hypertension, and an elevated serum creatinine, although often only the latter is present. A biopsy of the kidney usually reveals a cellular infiltrate of immunoblasts, lymphoblasts, and plasma cells. This form of rejection is typically responsive to antirejection therapy. **Chronic rejection** occurs late after transplantation and is felt to be humorally mediated, although good evidence for this is lacking. It may well be the result of progressive damage and ischemia from previous rejection episodes. Renal biopsy demonstrates vascular changes such as intimal proliferation, and interstitial fibrosis is seen as well as areas of atrophy and infarction. It is frequently not responsive to antirejection therapy, and it is important for the patient to undergo a biopsy to differentiate it from the unusual circumstance of a late acute rejection episode.

28. What is the impact of tissue typing and cross-matching with respect to rejection in renal transplantation?
Potential recipients as well as their donors undergo tissue typing to identify specific histocompatibility loci antigens (also referred to as human leukocyte antigens) that are located in the major histocompatibility complex on chromosome 6. Although a number of loci exist, the ones primarily tested for include HLA-A, HLA-B, and HLA-D. If a potential recipient has several possible living, related donors, then assuming all other circumstances are equal, the best matched donor would be chosen. Data clearly indicate that the recipient of a ''perfectly'' matched sibling's kidney enjoys better allograft survival than if transplanted from a lesser matched family member. Similarly, attempts are made to place cadaveric kidneys into the best matched recipients, although some controversy exists as to the exact benefit of matching in this setting, especially with the use of newer immunosuppressive agents. Data suggest that recipients of six antigen (two antigens at each of the loci mentioned above) matched kidneys do better than those receiving poorer matched kidneys, and it appears that the benefit of matching is seen in long-term survival rather than 1- and 2-year results. At the time of transplant, recipients are screened for the presence of preformed cytotoxic antibodies via cytotoxic crossmatches using recipient's sera and donor cells. A positive cross-match indicates the presence of antibodies and essentially precludes transplantation, thus preventing circumstances of hyperacute rejection.

29. How is rejection prevented and treated?
Although the ultimate goal is to induce a state of tolerance in recipients such that a foreign substance (transplanted kidney) will be accepted, and research is currently intensely focused in this area, the mainstay of rejection prevention and treatment is immunosuppressive medication. A number of procedures used to manipulate the immune system, including splenectomy, total lymphoid irradiation, thoracic duct drainage (depletion of lymph), and blood transfusions, have not been successful in inducing tolerance and have had adverse side effects. The principal immunosuppressive medications used for maintenance therapy to prevent rejection include **corticosteroids, azathioprine, and cyclosporine.** Corticosteriods are also used to treat rejection episodes, as are antilymphocyte preparations (both polyclonal and monoclonal). Antilymphocyte preparations have also been used for ''induction'' therapy prior to beginning maintenance immunosuppression in attempts to reduce rejection as well as side effects, especially those of cyclosporine.

Unfortunately, currently available immunosuppressive medications are not selective in their actives, exerting effects on many aspects of the immune system. Newer immunosuppressive agents, including OG-37-325 (cyclosporine G), FK506, rapamycin, RS 61443 (mycophenolate mofetil), mizoribine, brequinar sodium, 15-deoxyspergualin, and leuflonamide are being investigated in an attempt to reduce toxicities while maintaining adequate immunosuppression.

30. What are the side effects of immunosuppressive medications?
The principal side effect of immunosuppression in general is an increased susceptibility to infection, especially opportunistic and viral infections as well as malignancies, predominantly lymphoproliferative disorders. Specific toxicities of the commonly used immunosuppressive agents are listed in the following table.

Side Effects of Immunosuppressive Medications

Corticosteroids	**Azathioprine**
Hyperglycemia (diabetes)	Bone marrow suppression
Hyperlipidemia	Gastrointestinal disturbances
Cushingoid features	Hepatotoxicity
Obesity	Hair loss
Impaired wound healing	**Antilymphocytic Agents**
Aseptic necrosis (bone)	**Polyclonal**
Cataracts	Fever, chills
Hypertension	Leukopenia, thrombocytopenia
Peptic ulceration	Serum sickness
Growth retardation	Local phlebitis
Cyclosporine	**Monoclonal**
Nephrotoxicity	First (and often second) dose flu-like syndrome:
Hypertension	Fever, chills, tremors, headache, nausea,
Hyperkalemia	vomiting, and diarrhea
Hyperuricemia	Aseptic meningitis
Hepatotoxicity	Respiratory difficulties
Hirsutism	Pulmonary edema
Gingival hypertrophy	Hypotension
Tremors/seizures	

31. If the transplant kidney fails, does it have to be removed?

Kidneys that fail within the first few months are usually removed to prevent complications associated with ongoing rejection. Kidneys lost late are not usually removed, as they tend to cause fewer problems and the surgical removal is more difficult due to scarring. Once the transplant has failed, patients are tapered off the immunosuppressive medications to reduce adverse effects. Unless other complications have ensued, most patients with a failed allograft are candidates for retransplantation, although the success rate is slightly lower and it can be more difficult to find compatible donors if the patient has developed significant antibodies from the previous transplant.

BIBLIOGRAPHY

1. Agodoa LYC, Hold PJ, Port FK: U.S. Renal Data System, USRDS 1993 Annual Data Report. Bethesda, MD, The National Institutes of Health, National Institute of Diabetes and Digestive and Kidney Disease, March 1993.
2. Suranyi MG, Halloran PF, Hall BM: Recent developments in renal transplantation. In Gonick H (ed): Current Nephrology. St. Louis, Mosby, 1994, pp 385–463.

This text contains detailed descriptions of techniques and complications of hemodialysis and peritoneal dialysis:

3. Stone WJ, Hakin RM: Therapeutic options in the management of end-stage renal disease. In Jacobson HR, Striker GE, Klahr S (eds): The Principles and Practice of Nephrology. Philadelphia, B. C. Decker, 1991, pp 736–739.

Additional comprehensive reference texts on transplantation:

4. Brent L, Sells RA: Organ Transplantation: Current Clinical and Immunological Concepts. London, Bailliere Tindall, 1989.
5. Cerilli GJ: Organ Transplantation and Replacement. London, J. B. Lippincott, 1988.
6. Flye MW: Principles of Organ Transplantation. Philadelphia, W. B. Saunders, 1989.
7. Morris PT: Kidney Transplantation: Principles and Practice, 4th ed. Philadelphia, W. B. Saunders, 1994.

52. RENAL ARTERY DISEASE

Andrew C. Novick, M.D.

1. What are the causes of renal artery disease?

Renal artery disease is most commonly characterized by stenosis of the renal artery from atherosclerosis or fibrous dysplasia. These diseases account for approximately 65–70% and 25–30%, respectively, of all such renal lesions. There are three different varieties of fibrous dysplasia, termed intimal fibroplasia, medial fibroplasia, and perimedial fibroplasia, each with its distinctive histologic and arteriographic features and a different biologic history. Other less common disorders that can cause renal artery disease include arterial aneurysm, arteriovenous fistula, neurofibromatosis, arteritis, Takayasu's disease, and renal artery thrombosis or embolism.

2. How does renovascular disease differ from renovascular hypertension (RVH)?

RVH is an important correctable cause of hypertension with an estimated prevalence of approximately 0.5% among all patients with hypertension. It is important to differentiate between renovascular disease with RVH, because occlusive lesions of the renal artery do not always result in hypertension. The diagnosis of renovascular disease depends on angiographic demonstration of a stenotic lesion in the renal artery or its branches, whereas the diagnosis of RVH can be confirmed only in retrospect and implies permanent relief of hypertension after revascularization or removal of the affected kidney. The simultaneous occurrence of essential hypertension and coincidental renovascular disease is, in fact, more frequent than the occurrence of true RVH.

3. What are the clinical manifestations of RVH?

There is no single clinical manifestation that can reliably distinguish RVH from essential hypertension. Nevertheless, when taken in the aggregate, certain clinical manifestations are helpful in making this differential diagnosis. Patients with RVH are much more likely to have a short duration of hypertension, advanced retinopathy, azotemia, hypokalemia, alkalosis, or a bruit auscultated in the abdomen or flank. RVH is much less common in blacks than whites. In general, the most helpful clues to the diagnosis of RVH, in descending order of importance, have been:

1. An abdominal bruit with both systolic and diastolic components
2. An abrupt onset or exacerbation of hypertension with rapid progression
3. Onset of hypertension before age 30 or after age 55
4. Retinal vascular changes

4. What are the most useful screening tests for RVH?

Several screening tests are available for establishing the diagnosis of RVH in patients with suggestive clinical features.

1. The **rapid-sequence intravenous pyelogram** (IVP) is still occasionally used as a screening test for this disease. Findings suggestive of significant renal artery obstruction include (1) delay in the function of one kidney, (2) decrease in renal length of > 1.5 cm on the right or 1 cm on the left, (3) late hyperconcentration of contrast medium in one kidney, or (4) presence of ureteral notching due to collateral vessels. Its usefulness for RVH is limited by a high rate of false-positive and false negative studies.

2. **Isotope renography** with technetium or iodohippurate has not been a useful diagnostic test for RVH due to a large number of false-positive results. However, when an angiotensin-converting enzyme inhibitor (such as captopril) is added to the standard isotope renogram, the sensitivity and specificity increase considerably, especially for unilateral renal artery stenosis.

3. Recently, **duplex ultrasound scanning** of the renal arteries has become a useful noninvasive screening test for significant renal artery stenosis. When the arterial segment is

stenotic, there are alterations in laminar blood flow and the Doppler signal changes. While this technique is operator-dependent and time-consuming, initial reports indicate sensitivity and specificity rates of 80–90% in patients with renal artery stenosis.

4. **Renal arteriography** remains the gold standard for establishing the diagnosis of renal artery stenosis, and **intra-arterial digital subtraction arteriography** is the preferred method.

5. Developmental studies are in progress with **magnetic resonance angiography** as a potentially less-invasive technique for imaging the aorta and renal arteries.

5. How useful are plasma renin assays?

Differential renal vein plasma renin assays were formerly a popular test, proving the diagnosis of RVH with 90% accuracy when the renin level from the stenotic kidney is two or more times higher than the renin level from the normal contralateral kidney. However, the finding of nonlateralization with this test is very unreliable, since more than 50% of such patients are ultimately proved to have RVH. In patients with bilateral renal artery stenosis, renal vein renin ratios may be helpful in indicating which kidney is more severely affected.

Measurement of the peripheral plasma renin level is not reliable in identifying patients with RVH. However, the utility of this test can be significantly enhanced by administering an oral dose of captopril and obtaining a repeat plasma renin measurement 1 hour later. Captopril-stimulated peripheral plasma renin activity has become a useful noninvasive test for demonstrating the presence of renin-mediated or renovascular hypertension.

6. How often does renal artery disease cause renal failure?

Renal artery disease from atherosclerosis is now believed to be an important cause of chronic renal failure, and this has been termed **ischemic nephropathy.** Epidemiologic studies have shown that atherosclerotic renal artery disease is quite common in patients with generalized atherosclerosis obliterans, regardless of whether RVH is present. Studies on the natural history of atherosclerotic renal artery disease have made it possible to identify those patients in whom this disease poses a significant threat to overall renal function. This designation applies to patients with high-grade arterial stenosis affecting both kidneys or a solitary kidney. Intervention to restore normal renal arterial blood flow is indicated in such patients to prevent deterioration of renal function that may culminate in the need for dialytic replacement therapy.

7. What are the treatment options for patients with renal artery disease?
1. Medical antihypertensive therapy
2. Surgical revascularization or nephrectomy
3. Percutaneous transluminal angioplasty (PTA)

8. What is the appropriate treatment for RVH due to fibrous dysplasia?

In patients with fibrous dysplasia and suspected RVH, the need for interventive treatment (surgery or PTA) is guided by the specific type of disease, angiographic findings, and associated natural history. **Medical management** of hypertension is the preferred initial treatment for patients with medial fibroplasia, since loss of renal function from progressive obstruction is uncommon with this disease.

Interventive treatment in the latter category is reserved for patients whose blood pressure is difficult to control with multidrug antihypertensive therapy. Conversely, renal artery stenosis due to intimal fibroplasia or perimedial fibroplasia generally progresses and often eventuates in ischemic renal atrophy. Furthermore, these lesions tend to occur in younger patients and cause hypertension that may be difficult to control. Early interventive therapy in these groups is therefore indicated both to preserve renal function and to minimize the need for long-term antihypertensive medication.

The results of **PTA** in patients with main renal artery stenosis due to fibrous dysplasia are excellent and equivalent to those obtained with surgical revascularization. Therefore, PTA is the treatment of choice in such cases. However, as many as 30% of patients with fibrous dysplasia have branch renal arterial involvement, which increases the technical difficulty of PTA and often renders this procedure difficult or impossible to perform. Surgical renal revascularization remains the primary interventive treatment for such patients with branch renal artery disease.

9. How is RVH due to atherosclerosis treated?

In patients with atherosclerosis and suspected RVH, the indications for interventive therapy are more restrictive owing to their older age and the frequent presence of extrarenal vascular disease. In this group, more vigorous attempts at medical management are warranted and multidrug regimens to control blood pressure are often the preferred approach, particularly in patients with generalized atherosclerosis. Surgical revascularization and PTA are more appropriately reserved for patients whose hypertension cannot be controlled or when renal function is threatened by severe stenosis involving both kidneys or a solitary kidney.

In patients with atherosclerotic renal artery disease, the success rate of PTA has been excellent and comparable to that of surgical revascularization in patients with nonostial lesions. These lesions comprise only 15–20% of all atherosclerotic renal artery lesions, and PTA is the treatment of choice. In the more commonly encountered ostial atherosclerotic lesions, the results of PTA are less satisfactory. This group also comprises the majority of older patients who require relief of arterial obstruction for treatment of ischemic nephropathy. Surgical renal revascularization remains the primary interventive treatment for patients with ostial atherosclerotic RAD.

BIBLIOGRAPHY

1. Debatin JJ, Spritzer CE, Grist TM, et al: Imaging of the renal arteries: Value of MR angiography. AJR 157:981–990, 1991.
2. Hansen KJ, Tribble RW, Reavis SW, et al: Renal duplex sonography: Evaluation of clinical utility. J Vasc Surg 12:227–236, 1990.
3. Hayes J, Risius B, Novick AC, et al: Experience with percutaneous transluminal angioplasty for renal artery stenosis at the Cleveland Clinic. J Urol 139:488–492, 1988.
4. Kaylor W, Novick AC, Ziegelbaum M, Vidt D: Reversal of end-stage renal failure with surgical revascularization in patients with atherosclerotic renal artery occlusion. J Urol 141:486–488, 1989.
5. Libertino JA, Bosco PJ, Ying CY, et al: Renal revascularization to preserve and restore renal function. J Urol 147:1495–1497, 1992.
6. Nally JV, Black HR: State-of-the-art review: Captopril renography—Pathophysiological considerations and clinical observations. Semin Nucl Med 22:85–97, 1992.
7. Novick AC: Surgical correction of renovascular hypertension. Surg Clin North Am 68:1007, 1988.
8. Novick AC, Ziegelbaum M, Vidt DG, et al: Trends in surgical revascularization for renal artery disease: Ten years' experience. JAMA 257:498–501, 1987.
9. Olin JW, Melia M, Young JR, et al: Prevalence of atherosclerotic renal artery stenosis in patients with atherosclerosis elsewhere. Am J Med 188:46–51, 1990.
10. Schreiber MJ, Pohl MA, Novick AC: The natural history of atherosclerotic and fibrous renal artery disease. Urol Clin North Am 11:383–392, 1984.
11. Sos TA, Pickering PG, Sniderman KW, et al: Percutaneous transluminal renal angiography in renovascular hypertension due to atheroma or fibrous dysplasia. N Engl J Med 309:274–279, 1983.
12. Svetky LP, Himmelstein SI, Dunnick NR, et al: Prospective analysis of strategies for diagnosing renovascular hypertension. Hypertension 14:247–257, 1989.

53. AMBIGUOUS GENITALIA

Robert Kay, M.D.

1. How does the indifferent gonad become the testis or ovary?

The indifferent gonad begins at 6 weeks to become differentiated. The presence of the Y chromosome and genetic material in the short arm of the Y chromosome direct the gonad toward the testis. The absence of the Y chromosome directs the gonad into an ovary.

2. What hormones does the testis produce that are important in sexual differentiation?

Testosterone and müllerian-inhibiting substance.

3. How does testosterone affect sexual differentiation?

Testosterone stimulates the internal genitalia and the wolffian duct to develop. In the male, the wolffian duct becomes the epididymis, vas, and seminal vesicles. In the female, the wolffian duct becomes Gärtner's duct at one end and the epoöphoron at the other end near the ovary.

4. How are intersex states classified?

Classification of Intersex States

Disorders of genetic sex
    Turner's syndrome
    Mixed gonadal dysgenesis
    Kleinfelter's syndrome
    46XX male
Disorders of gonadal sex
    True hermaphroditism
    Pure gonadal dysgenesis
    Vanishing testis syndrome
Disorders of phenotypic sex
    Female pseudohermaphroditism
        Congenital adrenal hyperplasia
        Nonadrenal
            Maternal progestational agents
            Virilizing tumors of mother
    Male pseudohermaphroditism
        Abnormalities in androgen synthesis
        Abnormalities in androgen action
            Complete testicular feminization
            Incomplete testicular feminization
                Type 1. Reifenstein's, Lubs syndromes
                Type 2. 5α-reductase deficiency
        Persistent müllerian duct syndrome

5. What is the müllerian-inhibiting substance?

The müllerian-inhibiting substance is a hormone produced by the testis which suppresses the müllerian ducts. The müllerian structures in the female become the fallopian tube of the uterus and the upper third of the vagina. In the male, the müllerian duct regresses to the appendix testis on one end and the prostatic utricle on the other end.

6. What hormones in females lead to sexual differentiation?

In the female, androgen and müllerian-inhibiting factor are not produced. Therefore, the wolffian duct structures do not develop and the müllerian structures do develop. In a child who has no ovaries or testes, they will phenotypically develop as a female and the internal genitalia will be that of a female.

7. What is the most common cause of ambiguous genitalia in the newborn?
Congenital adrenal hyperplasia is the most common cause of ambiguous genitalia in the newborn, and it is the only cause that is potentially life-threatening (due to salt-wasting).

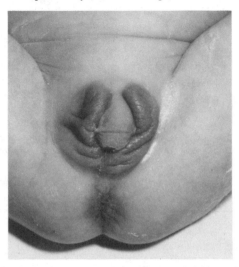

Ambiguous genitalia in newborn infant with congenital adrenal hyperplasia.

8. Describe the evaluation of ambiguous genitalia.

Evaluation of Ambiguous Genitalia

History	Genetic determination
Family history	Karyotype
Pregnancy (drugs, illness)	Biochemical
Physical examination	plasma 17-OH progesterone
Phallus size	Genitogram
Location of urethra	Ultrasound of pelvis
Labio-scrotal folds	Endoscopy
Palpable gonads	Laparoscopy or laparotomy
Excessive pigmentation	Gonadal biopsy
Rectal (presence of cervix)	

9. What causes masculinization of the male external genitalia?
Testosterone is converted by the enzyme 5α-reductase to become the active androgen, 5α-dihydrotestosterone. This androgen stimulates the indifferent external genitalia toward the male external genitalia.

10. At what gestational age does the male external genitalia develop?
By the end of the third month, the development is complete, with further growth of the phallus shortly before birth.

11. Which physical characteristic helps assess male differentiation in the newborn?
The palpable gonad is usually a testis and suggests male differentiation. Rarely, an ovary can be palpated with a large inguinal hernia, but in general, if a gonad is palpated, it is a testis.

12. What is the most common enzymatic defects in congenital adrenal hyperplasia?
21-Hydroxylase deficiency account for 90% of cases of congenital adrenal hyperplasia.

13. Can a blood test confirm congenital adrenal hyperplasia?
Plasma 17-hydroxyprogesterone is a sensitive marker for congenital adrenal hyperplasia.

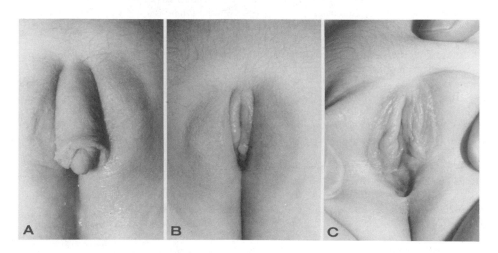

A, External genitalia of a child with late-onset congenital adrenal hyperplasia. Note virilization. **B** and **C,** External genitalia of the child following surgical repair.

14. How do children with 21-hydroxylase deficiency and 11β-hydroxylase deficiency differ clinically?
Children with 11β-hydroxylase deficiency may have hypertension secondary to a buildup of deoxycorticosterone (DOCA).

15. Are there nonadrenal factors that lead to virilization of the female newborn?
Yes. Maternal progestational agents taken in the first trimester of life or virilizing tumors in the mother may lead to virilization of the child.

16. Define true hermaphroditism?
True hermaphroditism is defined as having the presence of both ovarian and testicular tissue.

17. What is the karyotype of true hermaphroditism?
Although there is some geographical variation, approximately 50% of all true hermaphrodites are 46XX and 50% are divided between a mosaicism and 46XY.

18. What tumors are most often seen in the gonads of intersexual patients?
Gonadoblastoma and dysgerminoma.

19. Define male pseudohermaphroditism.
A male pseudohermaphrodite is a child with normal histologic testis and ambiguous external genitalia.

20. What causes male pseudohermaphroditism?
Androgen insensitivity at the end organ or an abnormality in the synthesis of androgens.

21. How do children with complete testicular feminization come to attention?
Patients with complete testicular feminization or total androgen insensitivity present either with a testis found during inguinal surgery or, more likely, during an evaluation of primary amenorrhea.

22. How are testosterone and luteinizing hormone levels affected in patients with complete testicular feminization?
Both are significantly elevated. Because the pituitary cannot detect testosterone due to total androgen insensitivity, gonadotropins are increased and stimulate the testis to release testosterone.

23. What do Reifenstein, Gilbert Dreyfus, Lubs, and Rosewater have in common?
These are all syndromes seen in patients with partial androgen insensitivity.

24. How do you determine the sex of rearing?
Although many factors must be considered, including age, fertility, anatomy, and endocrine status, the sex of rearing still should be determined by the ability of the child to function effectively in the sex that is chosen.

25. What is the second most common cause of ambiguous genitalia in the newborn?
Mixed gonadal dysgenesis.

26. What is the classic karyotype for mixed gonadal dysgenesis?
45XO/46XY.

27. Describe the internal genitalia in mixed gonadal dysgenesis.
The internal genitalia in mixed gonadal dysgenesis is almost always a testis on one side and a streak gonad on the other. On the side of the testis, the vas and epididymis may be normal, while on the side of the streak gonad, there usually are a fallopian tube and uterus.

28. Describe the Denys-Drash syndrome.
Denys-Drash syndrome refers to children with ambiguous genitalia, glomerulonephritis or other renal abnormalities, and Wilms' tumor.

BIBLIOGRAPHY

1. Aaronson, IA: Sexual differentiation and intersexuality. In Kelalis PP, King LR, Belman AB (eds): Clinical Pediatric Urology, 3rd ed. Philadelphia, W. B. Saunders, 1992.
2. Allen TD: Disorders of sexual differentiation. Urology 7:1, 1976.
3. Donahoe PK: The diagnosis and treatment of infants with intersex abnormalities. Pediatr Clin North Am 34:1333, 1987.
4. Donahoe PK, Ito Y, Morikawa Y, Hendren WH: Müllerian inhibiting substance in human testes after birth. J Pediatr Surg 12:323, 1977.
5. Griffin JE, Wilson JE: Disorders of sexual differentiation. In Walsh PC, Retik AB, Stamey TA, Vaughan ED Jr (eds): Campbell's Urology, 6th ed. Philadelphia, W. B. Saunders, 1992.
6. Jensen JC, Ehrlich RM, Hanna MK, et al: A report of 4 patients with Drash syndrome and a review of the literature. J Urol 141:1174, 1989.
7. Pagan RA: Diagnostic approach to the newborn with ambiguous genitalia. Pediatr Clin North Am 34:1019, 1987.
8. Sloan WR, Walsh PC: Familial persistent müllerian duct syndrome. J Urol 115:459, 1976.
9. Walsh PC, Madden JD, Harrod MJ, et al: Familial incomplete male pseudohermaphroditism, type 2: Reversed dihydrotestosterone formation in pseudovaginal perineoscrotal hypospadias. N Engl J Med 291:944, 1974.
10. White PC, New MI, Dupont B: Congenital adrenal hyperplasia. N Engl J Med 316:1519, 1987.

54. CRYPTORCHIDISM

Jonathan H. Ross, M.D.

1. Explain the difference between a cryptorchid testis and an ectopic testis.

A cryptorchid testis is a testis that is located along the normal path of descent but has failed to reach a dependent position in the scrotum. Ectopic testes descend normally through the external ring but are then misdirected to an ectopic site. Possible locations for ectopic testes include perineal, prepenile, transverse scrotal, femoral, and umbilical sites.

2. Where are most undescended testes located?

The inguinal canal.

3. What is the incidence of cryptorchidism at birth?

In term infants, 3.4%; in premature infants, 30%.

4. Can an undescended testis descend spontaneously?

Yes, but only in the first year of life (and most of those descend in the first 3 months). Approximately 74% of undescended testes in term infants and 95% of undescended testes in premature infants will descend spontaneously.

5. What is the normal mechanism of testicular descent?

Several theories exist, and normal descent may indeed be multifactorial. The most commonly proposed factors include:
1. Downward traction by the gubernaculum.
2. Differential growth of the body relative to the spermatic cord and gubernaculum.
3. Increased intra-abdominal pressure pushing the testis through the internal ring.
4. Development and maturation of the epididymis.
5. Endocrinologic factors.

6. Why is the finding of hypospadias in association with cryptorchidism significant?

It raises the possibility of intersex. A female with congenital adrenal hyperplasia may present with hypospadias and bilateral impalpable gonads, and a male with mixed gonadal dysgenesis may present with hypospadias and unilateral or bilateral undescended gonads. Of course, many children with hypospadias and cryptorchidism are not intersex patients.

7. What is a retractile testis?

A retractile testis is a normal testis. The term really describes a finding artificially created by the environment of the doctor's office. When a child is cold and frightened, the cremasteric reflex is activated, and the testis may be pulled out of the scrotum temporarily. Children with particularly active cremasteric reflexes (or children who are especially cold and frightened) may appear to have an undescended testis.

8. How can one distinguish a retractile testis from an undescended testis?

The following suggest the testis is retractile:
1. The parents report that when the child is relaxed (particularly in a warm bath), the testis is in the scrotum.
2. The testis can be milked into the scrotum and remains there, at least temporarily, without tension.
3. The hemiscrotum is well developed on the side in question.
4. Serial examination several months apart may clarify an equivocal case.
5. Hormonal therapy.

9. What is the most common treatment for an undescended testicle?
Orchiopexy.

10. What is hormonal therapy?
The administration of human chorionic gonadotropin (hCG), 5,000–10,000 units given in several injections over a period of 2–4 weeks, is used to stimulate descent without an operation. Gonadotropin-releasing hormone (GnRH) nasal spray has been used in Europe but it is not approved for use in the United States.

11. How successful is hormonal therapy?
There is widespread disagreement on this point. Reported success rates range from 6–70%. The true efficacy is probably in the range of 10–20%. Those series reporting higher success rates probably include a large number of patients with retractile testes which are known to "descend" in response to hCG.

12. What are the roles of MRI, CT, and ultrasound in localizing an impalpable testis?
Very limited. The differential diagnosis of an impalpable testis is an intra-abdominal testis or an absent testis. If an imaging study identifies an intra-abdominal testis, then an operation is indicated. Because of a significant false-negative rate with each of these studies, failure to demonstrate a testis does not prove that it is absent. Therefore, patients with a negative imaging study also require an operation. Because the imaging study will not alter the management of the patient, it is not indicated.

13. What biochemical test can be used to prove anorchia in a patient with bilateral impalpable testes?
Castrate levels of serum testosterone after hCG stimulation.

14. How do you definitively locate an impalpable testis?
Surgical exploration is the gold standard. Laparoscopy is also extremely effective, but occasionally a high intra-abdominal testis may not be visualized.

15. If a high intra-abdominal testis is discovered at laparoscopy, what are the options for management?
    1. Immediate orchiopexy, if the vessels are thought to be long enough to allow it.
    2. Laparoscopic ligation of the testicular artery, which stimulates enlargement of collateral vessels. Six months later, the testicular artery is divided and the testis brought down on a pedicle of collateral vessels. When described as a two-stage open procedure, this has been given the eponym "Fowler-Stephens" orchiopexy.
    3. Laparoscopic orchiectomy, if the testis is grossly abnormal, or if the patient is postpubertal and has a normal contralateral testis.

16. If blind-ending vessels and vas are discovered at laparoscopy, what should be done?
The finding of blind-ending vessels confirms anorchia, and nothing further need be done.

17. If a blind-ending vas is discovered at laparoscopy and the vessels are not identified, what should be done?
A blind-ending vas does not confirm the diagnosis of anorchia. The vessels must be identified. If they cannot, than an exploration is indicated to rule out a high intra-abdominal testis which was missed laparoscopically.

18. On laparoscopy, the vas and vessels are seen to enter the internal ring. Describe the management options.
If a hernia is present, then the patient probably has an undescended testis at the internal ring. These can move in and out of the abdomen (so-called **peeping** testis), accounting for the failure to

palpate them on physical examination. Palpation over the inguinal canal during laparoscopy may push the testis into the abdomen where it can be seen. In any case, an inguinal exploration is indicated.

If the testis is impalpable and the internal ring is closed, then the patient probably has a **vanishing** testis. This occurs when a testis descends beyond the internal ring and then is lost, probably to prenatal torsion. Some pediatric urologists believe that in this circumstance no exploration is needed. Others claim that an inguinal exploration is required to excise any atrophic remnant which may contain some viable seminiferous tubules with malignant potential.

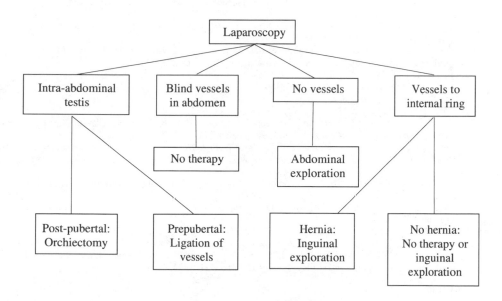

Management of an impalpable testis.

19. List four complications of an undescended testis.

1. **Testicular cancer** is approximately 10 times more common in undescended testes. The risk is greatest for intra-abdominal testes.

2. **Torsion** is more common in undescended testes.

3. A **patent processus vaginalis** (hernia) is present in nearly all cases, although it is rarely detected clinically.

4. **Infertility** may occur, particularly in patients with bilateral undescended testes, of whom approximately 70% are infertile.

20. What is the most common tumor in a cryptorchid testis?
Seminoma.

21. Is the contralateral testis at risk for tumor?
Yes. Twenty percent of tumors in patients with unilateral cryptorchidism occur in the contralateral testis. In a patient with bilateral cryptorchidism and a testis tumor, there is a 15% chance that a contralateral tumor will develop. If both testes are intra-abdominal, that risk is 30%.

22. What is the significance of testicular torsion of a cryptorchid testis in an adult?
More than 50% will be found to have a tumor. This diagnosis should be considered in a man with abdominal pain and an empty hemiscrotum.

23. Do patients with unilateral cryptorchidism have a normal contralateral testis?

No. There is a significant decrease in sperm density of the contralateral testis with a mild decrease in clinical fertility.

BIBLIOGRAPHY

1. Andrews PE, Malek RS: Unilateral cryptorchidism in adults. In Resnick MI, Kursh ED (eds): Current Therapy in Genitourinary Surgery. St. Louis, Mosby, 1992, pp 339–344.
2. Cendron M, Huff D, Keating MA, et al: Anatomical, morphological and volumetric analysis: A review of 759 cases of testicular maldescent. J Urol 149:570–573, 1993.
3. Gerber GS, Firlit CF: Anorchia. In Resnick MI, Kursh ED (eds): Current Therapy in Genitourinary Surgery. St. Louis, Mosby, 1992, pp 334–336.
4. Hadziselimovic F: Cryptorchidism. In Gillenwater JY, Grayhack JT, Howards SS, Duckett JW (eds): Adult and Pediatric Urology, 2nd ed. St. Louis, Mosby, 1991, pp 2217–2228.
5. Hrebinko RL, Bellinger MF: The limited role of imaging techniques in managing children with undescended testes. J Urol 150:458–460, 1993.
6. Joseph DB, Bauer SB: Bilateral cryptorchidism. In Resnick MI, Kursh ED (eds): Current Therapy in Genitourinary Surgery. St. Louis, Mosby, 1992, pp 344–346.
7. Kaplan GW: Unilateral cryptorchidism in children. In Resnick MI, Kursh ED (eds): Current Therapy in Genitourinary Surgery. St. Louis, Mosby, 1992, pp 336–339.
8. Kogan SJ: Treatment of cryptorchidism: An additional viewpoint. In Gillenwater JY, Grayhack JT, Howards SS, Duckett JW (eds): Adult and Pediatric Urology, 2nd ed. St. Louis, Mosby, 1991, pp 2229–2230.
9. Moore RG, Peters CA, Bauer SB, et al: Laparoscopic evaluation of the nonpalpable testis: A prospective assessment of accuracy. J Urol 151:728–731, 1994.
10. Rajfer J, Handelsman DJ, Swerdloff RS, et al: Hormonal therapy of cryptorchidism. N Engl J Med 314:466–470, 1986.
11. Tennenbaum SY, Lerner SE, McAleer IM, et al: Preoperative laparoscopic localization of the nonpalpable testis: A critical analysis of a 10-year experience. J Urol 151:732–734, 1994.
12. Turek PJ, Ewaslt DH, Synder HM III, et al: The absent cryptorchid testis: Surgical findings and their implications for diagnosis and etiology. J Urol 151:718–721, 1994.

55. SCROTAL MASS IN ADULTS

J. Patrick Spirnak, M.D.

1. What is the most common malignant scrotal mass?
Testicular cancer. It is the most common solid cancer in young adult males between ages 15 and 34 years.

2. What is the most common benign scrotal mass?
Hydrocele, occurring in an estimated 1% of adult males.

3. Define a hydrocele.
A hydrocele is a collection of serous fluid between the two layers of the tunica vaginalis.

4. What causes a hydrocele to form?
Any process that acts to stimulate increased production of serous fluid (e.g., tumor, inflammation, trauma) by the tunica vaginalis or to decrease the resorption of this fluid (e.g., inguinal surgery) by the scrotal lymphatics or venous system will result in hydrocele formation.

5. What is the characteristic physical finding of a hydrocele?
A smooth, cystic-feeling mass completely surrounding the testicle and not involving the spermatic cord is typical of a hydrocele. In addition, it readily transilluminates.

6. When is scrotal ultrasonography indicated in the evaluation of suspected hydrocele?
When a hydrocele is large and testicular palpation is not possible.

7. How are hydroceles treated?
Small asymptomatic hydroceles require no treatment other than patient reassurance. Surgical excision is recommended when the hydrocele is large and symptomatic.

8. Is aspiration ever indicated as a means of treatment?
Needle aspiration is a treatment option usually reserved for individuals who are poor surgical candidates. Unfortunately, fluid usually re-accumulates and the hydrocele recurs.

9. What is a spermatocele?
It is a sperm-containing cyst that usually arises from the head of the epididymis.

10. What causes a spermatocele to form?
A spermatocele may be idiopathic or due to ductal obstruction, usually caused by trauma or inflammation.

11. How does one differentiate a spermatocele from a hydrocele on physical examination?
A spermatocele is palpable as a cystic, nontender nodule usually arising superior to the testicle. Unlike a hydrocele, a spermatocele allows complete palpation of the entire testis.

12. When is surgical excision indicated?
Surgical excision is indicated when the spermatocele is large and symptomatic, or when it is socially embarrassing to the individual.

13. What is varicocele?
A varicocele is an abnormal dilation of the veins of the pampiniform plexus. It may be primary and due to a congenital anomaly of the venous valves, or secondary and due to any abdominal or retroperitoneal process obstructing the venous system.

14. Do varicoceles occur equally on right and left sides?
No. Clinical varicoceles occur more commonly on the left side.

15. Why are varicoceles more common on the left side?
The left testicular vein drains into the left renal vein and inserts at a 90° angle, whereas the right testicular vein inserts obliquely into the inferior vena cava.

16. Describe the physical findings of a large varicocele.
With the patient standing, a large varicocele appears as an irregular, worm-like mass beneath the scrotal skin overlying the spermatic cord. It is cystic on palpation and increases in size with a Valsalva maneuver. Primary varicoceles disappear when the patient is supine. Testicular atrophy may also be present.

17. Can a hernia ever present as a scrotal mass?
Yes. A large indirect inguinal hernia may contain small bowel located within the scrotum.

18. How can one differentiate an indirect inguinal hernia from other common causes of scrotal swelling?
Small indirect inguinal hernias are typically palpated when the patient coughs. Large hernias can usually be reduced with the patient supine. Hydroceles, spermatoceles, and testicular tumors do not change with a Valsalva maneuver and cannot be reduced.

19. What is the treatment of an inguinal hernia?
Surgical repair.

20. How does a testicular cancer usually present?
The typical patient will present with a painless testicular mass.

21. What is the treatment of a solid testicular mass?
Inguinal exploration with orchiectomy.

22. Is scrotal ultrasound ever indicated in the evaluation of a solid testicular mass?
Ultrasound is performed when the physical findings are inconclusive and one is unable to determine whether the mass is rising from the epididymis or from the testis.

BIBLIOGRAPHY

1. Donohue JP (ed): Testes Tumors. Baltimore, Williams & Wilkins, 1983.
2. Fournier GR, Laing FC, Jeffrey B, et al: High resolution scrotal ultrasound. J Urol 134:490, 1985.
3. Spirnak JP: Adult scrotal mass. In Resnick MI, Caldamone AA, Spirnak JP (eds): Decision Making in Urology. Toronto, B. C. Decker, 1985, pp 184.
4. Spirnak JP, Resnick MI: Hydrocele repair, the Lord procedure. Contemp Urol, 1989, p 55.
5. Zornow DH, Landes RR: Scrotal palpation. Am Fam Physician 23:150, 1981.

56. VARICOCELE

Anthony J. Thomas, Jr., MD

1. What is a varicocele?

A varicocele is a dilatation of the veins of the pampiniform plexus of the spermatic cord. The engorgement is caused by a lack of valves within the vein(s). The condition is apparent when the affected man is in the upright position. Approximately 15% of men have a varicocele, usually present from the time of puberty. Most affect the left testis, but they may be found on both sides or occasionally on the right side only.

2. What is the clinical significance of a varicocele?

In men with either unilateral or bilateral varicoceles, sperm quality may range from an azoospermic state to minimal or no change in semen. Some men with a unilateral varicocele may exhibit a measurable ipsilateral loss in testicular size. A varicocele rarely causes discomfort, but men who complain of testicular pain associated with this condition often describe it as a "heaviness or dull ache" on the affected side, particularly evident after long periods of standing or heavy exercise. Assuming the supine position and elevating the scrotum should quickly resolve pain due to a varicocele.

3. What methods are useful to identify a varicocele?

The most common method of identifying a varicocele is direct examination of the patient's scrotum when he is standing upright in a warm, well-lighted room. The veins of a moderate or large varicocele bulge outward above and often behind the affected testis. Smaller varicoceles may be palpable and increase in size when the patient performs a Valsalva maneuver. Using a simple, 5.3-MHz Doppler stethoscope over the suspected varicocele, the examiner can hear an audible rush of blood when the patient performs a Valsalva maneuver. When the patient is recumbent, the varicocele should collapse as the testis is elevated. Color Doppler ultrasound has been used to identify smaller, so-called subclinical varicoceles that are difficult to palpate. Some investigators question the clinical significance of this "subclinical" entity.

4. What causes the alterations in sperm quality associated with a varicocele?

Of the many theories, the most widely accepted is increase in testicular temperature. Laboratory studies have demonstrated an increase in arterial blood flow with experimentally produced varicoceles in rats. The temperature in both testicles increases, even in the presence of a unilateral varicocele.

5. Is any risk other than infertility or pain associated with varicocele?

No specific health risks are associated with a varicocele other than the possibility of impaired sperm quality, which does not affect all men with varicoceles. Some men have a smaller testis on the ipsilateral side, and an increased incidence of sperm antibodies has been noted in men with varicoceles. Sperm quality may gradually diminish over time. Varicocele has been noted to be a prominent finding in men who seek medical attention for secondary infertility.

6. If not all men with varicoceles are infertile, what are the indications for recommending correction?

1. **Impaired sperm quality.** Impairment may range from azoospermia associated with maturational arrest to mild impairment in concentration or motility. In men with severely atrophic, scarred testes or testicles that demonstrate Sertoli Cells Only by biopsy, correction of the varicocele will not improve semen parameters.

2. **Pain.** Although relatively uncommon, the type of pain, as mentioned above, is highly characteristic. A careful and thorough history should differentiate men who stand a good chance of pain relief from men with other causes for testicular pain.

3. **Cosmetic indications,** particularly in the presence of a large varicocele in an adolescent, most of whom are particularly conscious of their genitals and have a great desire to be "like everyone else."

4. **Failure of the affected testis to grow** compared with its contralateral partner in the young adolescent (see question 11).

7. Is there an optimal method or surgical approach to correct a varicocele?

Five techniques are used to obliterate a varicocele: (1) inguinal approach; (2) retroperitoneal approach; (3) subinguinal incision; (4) laparoscopic clipping; and (5) transvenous embolization. Each method can be effective in the proper hands. Most urologists are familiar with the inguinal incision and ligation. Special training is required for the laparoscopic technique. In the author's opinion, unless laparoscopy is done with sufficient frequency to maintain proficiency, it should not be used for varicocele obliteration, because it presents greater risks to the patient than the more standard surgical approaches. Inguinal and subinguinal incisions seem to provide the surgeon with the best chance of ligating all the major venous channels and collaterals (see figure below). Transvenous embolization should be done only by skilled interventional radiologists, but it is as effective and safe as surgery and has the major advantage of quick return to full activity.

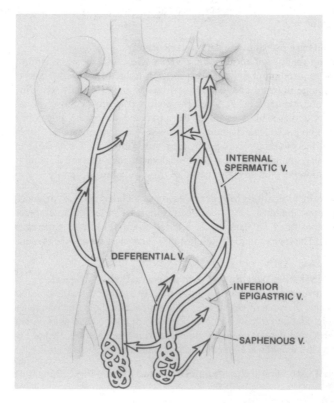

Possible venous pathways associated with varicocele.

8. Why do some varicoceles persist after surgery or embolization?

The estimated failure rate of varicocele surgery is 0–10%, depending on the series. The most obvious explanation is a missed vein that was not ligated or embolized. A number of collateral channels may be associated with the varicocele, and the spermatic cord must be scrutinized carefully at the time of surgery. Particularly large varicoceles often have posterior collateral veins that traverse the floor of the inguinal canal and enter the iliac vein below. Careful dissection of the cord, preserving the testicular artery, the vas deferens with its associated vessels, and the lymphatics minimizes failure. It is also helpful to place a Penrose drain beneath the cord and to lift upward, pulling the testis toward the incision to identify and ligate any perforating veins that travel toward the iliac or hypogastric veins. Failure of embolization procedures usually is due to the inability of the radiologist to catheterize a collateral vein because of the angle at which it branches from the main vein or because of its proximity to the testis.

9. What is the anticipated rate of improvement in sperm quality and fertility?

Rates of improvement in sperm quality and subsequent fertility vary depending on the investigator and the series size. Some report no improvement, whereas others report improvement in as many as 75% of patients. The true rate is probably somewhere between the two extremes. When the statistics from many large studies are combined, approximately two-thirds of patients showed some improvement in some of their semen parameters, and 40% established pregnancies with their spouses. Statistics vary with factors such as the partner's fertility potential, sperm–cervical mucus interaction, and frequency of intercourse.

10. What are the potential complications of varicocele surgery or embolization?

Major complications are rare with surgery but may include wound infection, hematoma, hydrocele, and even testicular atrophy. Hydroceles can be prevented by carefully preserving the lymphatic vessels that parallel the testicular artery and veins. Testicular atrophy may occur as a consequence of inadvertent or intentional ligation and division of the testicular artery. Of note, some investigators report routine ligation of the artery and vein in the retroperitoneum without subsequent atrophy. Routine ligation is not recommended, however, because the vasal artery and other small branches may be insufficient to sustain normal testicular function, even with no measurable change in size of the testis. Laparoscopy, particularly in less experienced hands, involves the risk of bowel injury by perforation or coagulation, major vascular injury, and even inadvertent ligation of the ureter, which may be mistaken for the spermatic vein. In experienced hands, laparoscopy appears as safe and effective as open surgery. Complications during and after percutaneous embolization are also related to the experience of the interventional radiologist. Occlusive balloons involve the risk of migration to the pulmonary arteries, but because of their small size, they may be tolerated without sequelae. Stainless steel coils, hot contrast, and concentrated dextrose solutions (70% dextrose) are suitable alternatives that remain popular and equally safe with some radiologists. Other complications of the percutaneous technique relate to venous access, which may result in deep vein thrombosis, venous perforation, adverse reaction to contrast material, or hematoma at the site of puncture.

11. If a varicocele is discovered during a routine school physical in an adolescent boy, should anything be done?

There is considerable controversy about whether to recommend correction or observation. Most urologists favor correction of the varicocele if the involved testis is significantly smaller than its contralateral mate of if the involved testis fails to grow normally as the boy is followed from year to year. Some evidence suggests that compensatory growth may occur after obliteration of the varicocele; for this reason alone, fertility potential may be greater if correction is immediate rather than delayed until the young man is trying to father children. Whether immediate correction alters fertility is yet to be completely proved, but at this point it seems a reasonable approach. It is not appropriate to request a semen sample from adolescent boys, nor is it wise to focus so much attention on scrotal contents that they perceive themselves as "sexually abnormal." If the testes are of equal size and growing normally, the young man needs to be seen only on a yearly basis to ensure that atrophy does not occur; if it does, correction is recommended. Prospective studies of boys and young men with varicoceles are in progress; it will be some time before an optimal answer is available.

BIBLIOGRAPHY

1. Comhaire F: The pathogenesis of epididymo-testicular dysfunction in varicocele: Factors other than temperature. Adv Exp Med Biol 286:281–287, 1991.
2. Constabile RA, Skoog S, Radowich M: Testicular volume assessment in the adolescent with a varicocele. J Urol 147:1348–1350, 1992.
3. Gorelick JI, Goldstein M: Loss of fertility in men with varicocele. Fertil Steril 59:613–616, 1993.
4. Howards SS: Subclinical varicocele (editorial). Fertil Steril 57:725–726, 1992.
5. Kondoh N, Meguro N, Matsumiya K, et al: Significance of subclinical varicocele detected by scrotal sonography in male infertility: A preliminary report. J Urol 150:1158–1160, 1993.
6. Laven JS, Haans LC, Mali WP, et al: Effects of varicocele treatment in adolescents: A randomized study. Fertil Steril 58:756–762, 1992.
7. McClure RD, Khoo D, Jarvi K, et al: Subclinical varicocele: The effectiveness of varicocelectomy. J Urol 145:789–791, 1991.
8. Mehan DJ, Andrus CH, Parra RO: Laparoscopic internal spermatic vein ligation: Report of a new technique. Fertil Steril 58:1263–1266, 1992.
9. Takihara H, Sakatoku J, Cockett AT: The pathophysiology of varicocele in male infertility. Fertil Steril 55:861–868, 1991.
10. Thomas AJ, Geisinger MA: Current management of varicoceles. Urol Clin North Am 17:893–907, 1990.
11. Witt MA, Lipshultz LI: Varicocele: A progressive or static lesion. Urology 42:541–543, 1993.

IV. Inflammation and Infection

57. ACUTE PYELONEPHRITIS

Bashir R. Sankari, M.D.

1. What is acute pyelonephritis?

Acute pyelonephritis is an acute infection of the renal parenchyma and collecting system. It is most commonly caused by a bacterial pathogen. *Escherichia coli* and other *Enterobacteriaceae* account for over 90% of the infections. Acute pyelonephritis is sometimes referred to as **upper urinary tract system infection** and should be differentiated from the more common, uncomplicated lower urinary tract infections such as cystitis.

2. What is the route of infection?

Two routes of infection exist. Ascending uriniferous spread is the most common. It is caused by retrograde ascent of bacteria from the bladder through the ureter to the renal pelvis and parenchyma. Colonization of the perineum with gut enterobacteria precedes the episode of acute pyelonephritis. The second route of infection is hematogenous spread and is less common. It is usually associated with other extrarenal foci of infection such as tuberculosis and staphylococcal septicemia.

3. Do any conditions predispose to acute pyelonephritis?

- Obstruction of the urinary collecting system
- Vesicoureteral reflux
- Renal calculi
- Neurogenic bladder
- Diabetes mellitus
- Altered host resistance (immunosuppression)
- Congenital anomalies
- Pregnancy
- Prolonged catheter drainage

4. Describe the clinical presentation of acute pyelonephritis.

Because acute bacterial nephritis is a parenchymal infection, it is most frequently associated with fever, chills, malaise, and pain in the flank, with or without radiation to the groin. Gastrointestinal symptoms are often present with nausea and vomiting and are mainly secondary to paralytic ileus. Lower urinary tract symptoms such as dysuria, urgency, and frequency are present in 50% of the cases. On physical examination, the hallmark finding is the presence of costovertebral angle tenderness on the affected side. Concurrent abdominal pain and tenderness and paralytic ileus may also occur, adding to the confusion and prompting consideration of other intra-abdominal processes such as appendicitis, diverticulitis, pancreatitis, and cholecystitis in the differential diagnosis.

5. What are the laboratory findings?

Urinalysis shows pyuria, bacteriuria, and gross or microscopic blood. The complete blood count reveals leukocytosis with predominance of neutrophils. The serum creatinine may be elevated due to the transient renal dysfunction and/or dehydration. Urine cultures are diagnostic, and the sensitivity study will identify the appropriate antibiotic therapy.

6. What is the spectrum of the disease?

Infectious Disease Processes in the Kidney
Acute pyelonephritis
Focal bacterial nephritis (lobar nephronia)
Multifocal bacterial nephritis
Renal abscess, perinephric abscess
Emphysematous pyelonephritis
Xanthogranulomatous pyelonephritis

Acute pyelonephritis can take a more or less complicated course depending on the severity of the infectious process, time of presentation, predisposing conditions, and promptness of effective therapy. As the route of infection is mostly ascending, many renal infections follow the lobar and lobular distribution of renal parenchyma and remain confined within the rigid capsule of the kidney. In the classic presentation of **acute pyelonephritis,** the whole kidney is enlarged with generalized inflammation and swelling. **Urosepsis** can result from the associated bacteremia. In its severe form, acute renal infection with heavy leukocyte infiltrate can be confined to a single renal lobe or multiple lobes, resulting in **acute focal** or **multifocal bacterial nephritis. Renal abscesses** can evolve from these lesions with progressive suppuration of the renal parenchyma. Rupture outside the renal capsule results in perinephric abscess collection.

In diabetic patients, fermentation of sugar by gas-forming organisms (such as *E. coli*) will result in carbon dioxide production which is visualized as air in the renal parenchyma, a condition referred to as **emphysematous pyelonephritis.** Patients with associated chronic stones (ammonium-magnesium-phosphate or struvite stones) related to infection with urea-splitting organisms such as *Proteus* and *E. coli* can develop **xanthogranulomatous pyelonephritis,** an atypical form of renal infection that is characterized by a cellular infiltrate of lipid-laden mononuclear macrophages (foam cells) on microscopic examination. Grossly, it has the shape of a mass lesion, which may be localized or diffuse, depending on the severity and the extent of disease, and is confused commonly with renal cell carcinoma.

7. Is radiologic investigation needed in the patient with acute pyelonephritis?
Radiologic investigation is important in acute pyelonephritis to rule out associated anomalies that have predisposed the patient for the infectious process and to define the pathologic process in complicated cases. Imaging studies become essential if the infectious process fails to improve despite appropriate therapy.

8. What is the best radiologic test in acute pyelonephritis?
No single study provides a uniformly diagnostic picture under all circumstances. The workup must be tailored to the anticipated abnormality and the clinical outcome of treatment, and it should be adjusted when further study is expected to provide additional useful information.

1. A simple **plain film** of the abdomen is useful to rule out air in the renal parenchyma. In addition, it may show radiopaque stones or shadowing of psoas muscle in perinephric or renal abscess.

2. **Intravenous pyelogram** (IVP) is usually negative in acute pyelonephritis. It may show only some delay in visualization and excretion of the contrast and swelling of renal parenchyma. IVP is very important to rule out congential anomalies, such as ureteropelvic junction obstruction or an obstructing stone in the ureter. The bladder film will help assess the wall of the bladder and rule out neurogenic bladder, and the postvoid film will rule out bladder outlet obstruction.

3. **Computed tomography (CT) scan with intravenous contrast** becomes important in defining the lobar or multilobar involvement of the infectious process when clinical circum-

stances justify the investigation. It helps in the diagnosis of renal abscess, perinephric abscess, and xanthogranulomatous pyelonephritis.

4. **Ultrasonography** is helpful in the diagnosis and followup of renal abscess and focal bacterial nephritis.

5. **Renal nuclear scan** with mercaptoacetyltriglycine (MAG-3) or diethylenetriamine pentaacetic acid (DTPA) is important to assess residual renal function when clinical condition warrant surgical intervention or ablation. Dimercaptosuccinic acid (DMSA) renal scan concentrates in the renal cortex and is a very good study in assessing cortical scar when indicated, such as in followup of children with vesicoureteral reflux.

9. How does acute pyelonephritis affect renal function?
With each kidney infection, there is a variable degree of structural damage, depending on the severity of infection and the promptness of therapy. Residual scarring with some loss of functioning tissue is the rule and is dependent upon the severity and chronicity of the infection.

10. Explain the treatment of acute pyelonephritis.
Treatment is usually indicated upon clinical suspicion and should be prompt, preferably in a hospital with intravenous antibiotics. Some uncomplicated cases can be treated as outpatients. The antibiotics used should cover the prevalent gram-negative pathogens (*Escherichia coli, Proteus, Pseudomonas,* and *Klebsiella*) and be adjusted according to culture and sensitivity results.

Empirically, one-drug therapy with a third-generation cephalosporin or uriedo penicillin is usually effective. Fluoroquinolones are good alternative agents and can be continued orally as outpatient therapy. In severe cases, two-drug therapies should be considered for synergistic effect. Though aminoglycocides are good gram-negative antimicrobials, their role is becoming limited due to their nephrotoxicity, ototoxicity, huge liabilities, and the ready availability of effective and safer alternative antimicrobial agents. Aminoglycosides plus ampicillin may be required for compromised hosts with nosocomial infections. If the patient does not improve within an acceptable time frame (3–5 days), despite appropriate therapy, further investigation should be done to rule out associated anomalies and conditions that require intervention, such as obstruction and renal abscess.

Acute pyelonephritis deserves 2 weeks of combined intravenous and oral antibiotics. Focal and multifocal bacterial nephritis requires up to 6 weeks of combined therapy depending on response. Emphysematous pyelonephritis requires an aggressive intravenous antibiotic course. If symptoms persist, percutaneous drainage and/or nephrectomy should be considered. Xanthogranulomatous pyelonephritis requires surgical intervention through either total or partial nephrectomy.

BIBLIOGRAPHY

1. Benson M, Lipuma JP, Resnick MI: The role of imaging studies in urinary tract infection. Urol Clin North Am 13:605–625, 1986.
2. Conway J: The role of scintigraphy in urinary tract infection. Semin Nucl Med 18:308–319, 1988.
3. Elder JS: Xanthogranulomatous pyelonephritis and gas forming infections of the urinary tract. AUA Update 3(2):lesson 31, 1984.
4. Hill GS: Renal infection. In Hill GS (ed): Uropathology. New York, Churchill Livingstone, 1989, pp 333–429.
5. Hudson MA, Weyman PJ, van der Vliet AH, Catalona WJ: Emphysematous pyelonephritis: Successful management by percutaneous drainage. J Urol 136:884–886, 1986.
6. Nosher JL, Tamminen JL, Amorosa JK, Kallich M: Acute focal bacterial nephritis. Am J Kidney Dis 11:36–42, 1988.
7. Schaeffer AJ: Renal infection. In Gillenwater JY, et al (eds): Adult and Pediatric Urology, 2nd ed. St. Louis, Mosby, 1991, pp 745–787.
8. Stoller ML, Kogan BA: Sensitivity of technetium-DMSA for the diagnosis of chronic pyelonephritis: Clinical and theoretical considerations. J Urol 135:977–980, 1986.

58. RENAL AND PERIRENAL ABSCESS

Nehemia Hampel, M.D.

1. What is an abscess?

An abscess is a focus of suppuration within an organ tissue or region of the body; it may be microscopic or macroscopic. Most abscesses are acute, but some may be chronic. Renal abscesses are located within the renal parenchyma, whereas perirenal abscesses are located within the perirenal fascia (Gerota's fascia).

2. What is the difference between renal and perirenal abscesses?

Renal abscesses are localized kidney lesions that are either intraparenchymal (cortical, medullary, or infected renal cyst) or confined to an obstructed renal calyx. Perirenal abscesses involve the perirenal space surrounded by the perirenal fascia of Gerota. Most perinephric abscesses are associated with renal abscess.

3. What is the significance of renal and perirenal abscesses?

The major risk is life-threatening urosepsis and septicemia. Because of their location in the retroperitoneum, renal and perirenal abscesses are difficult to diagnose. Poor prognosis is related to delay in diagnosis and to associated medical problems.

4. Describe the pathogenesis.

In the past the majority of renal and perirenal abscesses were caused by hematologic spread from skin or respiratory infections. Today many result from ascending infections from the lower urinary tract. Perinephric abscesses develop mainly from rupture of an intrarenal abscess. Usually Gerota's fascia confines abscess formation to the perinephric space, but the process may extend to adjacent cavities and structures. Preexisting renal disease is present in the majority of cases. Pyelonephritis and renal calculus disease are common causes. Vesicoureteral reflux and urinary tract infections in children as well as adults may result in renal or perirenal abscesses. Predisposing conditions include diabetes mellitus, urinary tract infection, urinary tract obstruction, nephrolithiasis, intravenous drug use, and immunosuppression.

5. What microorganisms are involved in renal and perirenal abscesses?

The infective organisms of renal and perirenal abscesses are the same. Hematogenous spread involves gram-positive organisms, most commonly *Staphylococcus aureus*. Ascending infection usually involves gram-negative bacteria, primarily strains of *Escherichia coli* and *Klebsiella* and *Proteus* spp. Other bacteria, including *Pseudomonas* sp., obligatory anaerobic bacteria, fungi, and *Mycobacterium tuberculosis*, are sometimes responsible. In about 25% of cases cultures are polymicrobial.

6. What are the significant symptoms and signs?

Renal abscess has an abrupt onset. Chills, fever, and localized costovertebral angle tenderness and pain are typical features. When the etiology is associated with lower urinary tract infection, urinary symptoms include increased frequency and urgency of urination and dysuria. Nausea and vomiting may be present, often causing the clinician to suspect intraperitoneal disease. Symptoms of perinephric abscesses are often insidious in nature. Usually patients are symptomatic for several weeks before seeking medical attention and have a confusing clinical presentation. Fever and malaise are often present. Most renal and perirenal abscesses are unilateral. Physical examination findings include flank and costovertebral angle tenderness. Scoliosis with concavity toward the side with abscess is common. In extensive renal abscesses or in perirenal abscesses, flank or abdominal mass and edema of the flank skin may be noticed. Extension of the thigh increases the pain secondary to stretching of the psoas muscle.

7. Which laboratory tests are helpful in evaluation?

Complete blood count usually shows marked leukocytosis with shift to the left in the acute abscess; in longstanding infection, however, leukocytosis may be moderate. With communication between the abscess cavity and the renal collecting system, urinalysis reveals leukocytes, and urinary culture is usually positive. Both findings also are present in renal and perirenal abscesses secondary to urinary tract infections. In hematogenous infection urinalysis may be negative. Depending on the associated renal involvement and abnormalities, levels of serum urea nitrogen and creatinine may be normal or elevated. Patients with diabetes who have an abscess often have hyperglycemia, ketoaciduria, and glycosuria. In addition to urine culture, blood cultures should be obtained to identify bacteriemia.

8. Which imaging studies are most helpful?

Plain radiography of the abdomen often shows a mass effect, and scoliosis with concavity toward the affected side is usually present. The renal size may be enlarged, and if the inflammation is extrarenal, the shadow of the psoas muscle is lost. Intravenous urography may suggest the pathology, but ultrasonography and particularly computed tomographic (CT) scanning are fundamental in the diagnosis of retroperitoneal abscesses and in establishing the location, size, and extension of the abscess. CT scan is more helpful than ultrasonography and should be obtained in every patient suspected of having retroperitoneal abscess. Renal arteriography and radionuclide scanning are seldom diagnostic.

9. What is the treatment of renal and perirenal abscesses?

Until culture and sensitivity test results are available, parenteral board-spectrum antimicrobial therapy should be directed against the wide range of parenteral pathogens. Usually a combination of aminoglycoside and broad-spectrum penicillin is a proper initial treatment. If staphylococcal infection is suspected, therapy should include a beta-lactamase–resistant penicillin. Antibacterial therapy should be adjusted according to culture results and clinical response. Parenteral therapy should be continued for 7–14 days and followed by several weeks of oral therapy. As a general rule, abscesses have to be drained. Only small, localized lesions with prompt response to antibiotic therapy can be managed conservatively. CT- or ultrasonography-guided percutaneous drainage can be used when the abscess is not loculated. If drainage appears to be inadequate, open surgical drainage should be performed promptly. Perirenal abscesses always should be treated with early and thorough drainage. Traditionally open drainage has been advocated. Recently, appropriate percutaneous drainage has been reported in selected cases. Rarely nephrectomy may be required to control extensive renal involvement.

10. What are the treatment outcomes?

In treatment experiences reported several decades ago, the mortality rate was about 50%. Early diagnosis with improved imaging modalities, particularly CT and ultrasonography, now leads to prompt treatment and improved rates of patient survival. More effective antimicrobial therapy and better supportive care also may contribute to the improvement. Currently, survival is expected to be 90% or better. Patients with less extensive renal abscesses have a better prognosis than patients with perirenal abscesses.

BIBLIOGRAPHY

1. Edelstein H, McCabe R: Perinephric abscess: Modern diagnosis and treatment in 47 cases. Medicine 67:118–131, 1988.
2. Fowler JE Jr, Perkias T: Presentation, diagnosis and treatment of renal abscesses: 1972–1988. J Urol 151:847–851, 1994.

3. Gerzof SG: Percutaneous drainage of renal and perirenal abscess. Urol Radiol 2:171, 1981.
4. Gerzof SG, Gale ME: Computed tomography and ultrasonography for the diagnosis and treatment of renal and retroperitoneal abscesses. Urol Clin North Am 9:185–193, 1982.
5. Gillenwater JY, Grayhack JT, Howards SS, Duckett JW (eds): Adult and Pediatric Urology, 2nd ed. Chicago, Year Book, 1991.
6. Thornbury JR: Acute renal infections. Urol Radiol 12:209–213, 1991.
7. Walsh PC, Retik AB, Stamey TA, Vaughan ED Jr (eds): Campbell's Urology, 6th ed. Philadelphia, W. B. Saunders, 1992.

59. RENAL TUBERCULOSIS

Lawrence M. Wyner, M.D.

1. How many people worldwide are infected with the tubercle bacillus?
Approximately 1 billion, of whom 10 million are Americans.

2. How many people worldwide develop clinical tuberculosis (TB) each year?
Approximately 10 million, of whom roughly 20,000 are Americans. The vast majority of cases arise from reactivation, often many years after the initial exposure.

3. How common is extrapulmonary TB in patients who have already been diagnosed with pulmonary TB?
About one-sixth of patients with pulmonary involvement develop tuberculous disease in other organs. This risk is doubled in patients with compromised immune function, poor nutrition, or poor living conditions.

4. What organs are most commonly involved in extrapulmonary TB?
Lymph nodes, intestine, bone, kidneys.

5. Renal TB cases represent what percentage of extrapulmonary TB?
Roughly 20%.

6. Are there any symptoms that suggest a diagnosis of renal TB?
Early in the disease process, patients present with vague, nonspecific symptoms, such as lethargy, malaise, low-grade fever, and weight loss. Urinary seeding of the bladder gives rise to frequency and dysuria. Flank pain and hematuria usually take years to develop, after considerable renal destruction and stricture formation have occurred.

7. Are there any characteristic physical findings in renal TB?
Because urinary seeding may affect any genitourinary organ, in males, thickening or coarseness of the epididymides or prostate or a "beaded" vas deferens may be seen. Upper abdominal bruits may indicate advanced renal destruction, with obliterative changes of the renal artery and its branches.

8. What does the urinalysis show in renal TB?
About 50% of patients have microscopic hematuria, and almost all have pyuria. Proteinuria is common, too.

9. What does "sterile pyuria" mean?
Actually, this is a misnomer, since the urine of patients with renal TB is loaded with tubercle bacilli! The phrase reminds us that a routine urine culture will not detect the tubercle bacillus and that special media are required to grow this organism. Remember also that at least 20% of patients with renal TB have a superimposed bacterial urinary tract infection, so that a positive routine urine culture does not rule out coexisting renal TB. Moreover, tetracycline and sulfa drugs are bacteriostatic for the tubercle bacillus, and ofloxacin and ciprofloxacin are mycobactericidal; thus, their use may result in false-negative urinary cultures for acid-fast bacteria. A minimum of three early morning urine specimens are recommended to culture these bacteria successfully.

10. What blood work is helpful in managing these patients?
Baseline renal and hepatic function should be assessed, since antibiotic therapy may cause liver

toxicity, and doses may need to be adjusted for renal insufficiency. The erythrocyte sedimentation rate also is useful in monitoring the response to treatment.

11. Is the tuberculin skin test usually positive in patients with renal TB?
Yes, in greater than 90%.

12. What are the characteristic intravenous pyelogram (IVP) findings of renal TB?
About half of the patients have renal calcifications on the KUB film. Although renal TB is a bilateral disease, typically one kidney is affected more severely. Contrast excretion is poor on the more involved side. The parenchyma is deformed and may be completely destroyed (autonephrectomy). The minor calyces are dilated and irregular, and intrarenal fistulae may be seen. The ureters may be straightened or strictured, and the bladder capacity is diminished. Infundibular stenosis is pathognomonic of renal TB. In children and in patients whose disease is diagnosed early, however, the IVP may be normal.

13. What are the characteristic ultrasound findings of renal TB?
A nonfunctioning kidney on IVP, with a normal appearance on ultrasound, should at least raise the suspicion of early renal TB, since diffuse parenchymal tuberculomas can account for this scenario. Later, with the development of profound calyectasis and contraction of the renal pelvis, the so-called "daisy sign" is seen—a ring of dilated calyces often without a demonstrable renal pelvis.

14. Describe the characteristic pathologic features of renal TB.
Hematogenous spread of tubercle bacilli to the kidneys from a primary infection site, usually the lungs, causes tuberculomas to develop in the glomerular capillaries. The organisms then spread along the nephron to the loop of Henle. Granuloma formation ensues, with caseous necrosis of the renal papillae and deformity of the collecting system.

15. List two consequences of chronic inflammation on the urothelium.
1. Stricture formation.
2. Squamous metaplasia, with resultant squamous cell carcinoma.

16. How is renal TB treated?
Isoniazid and rifampin are administered for 9 months. If the organism is resistant to one of these agents, either streptomycin and pyrazinamide, or ethambutol, is added. Always obtain a chest x-ray and sputum for acid-fast bacteria before beginning treatment. If there is concomitant pulmonary tuberculosis, the 9-month course of therapy should be adequate to treat both sites of infection.

17. What are the side effects of the antituberculous drugs?

Side Effects of Antituberculous Drugs

DRUG	SIDE EFFECTS
Isoniazid	Hepatotoxicity; urticaria; fever; neurotoxicity (may be alleviated by pyridoxine).
Rifampin	Hepatotoxicity; may decrease serum levels of other drugs that undergo hepatic metabolism (e.g., estrogens, warfarin, digoxin, oral hypoglycemics); orange discoloration of body fluids; thrombocytopenic purpura; flu-like syndrome; gastrointestinal upset
Streptomycin	Ototoxicity
Pyrazinamide	Gastrointestinal upset; gouty arthralgias
Ethambutol	Optic neuritis; gouty arthralgias

18. Is surgery ever indicated in the treatment of renal TB?
Very rarely, since effective antibiotics alone cure more than 95% of patients. However, for those with intractable pain or hypertension or with chronic bacterial infection proximal to a strictured ureteral segment, partial or total nephrectomy may be needed.

19. How are patients with renal TB followed up?
Compliance with the antibiotic regimen is crucial to ensure proper treatment and to prevent resistant organisms from developing. A medical social worker should be involved early, and the local public health department must be notified. Patients are no longer contagious after 2–3 weeks on antituberculous therapy. Urine for acid-fast bacilli should be obtained at 2–3 month intervals to assess both the adequacy of therapy and the possible emergence of resistant organisms.

20. What is the most common iatrogenic cause of TB?
BCG bladder instillation for treatment of superficial bladder cancer.

21. What is BCG?
BCG stands for bacille Calmette-Guérin, a live-attenuated TB vaccine which produces intense urothelial inflammation when administered intravesically, sometimes leading to granulomatous prostatitis. Acute BCG sepsis occurs when the tubercle bacillus enters the bloodstream (e.g., from an unrecognized traumatic catheterization).

22. Is there a key drug to use in the treatment of acute BCG sepsis?
Cycloserine. It inhibits growth of the tubercle bacillus within 24 hours. It is used in combination with isoniazid, rifampin, and ethambutol.

23. What is the major side effect of cycloserine?
It lowers the seizure threshold.

BIBLIOGRAPHY

1. Centers for Disease Control: Tuberculosis control laws—United States, 1993. MMWR 42(Nov 12): 42(RR–15):1–28, 1993.
2. Cos LR, Cockett ATK: Genitourinary tuberculosis revisited. Urology 20:111–117, 1982.
3. Dutt AK, Moers D, Stead WW: Short-course chemotherapy for extrapulmonary tuberculosis: Nine years' experience. Ann Intern Med 104:7–12, 1986.
4. Ehrlich RM, Lattimer JK: Urogenital tuberculosis in children. J Urol 105:461–465, 1971.
5. Gow JG: Genitourinary tuberculosis. In Walsh PC, Retik AB, Stamey TA, Vaughan ED (eds): Campbell's Urology, 6th ed. Philadelphia, W.B. Saunders Co., 1992, pp 951–981.
6. Kaufman JJ, Goodwin WE: Renal hypertension secondary to renal tuberculosis. Am J Med 38:337–344, 1965.
7. Lamm DL: Complications of bacillus Calmette-Guérin immunotherapy. Urol Clin North Am 19:565–572, 1992.
8. O'Sullivan DC, Murphy D, Conlon P, Walshe J: Hypercalcemia due to squamous cell carcinoma in a tuberculous kidney: Case report and review of pathogenesis. Br J Urol 73:106–107, 1994.
9. Pitchenik AE, Fertel D: Tuberculosis and nontuberculous mycobacterial disease. Med Clin North Am 76:121–171, 1992.
10. Scott RF, Engelbrecht HE: Ultrasonography of the advanced tuberculous kidney. S Afr Med J 75:371–372, 1989.
11. Simon HB, Weinstein AJ, Pasternak MS, et al: Genitourinary tuberculosis—Clinical features in a general hospital population. Am J Med 63:410–420, 1977.
12. Snider DE: Introduction. In: Fogarty International Center Workshop, National Institutes of Health, Bethesda, MD, 1988: Research towards global control and prevention of tuberculosis with an emphasis on vaccine development. Rev Infect Dis 11 (suppl 2): S336–S338, 1989.
13. Weinberg AC, Boyd SD: Short-course chemotherapy and role of surgery in adult and pediatric genitourinary tuberculosis. Urology 31:95–102, 1988.

60. RETROPERITONEAL FIBROSIS

Ernest E. Hodge, M.D.

1. What is retroperitoneal fibrosis?

Retroperitoneal fibrosis is the formation of a fibrotic plaque that is usually centered over L4 and L5 and extends caudally to the sacral promontory and cephalad to the renal hilum. The lateral margins of extent are typically the outer edges of the psoas muscle. Occasionally, the fibrotic plaque extends caudally along the iliac vessels.

2. Does retroperitoneal fibrosis extend to other areas?

Yes. It has been associated with mediastinal fibrosis, mesenteric fibrosis, sclerosing cholangitis, Reidel's fibrosing thyroiditis, and fibrotic orbital pseudotumors.

3. What are the causes of retroperitoneal fibrosis?

Retroperitoneal fibrosis is idiopathic in two-thirds of cases. Numerous causes have been reported for the other one-third of patients, including drugs, especially methysergide (which was commonly used to treat migraine headaches and accounts for approximately 10% of all cases of retroperitoneal fibrosis), malignancies, infections, radiation, and other inflammatory conditions.

Causes of Retroperitoneal Fibrosis

Idiopathic	Malignancies
Drugs	Primary (lymphoma, sarcoma, etc.)
Amphetamines	Metastatic
Analgesics (phenacetin)	Inflammatory lesions
Beta blockers	Inflammatory bowel disease
Methyldopa (Aldomet)	Other GI tract infections (diverticulitis, etc.)
Lysergic acid diethylamide (LSD)	Biliary tract disease
Methysergide (Sansert)	Endometriosis
Other ergot alkaloids (bromocriptine, etc.)	Sarcoidosis
Reserpine	Periarteritis
Haloperidol	Perianeurysms (aortic or iliac)
Infections	Collagen vascular disease
Chronic urinary tract infections	Autoimmune diseases
Gonorrhea	Urinary extravasation
Syphilis	Hemorrhage (trauma, Henoch-Schönlein, etc.)
Tuberculosis	Previous intraabdominal surgery
Radiation	

4. Is there an explanation for idiopathic retroperitoneal fibrosis?

Many believe that it is the result of an immunologic response to the leakage of material from diseased (atherosclerotic) blood vessels, although the true etiology is unknown.

5. How often does retroperitoneal fibrosis occur?

Retroperitoneal fibrosis is uncommon, with a prevalence of approximately 1/200,000 population. It is usually diagnosed between ages 30 and 60, and idiopathic retroperitoneal fibrosis occurs twice as commonly in males as females.

6. Name the consequences of retroperitoneal fibrosis.

The most common sequelae is obstructive uropathy secondary to ureteral compression. However, intestinal, venous, and, less commonly, arterial and biliary obstruction also occur.

7. What clinical symptoms do patients experience?

Most patients generally present with vague symptoms including low back pain, malaise, anorexia, and weight loss. Occasionally, patients may exhibit low-grade fever and symptoms specifically related to areas of obstruction, i.e., lower extremity edema from venous obstruction.

8. Are there any abnormal laboratory values associated with retroperitoneal fibrosis?

While there are no specific laboratory values associated with retroperitoneal fibrosis, approximately 60–90% of patients have an elevated erythrocyte sedimentation rate, a nonspecific indicator of inflammation. Anemia and leukocytosis may also be present as well as varying degrees of azotemia.

9. Which radiographic studies best demonstrate retroperitoneal fibrosis? What are the findings?

Historically, the **intravenous urogram** has been used to identify the findings of retroperitoneal fibrosis, which include long narrowed segments of the ureter with medial deviation of the middle third of the ureters and hydronephrosis. However, the medial deviation is not always present in retroperitoneal fibrosis, and as many as 20% of individuals with normal urinary tracts have medial deviations of the ureters on an intravenous urogram. More recently, **computed tomography** (CT) and **magnetic resonance imaging** (MRI) have been used to better delineate retroperitoneal fibrosis, which is seen as a mass encompassing the vena cava and aorta.

10. Are the radiographic findings sufficient to diagnose the cause?

No. Although MRI may in a few cases, radiographic imaging currently does not allow differentiation between malignant and benign causes of retroperitoneal fibrosis. A firm diagnosis and a differentiation between malignant and benign retroperitoneal fibrosis require multiple deep biopsies of the mass.

11. Is a percutaneous biopsy adequate?

The dispersed nature of the cellular infiltrate in malignant retroperitoneal fibrosis often requires multiple deep surgical biopsies. The tissue obtained with percutaneous biopsies is often inadequate.

12. What is the gross appearance of retroperitoneal fibrosis?

Grossly, the fibrotic plaque is grayish white and has a firm, woody consistency.

13. How about the microscopic appearance?

Early in the disease process, histologic examination of the plaque reveals a cellular immature fibrotic process with many inflammatory cells (primarily lymphocytes and plasma cells) and fibroblasts. Later, as the plaque matures, it becomes relatively acellular and is composed primarily of dense hyalinized collagen. This progresses from the medial aspect of the plaque laterally, and thus biopsies from the lateral edges may still show a relatively cellular picture late in the disease.

14. How is retroperitoneal fibrosis treated?

The treatment is dictated by the underlying cause. If medication such as methysergide is thought to be responsible, cessation of the medication often will result in resolution. Malignancies are treated according to their cell type. Idiopathic retroperitoneal fibrosis often responds to corticosteroids and/or additional immunosuppressive medications. However, especially in advanced disease, the patient often requires surgical intervention to free up the ureters and other structures to alleviate obstruction.

15. Are steroids alone really effective therapy?

Yes. Although for a number of years, steroids were thought to be indicated as adjunctive therapy to surgery or used only in patients who were poor surgical risks, recent reports describing significant improvement with steroids warrants an attempt at initial medical therapy, with surgery being reserved for medical failures. The patient may require temporary relief of ureteral obstruction with ureteral stents or percutaneous nephrostomies in the early course of treatment.

16. What is the prognosis following treatment for retroperitoneal fibrosis?
Assuming that irreversible renal damage has not occurred secondary to long-standing obstruction, the prognosis is good for patients who have been treated for retroperitoneal fibrosis. However, patients have experienced relapses of the disease ranging from a short interval to many years following therapy and thus must have lifelong careful follow-up with ultrasound.

BIBLIOGRAPHY

1. Amis ES Jr: Retroperitoneal fibrosis: Review article. AJR 157:321–329, 1991.
2. Cedron M, Payne CK, Pollack HM: Diseases of the retroperitoneum. In Gillenwater JY, Grayhack JT, Howards SS, Duckett JW (eds): Adult and Pediatric Urology, 2nd ed. St. Louis, Mosby Yearbook, 1991, pp 917–931.
3. Hodge EE: Operations of the ureter. In Novick AC, Streem SB, Pontes JE (eds): Stewart's Operative Urology, 2nd ed. Baltimore, Williams & Wilkins, 1989, pp 369–373.
4. Hughes D, Buckley PJ: Idiopathic retroperitoneal fibrosis is a microphage-rich process: Implications for its pathogenesis and treatment. Am J Surg Pathol 17:482–490, 1993.
5. McDougal WS, MacDonell RC Jr: Treatment of idiopathic retroperitoneal fibrosis by immunosuppression. J Urol 145:112–114, 1991.
6. Persky L, Kursh ED, Feldman S, Resnick MI: Diseases of the retroperitoneum: Retroperitoneal fibrosis. In Walsh PC, Retik AB, Stamey TA, Vaughan ED Jr (eds): Campbell's Urology, 6th ed. Philadelphia, W.B. Saunders, 1992, pp 595–613.

61. INTERSTITIAL CYSTITIS

David S. Sandock, M.D., and Elroy D. Kursh, M.D.

1. What is interstitial cystitis?
Interstitial cystitis is a noninfectious inflammation of the bladder. It is not a specific disease, but rather a symptom complex or bladder syndrome. These patients have irritative voiding symptoms (i.e., urgency, frequency, nocturia, dysuria) secondary to a decreased bladder capacity and pain related to bladder filling (usually somewhat relieved with bladder emptying). Urine culture and cytologic findings must be negative, and there should not be any other urologic abnormality that might account for the patient's symptoms.

2. What is the etiology of interstitial cystitis?
The etiology of interstitial cystitis is unknown. Many theories have been proposed: infection, lymphatic congestion, neuropathy, deficient protective bladder lining, psychologic abnormalities, immunologic abnormalities, and secondary to toxic substances in the urine. While none of these has been proven, the current most-accepted premise is that interstitial cystitis is due to a deficiency in the glycosaminoglycan lining of the bladder transitional cell epithelium, which allows the constituents of normal urine to leak into the bladder wall and establish the inflammation.

3. Who is affected by interstitial cystitis?
Most patients are reproductive-age women. Interstitial cystitis is much more common in women than men (by at least 10 times) and is rare in children and the elderly. Affected patients may have minimal symptoms for several years prior to an abrupt worsening of their symptoms. In most patients, the disease generally stabilizes at some time. Many find that they can live with the symptoms once they realize they do not have cancer.

4. How does one make a diagnosis of interstitial cystitis?
Interstitial cystitis is a diagnosis of exclusion. There is no absolute test to confirm the diagnosis. If a patient has urgency, frequency, nocturia, suprapubic pain related to bladder filling, positive findings at cystoscopy, combined with negative urine culture and cytologic results, a presumptive diagnosis of interstitial cystitis is made.

5. How is cystoscopy performed?
Cystoscopy must be performed under general or spinal anesthesia and accompanied by distention of the bladder with fluid (**hydrodistention**). Hydrodistention is accomplished by filling the bladder to capacity under the force of gravity only, with the water source at 80–100 cm above the patient's bladder. Hydrodistention is both diagnostic and therapeutic.

6. What are the typical findings on cystoscopy?
The most common initial finding at cystoscopy is that the patient has a markedly reduced bladder capacity; however, this is not diagnostic. The two findings indicative of interstitial cystitis are **glomerulations** and **Hunner's ulcers.** Glomerulations are typically round submucosal hemorrhages and should be viewed in several different quadrants of the bladder. Hunner's ulcers are salmon-pink ulcerations in the bladder mucosa and are less commonly seen. The presence of either glomerulations or Hunner's ulcers is required for a diagnosis of interstitial cystitis.

7. What is the differential diagnosis?
- Infections of the bladder (bacterial cystitis, viral cystitis, tuberculous cystitis, malacoplakia)
- Infections of the urethra (urethritis, urethral syndrome)

- Malignant processes (carcinoma-in-situ, transitional cell carcinoma of the bladder)
- Other inflammatory diseases of the bladder (e.g., radiation- and cyclophosphamide-induced cystitis)

8. Is a bladder biopsy indicated?

Although it is somewhat controversial, biopsy is not necessary for the diagnosis of interstitial cystitis. The main indication for biopsy is to rule out carcinoma-in-situ rather than to confirm a diagnosis of interstitial cystitis. The decision to biopsy should be based on the urologist's suspicion of the presence of a malignant process. There are no pathognomonic findings of interstitial cystitis on biopsy, but when examined, the biopsy material may demonstrate submucosal edema, mast cell infiltrates, perineural inflammation, or fibrosis.

9. What medical treatments are available for interstitial cystitis?

Before any treatment is started, reassurance is imperative. Once the diagnosis is made, the patient must be made aware that even though the symptoms are annoying, there is no increased risk of cancer. An important role of the physician is to provide encouragement and to help the patient cope with the bothersome symptoms. Treatment options range from medical to surgical and may be local or systemic in nature. The usual first treatment is hydrodistention, since this is part of the diagnostic work-up. Hydrodistention offers relief for approximately 50–60% of patients.

The next line of therapy consists of serial **local instillations** of various chemical agents, such as dimethylsulfoxide (DMSO) or heparin, into the bladder. DMSO is an anti-inflammatory agent and supposedly works by degranulating bladder mast cells. Heparin is a naturally occurring glycosaminoglycan and may help restore the protective glycosaminoglyian layer of the bladder.

Patients may also be given a trial of **systemic agents** such as subcutaneous heparin, oral amitriptyline or sodium pentosan polysulfate. Amitriptyline does not cure interstitial cystitis but helps the patient function better with the irritative symptoms. Sodium pentosanpolysulfate is a highly sulfated polysaccharide which augments the bladder surface defense mechanisms. All of these therapies have moderate short-term success but rather disappointing long-term success. Nonmedical therapies, such as biofeedback and bladder retraining, have also had limited success.

10. Does surgery have a role in treatment?

The most severe cases may come to surgery. Options range from cystitis (dissecting the bladder free of its nervous and vascular supply) and augmentation cystoplasty (enlarging the bladder by adding a segment of intestine) to complete urinary diversion. Only the last method is nearly 100% effective.

BIBLIOGRAPHY

1. Hanno P, Levin R, Monson F, et al: Diagnosis of interstitial cystitis. J Urol 143:278, 1990.
2. Parsons CL: Interstitial cystitis. In Kursh E, McGuire E (eds): Female Urology. Philadelphia, J.B. Lippincott, 1994, pp 421–438.
3. Parsons CL, Lilly J, Stein P: Epithelial dysfunction in non-bacterial cystitis (interstitial cystitis). J Urol 145:732, 1991.

62. PROSTATITIS

Kurt H. Dinchman, M.D.

1. What is prostatitis?
Prostatitis is a syndrome that presents with symptoms consistent with inflammation and/or infection of the prostate gland, including terminal dysuria, dysfunctional voiding, perineal pain, increased frequency of urination, and pain with ejaculation.

2. How is prostatitis classified?
Prostatitis is classified as bacterial or nonbacterial.

3. What is prostadynia?
Patients with prostadynia have symptoms consistent with prostatitis, but cultures of prostatic secretions are negative and white blood cells are absent.

4. How does acute bacterial prostatitis differ from chronic bacterial prostatitis?
Acute bacterial prostatitis is usually a febrile illness of sudden onset, characterized by severe irritative symptoms, positive urine cultures, and a boggy, enlarged, and tender prostate on physical examination.

Chronic bacterial prostatitis is characterized by persistent bacterial infections with inflammatory cells in prostatic secretions despite multiple regimens of prolonged antibiotic therapy. Patients typically have a long history of irritative symptoms, along with mild obstructive voiding.

5. How is prostatitis diagnosed?
It is difficult to diagnose prostatitis unless it is the acute bacterial variety. It is difficult to differentiate among chronic bacterial prostatitis, nonbacterial prostatitis, and prostadynia, because symptoms and physical findings may be similar.

6. What is the role of examination of prostatic secretions?
Prostatic secretions obtained by prostatic massage may reveal white blood cells from the initially voided specimen; bacterial may be seen in acute prostatitis.

7. What are segmented cultures?
Segmented cultures are quantative cultures aimed at localizing bacteria to a particular segment of the urinary tract. Usually four segments are cultured. The first segment called VB_1, is the first voided 10 ml of urine. A positive VB_1 culture indicates urethritis and/or prostatitis. A positive VB_2 (midstream urine) culture indicates cystitis. EPS, or expressed positive cultures of VB_3 (first 10 ml of urine voided after prostatic massage), and expressed prostatic secretions (ESP) indicate prostatic infection.

8. What is the most common pathogen in prostatitis?
Escherichia coli by far is the most common. Other agents include *Enterobacter, Proteus, Klebsiella,* and *Pseudomonas* spp.

9. What are the most commonly used antibiotic agents in the treatment of prostatitis? Why?
The most commonly used agent is trimethoprim-sulfamethoxazole, given orally in a dose of 160–180 mg twice a day. In a sulfa-allergic patient, ciprofloxacin (a fluoroquinolone), 500 mg twice a day, is also an excellent choice. Both are superior to other agents because of their 2:1–3:1 concentration in prostatic tissue vs. serum.

10. How do treatment plans differ between acute and chronic prostatitis?

Acute prostatitis often presents with systemic manifestations. The involved pathogen is usually a gram-negative agent and may require parenteral administration of antibiotics, such as an aminoglycoside and ampicillin, followed by a 4-week regimen of oral antibiotics to avert chronic bacterial prostatitis. Chronic bacterial prostatitis may require a prolonged antibiotic schedule. Patients often have prostatic calculi, which may harbor bacteria that present a potential for reinfection; chronic suppression may be required.

11. How is nonbacterial prostatitis treated?

Because no pathogen is isolated, a regimen of a broad-range antibiotic, such as doxycycline, may be tried. Patients with unsatisfactory results may be managed with anti-inflammatory agents.

12. How is prostadynia treated?

Prostadynia is by far the most difficult prostatic syndrome to treat; no infectious or inflammatory process is established. Patients are counseled on the nature of the syndrome, and treatment with an α-adrenergic agent and muscle relaxants, such as diazepam, has proved to be marginally successful.

13. What are the other forms of prostatitis?

Gonococcal prostatitis   Mycotic prostatitis
Tuberculous prostatitis   Nonspecific granulomatous prostatitis
Parasitic prostatitis

14. What is a prostatic abscess? How is it treated?

A prostatic abscess is a life-threatening infection of the prostate seen in immunocompromised patients, such as those with diabetes and renal failure. Treatment consists of immediate surgical drainage, including transurethral methods and wide-spectrum parenteral antibiotics.

BIBLIOGRAPHY

1. Gillenwater JY, Grayhack JT, Howards SS, Duckett JW (eds): Adult and Pediatric Urology, 2nd ed. Chicago, Year Book, 1993.
2. Walsh PC, Retik AB, Stamey TA, Vaughan ED Jr (eds): Campbell's Urology, 6th ed. Philadelphia, W.B. Saunders, 1992.
3. Seidman EJ, Hanno PM (eds): Current Urologic Therapy. Philadelphia, W.B. Saunders, 1994.

63. URINARY TRACT INFECTION IN ADULT FEMALES

David S. Sandock, M.D., and Elroy D. Kursh, M.D.

1. What is a urinary tract infection (UTI)?

A UTI is an inflammation of the urinary tract secondary to an infectious agent. This is most commonly due to bacteria, and a urine culture colony count of 10^5 colony-forming units (cfu)/ml is considered to be a significant infection. Bacteria in the urine without symptoms is referred to as asymptomatic bacteriuria. Bacteriuria $< 10^5$ cfu/ml may be a contamination or colonization and is generally not referred to as an infection.

2. How are UTIs classified?

UTIs may be classified as complicated or uncomplicated; upper tract or lower tract; first infection, recurrent infection, or resistant infection. They may also be classified by the type of infecting organism.

An uncomplicated UTI implies an infection with no associated fever in a patient with a normal urinary tract. A complicated UTI implies that the infection will be more difficult to treat, as in the case of a patient with a urinary tract abnormality or pyelonephritis. Upper tract UTI generally refers to an infection of the kidney, or pyelonephritis. Lower tract UTI refers to infections of the bladder (cystitis) or urethra (urethritis). The infecting organism may be bacterial, fungal, or viral.

Most infections in adult females are uncomplicated, lower tract, bacterial cystitis.

3. What are the classic symptoms and signs of acute cystitis and pyelonephritis?

Patients with **acute bacterial cystitis** experience dysuria, frequency, urgency, cloudy foul-smelling urine, pyuria (urinalysis reveals white blood cells), bacteriuria (urinalysis reveals bacteria), and sometimes hematuria. Patients with **pyelonephritis** generally have a fever (>38.0°C), chills, flank pain, flank tenderness, as well as the signs and symptoms of cystitis. Patients may also have nausea and vomiting.

4. How does one diagnose a UTI?

1. Clinical signs and symptoms
2. Microscopic examination of the urinary sediment
3. Quantitative urine culture

5. How should the urine specimen be obtained for culture?

In most cases, a clean-catch, midstream, voided urine sample is adequate. If this is not possible or appears contaminated, a straight catheterization or suprapubic aspiration is necessary.

6. What are the most common pathogens in female UTIs?

Escherichia coli is responsible for 70–85% of community-acquired UTIs in reproductive-aged women. *Staphylococcus saprophyticus* is the second most common pathogen, accounting for 10–20%. The remainder are caused mostly by gram-negative enteric bacilli.

7. What is the most common route of infection in female UTIs?

Ascending infection from the urethra is the most common route of entry of bacteria into the urinary tract. Because of the relatively short female urethra and a tendency for the vagina and perineum to be colonized with enteric organisms, women are especially susceptible to this route of entry. Less common routes include hematogenous (i.e., tuberculosis) and lymphatogenous as well as direct extension from another organ (i.e., inflammatory bowel disease, fistulas).

8. Describe the treatment for a UTI in an adult female.

After a culture is sent, the patient with **acute bacterial cystitis** should be started empirically on a short course (3–5 days) of a broad-spectrum antibiotic which covers most enteric pathogens (e.g. trimethoprim-sulfamethoxazole, nitrofurantoin, or amoxicillin/clavulanate). Because **pyeloneph-ritis** may lead to renal damage if untreated, patients should be started on broad-spectrum antibiotics immediately. Some patients with minimal symptoms may be treated as outpatients, although most should be hospitalized to administer intravenous antibiotics. In cases of pyeloneph-ritis, a urine culture must be done prior to the first antibiotic dose. Hydration should be encouraged in all cases.

9. Describe the treatment for recurrent UTI in the adult female.

Recurrent UTIs may be classified as frequent ≥3/year) and infrequent (<3/year). In general, **infrequent recurrent UTIs** may be treated as new infections, and each episode treated with a short course of antibiotics.

   Women with **frequent recurrent UTIs** are candidates for low-dose prophylactic (suppres-sive) antibiotics for a period of approximately 6 months. Commonly used agents include single daily doses of nitrofurantoin (50–100 mg) or trimethoprim-sulfamethoxazole (80/400 mg). Most of these infections are secondary to colonization of the urethra or vulva. Not only does a course of suppressive antibiotics prevent recurrences, but it generally leads to resolution of the colonized area. Women with recurrent urinary tract infections should have further evaluation of the urinary tract.

10. What are the complications of untreated UTIs?

An untreated, uncomplicated UTI may lead to vesicoureteral reflux, ascending infection with resultant pyelonephritis, possible renal parenchymal damage, and, in rare cases, sepsis and death.

11. What is bacterial adherence?

Some bacteria have a greater ability than others to adhere themselves to the bladder urothelium. This is bacterial adherence and is due to the fimbriae, or finger-like projections, that the bacteria possess, although not all bacteria possess fimbriae. Type 1 fimbriae are present on nearly all *E. coli* species and adhere to vaginal and buccal mucosa but not to urothelium. Type 2 fimbriae, or P fimbriae, adhere very well to urothelium and are present on only some species of *E. coli*. P fimbriae adhere to P^+ blood group antigens expressed on both erythrocytes and uroepithelial cells in P^+ patients. Bacteria with P fimbriae are more likely to adhere, colonize, and therefore cause a UTI. P fimbriae bacteria are also much more likely to cause pyelonephritis than type 1 fimbriae bacteria. Approximately 30% of women have the P^+ blood group antigen.

12. When is a more thorough evaluation necessary? What workup should be performed?

If a structural or functional abnormality of the urinary tract is suspected on the basis of a poor response to treatment, recurrent infections, or unusual organisms in the urine culture, a workup is necessary.

   The usual first study of the workup is the intravenous urogram. This study delineates the anatomy of the urinary tract, provides information about renal function, and reveals the presence of urinary calculi. Additional studies, such as renal ultrasound, computed tomography, renal scintigraphy, voiding cystourethrography, cystoscopy, and retrograde ureteropyelography may be performed depending on the results of the intravenous urogram.

13. Should UTIs be treated in pregnancy?

Yes. All bacteriuria, symptomatic or asymptomatic, should be treated with a course of the appropriate antibiotic.

14. What antibiotics are considered safe during pregnancy?

An aminopenicillin, cephalosporin, or nitrofurantoin.

15. What is honeymoon cystitis?

Honeymoon cystitis, or postcoital cystitis, refers to the increased incidence of acute bacterial cystitis after sexual intercourse. It is thought to be secondary to the continuous massage of the urethra during intercourse, which facilitates urethral colonization and retrograde entry of bacteria into the bladder. Its incidence is dramatically decreased by postcoital voiding or single-dose postcoital antibiotic prophylaxis.

BIBLIOGRAPHY

1. Norrby S: Short term treatment of uncomplicated lower urinary tract infections in women. Rev Infect Dis 12:458, 1990.
2. Stamey T: Pathogenesis and Treatment of Urinary Tract Infections. Baltimore, Williams & Wilkins, 1980.
3. Stamm W, McKevitt M, Johnson J: Urinary tract infections: From pathogenesis to treatment. J Infect Dis 159:400, 1989.

64. URINARY TRACT INFECTIONS IN CHILDREN

Jack S. Elder, M.D.

1. What is a urinary tract infection?

A urinary tract infection (UTI) is a bacterial infection in the urine. The number of bacteria that must be present to cause a significant urinary infections is 10,000 to 100,000 colony/forming units/ml of voided urine. The infection may involve the kidney, termed pyelonephritis, or the bladder, termed cystitis.

2. What is the incidence of bacteriuria in boys and girls?

Childhood UTIs are more common in girls, except during the first few months of life, when they are more common in boys. Between 0.03% and 1.2% of boys develop a UTI during school years; 3% to 5% of girls develop a UTI during this time.

3. How is the diagnosis of a UTI made?

The diagnosis of UTI usually is made from urinalysis and urine culture. In infants and in children who are not toilet trained, a clean bag is placed over the genitalia, which have been washed. This "bag specimen" may be unreliable because of bacterial contamination of the bag itself or contamination from bacteria that have colonized the skin. If the urinalysis from a bag specimen shows significant pyuria, if only one organism is cultured, and if the child is symptomatic, then the bag specimen may be considered to be reliable. However, if any of these three criteria is not met, one may **not** conclude that the child has a UTI. Instead, the infection should be confirmed with either a catheterized urine specimen or a suprapubic tap.

In older patients, diagnosis of a UTI usually is based on a voided specimen, which should grow at least 10,000 and preferably 100,000 colonies of a single organism.

4. At what ages are UTIs most commonly diagnosed?

In boys UTIs are most common between birth and 6 months, whereas in girls the peak incidence is 2–3 years.

5. What are the typical symptoms and signs of UTIs?

Urinary tract infections may be subclassified into cystitis and pyelonephritis. Typically, children with cystitis have dysuria, urgency, frequency, suprapubic pain, and often have incontinence also. An associated symptom is malodorous urine. In some cases the only manifestation of a UTI may be day and night incontinence or nocturnal enuresis.

Pyelonephritis refers to a renal infection. Typical symptoms include fever and upper abdominal or flank pain localized to the side of the infection; some may experience malaise, nausea, vomiting and diarrhea.

6. What are typical symptoms of UTIs in infants?

Approximately 66% have fever, 55% have irritability, 40% exhibit poor feeding, 35% have vomiting, and 31% have diarrhea; abdominal distention and jaundice occur in < 10% of patients.

7. How accurate is urinalysis in the diagnosis of a UTI?

Although pyuria, nitrites, and leukocyte esterase are helpful in indicating that a UTI is present, a positive urine culture is necessary to confirm the diagnosis.

8. What is the Griess test?

This test refers to the reagent for the detection of nitrites in solution. Given adequate contact, bacteria convert nitrate normally present in the urine to nitrite. Reagent paper is impregnated with sulfanilic acid and alpha-naphthylamine. In the presence of nitrites, a diazotization reaction occurs, causing the two substances to form a red azo dye. A positive colorimetric reaction implies the presence of bacteria in the urine. Approximately 4 hours is necessary for conversion of nitrate to nitrite. Thus, the first morning urine is the only reliable specimen for this test. The test has a specificity of 92–100% but a sensitivity of 35–85%.

9. What is the leukocyte esterase reaction?
The esterase enzyme, which is released by polymorphonuclear leukocytes, acts on an ester substrate on a test strip to produce the indoxyl compound. Two indoxyl molecules in the presence of oxygen will form indigo, a dark blue shade. The leukocyte esterase activity can thus be substantiated by a positive blue reaction.

10. What is the route of entry for children with cystitis?
The urethra. The bacteria causing cystitis come from stool flora. In uncircumcised males, bacteria that have colonized the glans often are the source of bacteriuria.

11. In children with pyelonephritis, what is the source of bacteria?
Pyelonephritis results from an ascending infection from the bladder, and the bacteria come from the stool flora.

12. What host factors normally resist UTI?
An acidic urine pH, high or low urine osmolality, and high urea and organic acid content resist bacterial growth. Furthermore, the ability of the bladder to empty completely helps resist bacterial colonization of the bladder. Polymorphonuclear leukoyctes are present in the bladder mucosal surface, which also resist infection.

13. What is bacterial adhesion?
Certain strains of urinary pathogens contain bacterial surface elements called fimbriae (pili), which recognize specific receptors on the epithelial cells. These fimbriae are nonflagellar, proteinaceous appendages that protrude from the bacterial cell surface like tiny hairs. The pili are classified into their ability to agglutinate erythrocytes of different animal species and by sugars that can block this hemagglutination.

Bacterial adhesion may be divided is divided into mannose-sensitive (inhibited by mannose) and mannose-resistant (adhesion not inhibited by mannose). Mannose-sensitive adhesion is mediated by type 1 fimbriae, which agglutinate guinea pig erythrocytes. Type 1 fimbriae are present on most *E. coli* strains, pathogens as well as nonpathogens. Type 2 pili or fimbriae agglutinate human erythrocytes and are mannose-resistant. An example of type 2 pili is P fimbriae, which interacts with a uroepithelial cell receptor that contains a gal-gal disaccharide, which is part of the oligosaccharide chain of the P blood group antigens. *E. coli* with P fimbriae have been identified within 90% of organisms causing pyelonephritis but < 20% of *E. coli* causing cystitis.

14. What host factors predispose to the development of UTIs?
Age: It is known that during the first few weeks of life, all babies have an increased incidence of UTIs. During this time the periurethral area of healthy girls and boys is massively colonized with aerobic bacteria, particularly *E. coli,* enterococci, and staphylococci. This colonization decreases during the first year and is unusual in children who do not get recurrent UTIs beyond the age of 5 years.

Voiding dysfunction: Urinary tract infections in girls are particularly common around 2–3 years of age, the peak age of toilet training, presumably because of mild voiding dysfunction that occurs during that time. In children with bladder instability that causes diurnal incontinence beyond the age of 3–4 years, there is a tendency not to empty the bladder completely, leaving residual urine, which also predisposes to UTI.

Vesicoureteral reflux: When urine is transported to the bladder, normally the urine remains in the bladder until it is voided, because a physiologic flap valve prevents it from returning back to the ureter and kidney. Children with reflux have an increased incidence of UTI.

Genitourinary anomalies: Several genitourinary anomalies that cause urinary stasis predispose the child to UTI: ureteropelvic junction obstruction, ureterovesical junction obstruction, retrocaval ureter, ureterocele, and posterior urethral valves.

Sex: Except for the newborn period, girls are more susceptible to UTIs than boys, presumably because the urethra is much shorter in the female.

Fecal colonization: As indicated above, the presence of urinary pathogens in the periurethral area predisposes the child to UTIs.

Chronic constipation: Some children with constipation are predisposed to UTIs because the dilated rectum interferes with voiding and may cause mild retention of urine.

Retention of foreskin: Uncircumcised male infants are much more likely to develop a UTI than boys who are circumcised, because bacteria seem to colonize the glans under the foreskin.

Host receptor activity: Uroepithelial cells from infection-prone girls and women bind *E. coli* more avidly than do cells from nonsusceptible girls. Glycolipids characterizing the P blood group system are found in host uroepithelial cells and may serve as bacterial receptors. The P blood group phenotype has been found in 90% of girls with recurrent pyelonephritis.

Immune status: Girls with a normal urinary tract and recurrent UTIs have significantly lower baseline levels of urinary IgA and a blunted response to infection. Lower baseline levels of immunoglobulins in the perineum may diminish the ability to develop a response to infection.

15. At what age are uncircumcised boys more likely to have a urinary tract infection?
They are 10–15 times more likely to have a UTI during the first year of life.

16. What is acute hemorrhagic cystitis?
Hemorrhagic cystitis refers to the passing of blood in the urine during a UTI. In children this condition may be caused by adenovirus 11. In one series of infants in children with acute hemorrhagic cystitis, 17% had an adenovirus, 17% had *E. coli,* and the remainder had no infectious agent isolated from their urine.

17. How does pyelonephritis cause renal scarring?
When a UTI is initiated, renal damage may occur by a direct effect of the bacteria, ischemia with reperfusion damage, and/or an inflammatory response. The bacteria may have a direct effect by bacterial adhesion, which brings the bacteria closer to the cell. Bacterial endotoxin is then concentrated adjacent to the cell, which activates the complement system. In addition, ischemic damage may result when the purine pool is consumed during anoxia due to anaerobic metabolism; during reperfusion the remaining hypoxanthine pool is metabolized to xanthine. In the presence of xanthine oxidase, xanthine is converted to uric acid and superoxide. Superoxide can be converted to peroxide and hydroxyl radicals, both of which are damaging to cells. Within 10 minutes after renal infection occurs, marked granulocyte aggregation may occur, which leads to capillary obstruction. During the inflammatory response, endotoxin causes complement activation, which leads to phagocytosis. This respiratory burst causes the release of superoxide and the formation of peroxide and hydroxyl radicals. All tissues in the body contain superoxide dismutase to degrade rapidly the superoxide. However, urine does not contain superoxide dismutase and thus the hydroxyl radicals act unopposed in the urine.

18. How long should a child with a UTI be treated?
Treatment depends on the age of the child and severity of the illness. In general, in children with a febrile UTI, treatment for 10–14 days is mandatory, whereas for cystitis, treatment for 5–7 days should suffice.

19. How is pyelonephritis diagnosed?
Pyelonephritis may be diagnosed on clinical factors, including fever, malaise, abdominal or flank pain, and irritability. In infants, irritability or poor feeding may be the only sign. The most accurate way of diagnosing true pyelonephritis with renal parenchymal infection is to perform a DMSA renal scan.

20. Which children should undergo radiologic evaluation for a UTI?
A UTI often is the first manifestation of a child's underlying anatomic or functional urinary tract abnormality. Approximately 30% of all children who have bacteriuria, and almost 50% of those under the age of 3 years, have abnormal radiologic studies of the urinary tract. Vesicoureteral reflux is most common. Radiologic investigation is recommended for all children under the age of 5 years with UTI, all boys irrespective of age, all girls with pyelonephritis, and following a second UTI in girls over 5 years old.

21. What does the radiologic evaluation for a UTI consist of?
The initial study is a voiding cystourethrogram to determine whether reflux or a structural abnormality of the lower urinary tract is present. Next, a renal ultrasound should be obtained to determine whether any upper urinary tract abnormalities are present. If both studies are negative, then no further evaluation is necessary at that time. However, if either study shows an abnormality, then further evaluation with an intravenous urogram or renal scan is necessary.

22. How is the child with a UTI managed following antimicrobial therapy, assuming the radiologic evaluation is normal?
The child should have a follow-up urinalysis and/or culture 1–2 weeks following treatment of the infection. In addition, attention to factors predisposing the child to a UTI (e.g., infrequent voiding, hygiene) should be reviewed with the child and family.

23. What is the management for children with recurrent UTI, assuming the radiologic evaluation is normal?
A child who has more than 2 or 3 UTIs in a period of 12 months should be managed with antimicrobial prophylaxis. In general, this consists of either trimethoprim-sulfamethoxazole, trimethoprim alone, or nitrofurantoin. These drugs are chosen because they have little effect on the stool's bacterial flora. In contrast, medication such as amoxicillin and cephalosporins cause alteration of the flora in the stool. The dosage for prophylaxis is 1/4 to 1/3 of the normal daily dose used for treatment of a UTI.

24. At what age is a child at greatest risk for renal damage from a UTI?
The child is most likely to develop renal scarring from a UTI during the first year of life. However, renal scarring may occur from pyelonephritis at any age, particularly if the infection is not treated promptly.

25. When should nitrofurantoin and sulfa derivatives be avoided?
These medications should not be administered if the patient is allergic to them. In addition, they should be avoided during the first 2 months of life. Sulfonamides displace protein-bound bilirubin and may interfere with bilirubin excretion, exacerbating neonatal physiological jaundice. Nitrofurantoin may cause hemolytic anemia because of glutathione instability in the erythrocyte during the first 2 months of life.

26. Which drugs should be used for the treatment of cystitis?
Trimethoprim-sulfamethoxazole, amoxicillin, ampicillin, cephlosporins, and nitrofurantoin often are used. Treatment should be initiated promptly, but the long-term course of therapy should depend on the results of the sensitivity studies.

27. Which drugs should be used in pyelonephritis?
As with cystitis, treatment should be initiated promptly pending sensitivity studies. In neonates or young infants, those with a complicated UTI (e.g., obstructive hydronephrosis, sepsis, stone disease, abnormal urinary tract), or vomiting, intravenous therapy with an aminoglycoside and cephalosporin or ampicillin is necessary. Otherwise, oral antibiotic therapy with trimethoprim-sulfamethoxazole, amoxicillin, or cephalosporin is satisfactory. Nitrofurantoin should not be given to children with pyelonephritis because tissue levels of the drug in the kidney are low.

28. What is the difference between a relapse and reinfection?
A relapse or persistent UTI refers to a recurrent infection with the same species and strain of organism. Most occur within a week of cessation of therapy. A reinfection refers to recurrent infection with a different organism and is more likely to appear weeks after therapy has ended.

29. What are causes of persistent UTIs?
If the UTI recurs with the same organism following the resolution of bacteriuria and cessation of antibiotics, this suggests that a source of infections may be present within the urinary tract. Causes may include an infected renal calculus, an infected calyceal diverticulum, an infected nonrefluxing ureteral stump following nephrectomy for pyonephrosis, an infected urachal cyst, or an infected necrotic papilla from papillary necrosis. These conditions are rare.

BIBLIOGRAPHY

1. Bourhier D, Abbott GD, Maling TMJ: Radiological abnormalities in infants with urinary tract infections. Arch Dis Child 59: 620, 1984.
2. Burbige KA, Retik AB, Colodny AH, et al: Urinary tract infection in boys. J Urol 132: 541, 1984.
3. Caldamone AA, Dobkin SF: Prompt treatment, probing follow-up study: Keys to managing pediatric UTI. Contemp Urol, December 1989, p 49.
4. deMan P, Jodal U, Lincolin K, Svanborg-Eden C: Bacterial attachment and inflammation in the urinary tract. J Infectious Dis 158: 29, 1988.
5. Ginsburg CM, McCracken GH, Jr: Urinary tract infections in young infants. Pediatrics 69: 409, 1982.
6. Lowe FC, Brendler CB: Evaluation of the urologic patient. In Walsh PC, Retik AB, Stamey TA, Vaughan ED Jr (eds): Campbell's Urology, 6th ed. Philadelphia, W.B. Saunders, 1992, p 307.
7. O'Regan S, Yasbeck S, Schick E: Constipation, bladder instability, urinary tract infection syndrome. Clin Nephrol 23: 152, 1985.
8. Roberts JA: Vesicoureteral reflux and pyelonephritis in the monkey: A review. J Urol 148: 1721, 1992.
9. Shortliffe LMD: Urinary tract infections in infants and children. In Walsh PC, Retik AB, Stamey TA, Vaughan ED Jr (eds): Campbell's Urology, 6th ed. Philadelphia, W.B. Saunders, 1992, p 1669.
10. Smith EM, Elder JS: Double antimicrobial prophylaxis in girls with breakthrough urinary tract infections. Urology 43: 708, 1994.
11. Spencer JR, Shaffer AJ: Pediatric urinary tract infections. Urol Clin North Am 13: 661, 1986.
12. Wiswell TE, Roscelli JD: Corroborative evidence for the decreased incidence of urinary tract infections in circumcised male infants. Pediatrics 78: 96, 1986.

65. EPIDIDYMITIS

Kenneth W. Angermeier, M.D.

1. Define acute epididymitis.
Acute epididymitis is inflammation, pain, and swelling of the epididymis of less than 6 weeks' duration.

2. What is believed to be the most common route of infection in acute epididymitis?
Most cases of epididymitis are believed to occur as a result of ascending infection from the urethra, prostate, or urinary bladder. Infected urine or secretions may enter the ejaculatory ducts and ascend the vas deferens to reach the epididymis.

3. Which microorganisms most commonly cause acute epididymitis?
In men under the age of 35 years, urethritis due to *Chlamydia trachomatis* and *Neisseria gonorrhoeae* is relatively common and accounts for the majority of cases of epididymitis in this age group. In men over the age of 35 years, bacteriuria due to progressive bladder outlet obstruction is more prevalent. In this setting, epididymitis is more often due to coliform bacteria, with *Escherichia coli* the most common.

4. What are the typical signs and symptoms of acute epididymitis?
Predisposing factors include recent severe physical strain, sexual activity or exposure to sexually transmitted disease, or a history of urethral instrumentation. The most common complaint is rapidly progressive scrotal swelling and pain, which may radiate up the spermatic cord to the lower abdomen. The overlying scrotal skin may be reddened, and the inflammatory process may give rise to a reactive hydrocele. After a period of time, the indurated, enlarged epididymis may be indistinguishable from the testis, forming one large inflammatory mass. Fever is often significant. A urethral discharge or evidence of urinary tract infection may be present. Rectal examination may demonstrate changes consistent with prostatitis. Prostatic massage should not be performed, as it may exacerbate the epididymitis.

5. What laboratory studies may help to identify the causative organism?
If a urethral discharge is present, a Gram stain may reveal the presence of intracellular gram-negative diplococci consistent with *N. gonorrhoeae*. If only white blood cells are seen, the most likely diagnosis is nongonococcal urethritis; the most common organism is *C. trachomatis*. A urinalysis and mid-stream urine culture are routinely performed to identify urinary tract infection as a result of coliform bacteria.

6. What other conditions are included in the differential diagnosis of acute, painful scrotal swelling?
The most important condition that must be excluded in making the diagnosis of acute epididymitis is testicular torsion, because delayed diagnosis may result in testicular loss. In adult men epididymitis is more common than torsion, but the latter must be considered in each instance. With torsion, the testicle is often retracted and may have a firm consistency. The spermatic cord may be thickened and difficult to palpate superior to the testicle. Early in its course, the epididymis may be palpated anterior to the testicle; however, subsequent swelling and inflammation may make this difficult. Doppler ultrasound or radionuclide scanning may provide useful information with regard to testicular blood flow but should not delay surgical exploration of possible torsion. Other less common conditions in the differential diagnosis include torsion of the testicular or epididymal appendages, testicular tumor, and trauma.

7. What are the potential complications of acute epididymitis?
An epididymal or scrotal abscess may evolve and require operative drainage. Infrequently an abscess may result in destruction of the testicle.

8. What is the treatment of acute epididymitis?
General measures include bed rest, scrotal elevation and support, and initially an ice bag to the scrotum to minimize swelling. Patients with acute epididymitis due to sexually transmitted urethritis often may be managed on an outpatient basis. Parenteral ceftriaxone is often administered initially, followed by a 14–21 day course of tetracycline or doxycycline. Sexual partners should be identified and treated. Patients with acute epididymitis secondary to coliform bacteriuria should be promptly treated with broad-spectrum antibiotics. If the infection is severe, hospitalization should be considered and parenteral therapy initiated. In less severe cases, outpatient treatment with trimethoprim-sulfamethoxazole or ciprofloxacin for 28 days is often effective.

9. In which patients with acute epididymitis is subsequent urinary tract evaluation indicated?
Patients with epididymitis due to urethritis infrequently have underlying urologic abnormalities. Men with epididymitis as a result of bacteriuria often have structural abnormalities of the urinary tract and should undergo radiographic and endoscopic evaluation.

10. Are there any special considerations when acute epididymitis occurs in children?
Younger boys usually have epididymitis as a result of bacteriuria, and structural urologic abnormalities are common. One possibility is the presence of an ectopic ureter draining into the epididymis. Conditions causing lower tract obstruction, such as unrecognized posterior urethral valves, also may lead to recurrent infection. Radiographic and endoscopic evaluation is essential.

11. What is chronic epididymitis?
Chronic epididymitis may develop after recurrent episodes of epididymitis; it is characterized by scarring and induration of the epididymis. Occlusion of epididymal tubules is not uncommon. Some patients may develop recurrent episodes of scrotal discomfort, although this is not always the case. On palpation the epididymis is thickened, mildly enlarged, and easily distinguished from the testicle. Tenderness may or may not be present during examination.

12. What are the complications of chronic epididymitis?
If chronic epididymitis is bilateral, infertility may result from diffuse scarring and occlusion of the epididymal tubules.

13. How is chronic epididymitis treated?
If clinical findings suggest that an exacerbation of chronic epididymitis is due to an infectious etiology, antibiotic therapy should be initiated. If discomfort or epididymal infection continues to occur in the setting of diffuse epididymal fibrosis, epididymectomy may be indicated.

BIBLIOGRAPHY

1. Berger RE: Sexually transmitted diseases. In Walsh PC, Retik AB, Stamey TA, Vaughan ED Jr (eds): Campbell's Urology, 6th ed. Philadelphia, W.B. Saunders, 1992, pp 830–832.
2. Berger RE, Alexander ER, Harnish JP, et al: Etiology, manifestations and therapy of acute epididymitis: Prospective study of 50 cases. J Urol 121:750, 1979.
3. Meares EM: Nonspecific infections of the genitourinary tract. In Tanagho EA, McAninch JW (eds): Smith's General Urology. Norwalk CT, Appleton & Lange, 1992, pp 228–231.

66. SCROTAL ABSCESS

Donald R. Bodner, M.D.

1. What are the normal contents of the scrotum?

The scrotum is a cutaneous pouch that contains the testis, the epididymis, and the spermatic cord structures. It is divided into two compartments by a septum that is manifest on the scrotal skin as the median raphe.

2. What are the layers of the scrotum and spermatic cord?

The scrotum is a continuation of the abdominal wall. The layers include the scrotal skin; dartos layer, immediately below the skin of which is a continuation of Colles' fascia; external spermatic fascia (continuation of external oblique aponeurosis); cremasteric muscle and fascia (internal oblique muscle); internal spermatic fascia (continuation of transversalis fascia); and tunica vaginalis.

3. How do superficial scrotal abscesses arise?

When superficial scrotal abscesses arise, they generally present as infected hair follicles and infections of scrotal lacerations or minor scrotal surgeries.

4. How do primary intrascrotal abscesses arise?

Intrascrotal abscesses usually arise from bacterial epididymal orchitis. The presumed mechanism includes retrograde passage of bacteria down the vas deferens into the epididymis or via lymphagenous or hematogenous spread to the epididymis. Neurogenic bladder, chronic catheter usage, instrumentation of the lower urinary tract and neglected epididymitis are risk factors for scrotal abscesses. Patients often have a urinary tract infection with the same organism found in the abscess.

5. How is a scrotal abscess diagnosed?

Scrotal abscess is diagnosed by inspection and palpation of the scrotum. Scrotal ultrasonography is helpful in diagnosing an abscess when an inflammatory mass is present in the scrotum. Ultrasonography also localizes the involvement of the abscess to the scrotal wall, epididymis, and/or testicle.

6. What is the treatment of a scrotal abscess?

An intrascrotal abscess, regardless of the cause, requires surgical drainage. All abscess cavities must be opened and drained, including the testicle if it is involved. The cavity should be left open and packed. If the contralateral testicle is normal, orchiectomy may be the most expeditious treatment. Epididymal function is often destroyed by the abscess. Broad-spectrum antibiotic coverage is also used, although primary treatment is surgical drainage.

7. What is Fournier's gangrene?

Jean Alfred Fournier, a French venereologist, reported five patients with unexplained gangrene of the penis and scrotum in 1882. Today Fournier's gangrene refers to any gangrenous, infectious process involving the external genitalia and perineum. It is rarely idiopathic and often arises from an infection involving the urinary tract or from direct extension from a perirectal source.

8. How is Fournier's gangrene diagnosed?

Physical examination is diagnostic. Early in the disease physical findings may be limited to swelling and erythema of the penis and scrotum. As the disease progresses, crepitus may overly the skin, extending up the abdominal wall along the distribution of Colles' fascia. A foul, feculent odor is often present and indicates an anaerobic infection.

9. What is the treatment of Fournier's gangrene?

Aggressive, broad-spectrum intravenous antibiotics, including coverage of both aerobic and anaerobic organisms, and early, wide surgical debridement are required, because mortality from this infection approaches 50%.

BIBLIOGRAPHY

1. Fuchs EF: Scrotal abscess. In Resnick MI, Kursh ED (eds): Current Therapy in Genitourinary Surgery, 2nd ed. St. Louis, Mosby, 1992, p 392.
2. Kearney GP, Carling PC: Fournier's gangrene: An approach to its management. J Urol 130:695–698, 1983.
3. Spirnak JP, Resnick MI, Hampel N, et al: Fournier's gangrene: Report of 20 patients. J Urol 131:289–291, 1984.

67. GONOCOCCAL AND NONGONOCOCCAL URETHRITIS

Allen D. Seftel, M.D.

1. What is acute urethritis?
Acute inflammation of the male urethra.

2. What are its causes?
In the older man, usually 50 or above, it is most commonly due to prostatitis. In the younger man between ages 15 and 40, acute urethritis is most commonly due to a sexually transmitted disease.

3. Which sexually transmitted diseases are implicated in acute urethritis?
Most commonly these are divided into two groups: nongonococcal urethritis and gonococcal urethritis.

4. What diagnostic tests distinguish between nongonococcal and gonococcal urethritis?
The urethral discharge should be examined both stained and unstained. If the unstained wet preparation typically shows 4–5 leukocytes/ high-powered field, the Gram stain will distinguish between nongonococcal and gonococcal urethritis. If the smear shows polymorphonuclear leukocytes containing gram-negative cocci, then the smear is considered positive and diagnosed as gonococcal urethritis, with 95% accuracy. A standard urine culture should also be obtained. Also, the smear can distinguish between trichomoniasis and other types of diseases as well.

5. How is nongonococcal urethritis treated?
Tetracycline or doxycycline may be helpful for all of the organisms except the trichomonads. Ciprofloxacin is also good for chlamydiae. Trichomoniasis is best treated with metronidazole. The sexual partner must be treated as well. Treatment for gonorrhea is with aqueous procaine penicillin or intramuscular ceftriaxone. Another possible treatment for gonorrhea is oral penicillin combined with probenecid, or another alternative is spectinomycin.

6. Are there long-term complications of these infections?
These infections could theoretically result in urethral stricture disease or perhaps infertility due to blockage of either the prostatic passage way or the urethra. Other long-term sequelae are unusual and rare.

68. SEXUALLY TRANSMITTED DISEASES

Allen D. *Seftel,* M.D.

SYPHILIS

1. What is syphilis?
Primary syphilis is a sexually transmitted genitourinary infection caused by the spirochete *Treponema pallidum.*

2. When does it occur?
Usually 2–4 weeks after sexual exposure.

3. How does it present?
It is usually a painless, papule or pustule (chancre) on the glans, corona, foreskin, shaft, or even the pubic area or scrotum. It breaks down to form an indurated, small punched-out ulcer.

4. What are the signs of syphilis?
The patient usually presents because of a painless penile sore. The ulcer is deep, has indurated edges, and a clean base.

5. How is the diagnosis made?
A diagnosis is made by finding the pathogenic spirochetes in the discharge from the ulcer on darkfield examination. Serologic tests for syphilis may remain negative for 1–3 weeks or longer after the appearance of the chancre.

6. What are the complications of syphilis?
Urologic complication of syphilis are rare.

7. How do you treat syphilis?
Penicillin is the first-line therapy. Patients allergic to penicillin should be given tetracycline. Alternatively, erythromycin is a third choice.

8. What is the prognosis?
The prognosis is excellent, if treated. Untreated syphilis may progress to neurosyphilis.

CHANCROID

9. What is chancroid?
A soft chancre. The infecting organism is *Haemophilus ducreyi,* a short, nonmotile, gram-negative streptobacillus that usually occurs in chains. The incubation period is 1–5 days.

10. How does chancroid present?
Macroscopically, one or several small penile ulcers are present, which are usually painful.

11. What are the clinical findings?
A few days after sexual exposure, one or more painful, dirty-appearing ulcers may be noted, and they gradually enlarge. Often, the inguinal nodes are involved and become large and tender. About 50% of patients usually have a fever, malaise, and headache.

12. What are the laboratory findings?
A smear with Gram's stain may show the *H. ducreyi* organism in 50% of cases. Culture is usually

more successful, and skin tests, known as the Ducrey test, are positive in about 75% of cases and remain positive for life. Biopsy of the lesion is diagnostic in all cases.

13. Complications?
Genitourinary complications of this organism may include phimosis and paraphimosis or, infrequently, destruction of penile or scrotal tissue.

14. Treatment?
Tetracycline, 500 mg every 6 hours for 10 days. Alternatively, erythromycin or trimethoprim-sulfamethoxazole may be used. Penicillin is usually not effective.

LYMPHOGRANULOMA VENEREUM (LGV)

15. What organism causes LGV?
Chlamydia trachomatis.

16. How does the disease present?
This disease is characterized by a transient genital lesion, followed by lymphadenitis and, at times, in females or homosexual men, rectal stricture. In men, the lymphatics of the inguinal or subinguinal nodes may become matted or infected.

17. What are the signs and symptoms?
The penile lesion develops 5–21 days after sexual exposure. It heals spontaneously and rapidly and is often not seen. The lesion may be papular or vesicular, although only a superficial erosion may occur. A few days or weeks later, painful enlargement of the inguinal nodes develops because the primary lesion is so often missed. This may be the initial symptom.

18. Are there laboratory findings?
There may be a leukocytosis. The intradermal Frei and complement fixation tests, if positive, are pathognomonic for present or past LGV. Specific immunofluorescence tests for antibodies can be performed.

19. What are the complications of this disease?
If untreated, multiple sinuses may develop from the involved lymph nodes. Elephantiasis of the genitalia can occur if lymphatic drainage is severely obstructed. Proctitis or rectal stricture may occur occasionally in women and rarely in men.

20. How is it treated?
Tetracycline and erythromycin are usually effective. Sulfamides can often control a secondary infection.

21. How are the complications treated?
Aspiration of infected or fluctuant lymph nodes is indicated. Draining sinuses may have to be excised. Rectal stenosis may require surgical measures.

22. What is the prognosis?
The prognosis is excellent. Only the late complications present with some difficulties.

GRANULOMA INGUINALE

23. What is granuloma inguinale?
It is a sexually transmitted chronic infection of the skin and subcutaneous tissues of the genitalia, perineum, or inguinal areas with an incubation period of 2–3 months. The infectious agent is *Calymmatobacterium granulomatis,* a bacterium related to *Klebsiella pneumoniae.*

24. What are the signs of this disease?
The first sign is an elevation on the skin on the genitals, perineum, or groin, which finally breaks down into a superficial painful ulcer that spreads and becomes quite extensive. The base of the ulcer is usually covered by pink granulation tissue that easily bleeds. There is usually a purulent discharge if a secondary infection occurs.

25. Describe the laboratory findings.
Identification of the ''Donovan body'' in large monocytes on a stained smear makes the diagnosis. Scrapings from the base of the lesion are placed in the slide, fixed in air, and stained. Wright and Giemsa staining techniques are both adequate. In case of doubt, a biopsy may be performed. Complement fixation and skin sensitivity tests are not dependable and not readily available.

26. What are the complications?
Secondary infection may cause deep ulceration and tissue destruction. Sinuses may result. Marked phimosis may occur, and a rectal stricture may occur as well.

27. How is it treated?
Tetracycline and ampicillin have proved to be effective in a high percentage of cases.

28. What is the treatment of secondary complications?
Secondary infection is effectively combatted in most cases by the drugs used to cure the primary disease. Rectal stricture may require surgery.

29. What is the prognosis?
There are few serious complications, and antibiotics are usually quite effective in treatment. The prognosis is good.

ANOGENITAL HERPES

30. What is anogenital herpes?
Anogenital herpes is usually due to recurrent herpesvirus type 2 and is characterized by grouped vesiculopustular lesions. There may be secondary adenopathy in the groins. Anogenital herpes can be a painful recurrent condition that may have an association with cervical carcinoma.

31. What are the treatments?
Acyclovir ointment (5%) or oral tablets may be helpful for primary attacks or in reduction of severity of occurrences.

V.   Trauma

69. RENAL TRAUMA

J. Patrick Spirnak, M.D.

1. What are the three most common causes of blunt renal trauma?
Motor vehicle accidents, falls, and sports injuries.

2. Blunt trauma causes what percentage of civilian renal injuries?
An estimated 60–90% of all renal injuries occur as a result of blunt trauma.

3. What common clinical findings suggest the presence of a renal injury?
  1. Evidence of flank trauma (i.e., rib fracture, flank ecchymosis)
  2. Gross hematuria
  3. Microscopic hematuria and systolic blood pressure < 90 mm Hg

4. Do all adults with microscopic hematuria and blunt abdominal trauma require a radiographic evaluation of the urinary tract?
No. Adult patients who present with microscopic hematuria, no other associated injuries, and who have stable vital signs do not require urologic evaluation. Patients with microscopic hematuria and shock or other associated injuries requiring hospitalization should undergo radiographic evaluation consisting of either an excretory urogram (IVP) or computed tomography (CT) scan of the abdomen. In many trauma centers, the abdominal CT has replaced the IVP as the initial study of choice, as it is more sensitive in identifying renal injuries and also detects other abdominal injuries.

5. Are the indications for urologic evaluation the same in pediatric patients?
Children under age 16 with any degree of hematuria should still undergo radiographic evaluation.

6. Why are the indications for urologic evaluation different in children?
The pediatric kidneys are at higher risk to sustain renal injury. They are less well protected, more mobile, and relatively larger than adult kidneys. A congenital anomaly is also more likely in these patients.

7. Does the degree of hematuria correlate with the severity of blunt renal injury?
No. Patients with renal contusions may present with gross hematuria, while renal pedicle injuries may occur in the absence of hematuria.

8. How should the trauma IVP be performed?
Stable patients are taken to the radiology department, where a high-dose IVP with nephrotomograms will adequately assess the kidneys in up to 90% of patients. Patients who are unable to be transported from the emergency department receive a bolus of intravenous contrast (1 ml/lb body weight up to a maximum of 150 ml), followed by serial abdominal films at 1, 5, and 10 minutes.

9. What is the purpose of the IVP?
The purpose of the trauma IVP is to identify and stage the extent of renal injury (in order to formulate a rational treatment plan) and to document the presence of two functioning kidneys.

10. What is a minor renal injury?
A minor renal injury occurs in up to 90% of all renal trauma patients and includes renal contusion and shallow lacerations limited to the renal cortex.

11. How are minor renal injuries treated?
Patients with minor injuries associated with gross hematuria are hospitalized and placed at bedrest until the urine clears. Patients with microscopic hematuria and a normal IVP require no further evaluation.

12. What is a major renal injury?
Major renal injuries can be classified into pedicle and nonpedicle injuries. Major renal lacerations extend through the corticomedullary junction. If the collecting system is entered, urinary extravasation may be present. Multiple major lacerations will result in a shattered kidney. Pedicle injuries consist of tears or occlusion to segmental or major vascular structures.

13. How are major renal injuries treated?
The treatment of major blunt renal injuries is controversial. Most stable patients with major renal injuries receive a CT scan to better assess the severity of the injury. Stable patients are hydrated, placed at bedrest until the urine clears, and closely monitored for changes in vital signs that indicate progressive bleeding. Blood transfusions are given as needed, and broad-spectrum antibiotics are administered. Patients with persistent vascular instability despite adequate resuscitative efforts undergo surgical exploration.

14. Does the presence of urinary extravasation require surgical intervention?
The presence of urinary extravasation confirms the diagnosis of major renal injury. Extravasation alone does not require surgical intervention.

These patients are closely observed for signs of sepsis or persistent extravasation which would require surgical exploration and drainage. In addition, it is important to visualize the ureter, as disruption of the ureteropelvic junction can occur and requires immediate exploration and repair.

15. Describe the radiographic findings of renal artery thrombosis.
On IVP, the involved kidney is nonvisualized. The most common CT finding is nonenhancement of the renal parenchyma.

16. What is the treatment of renal pedicle injuries?
Pedicle lacerations require prompt surgical exploration. Branch vessel occlusion is observed. Bilateral complete renal artery thrombosis requires immediate exploration and revascularization. The treatment of unilateral injuries is controversial. If the contralateral kidney is normal, opinion divides between attempted revascularization or observation. If observation is elected, these patients must be followed closely and their blood pressures monitored. If renal vascular hypertension develops, nephrectomy is performed.

17. What is the treatment of renal gunshot wounds?
All patients with penetrating abdominal gunshot wounds have sustained at least one injury to an abdominal viscera; therefore, surgical exploration is required. If the IVP or CT scan indicates the presence of a renal parenchymal injury, renal exploration, debridement, and reconstruction are performed.

18. Is observation ever indicated in patients with renal gunshot wounds?
If the missile has not penetrated the peritoneal cavity (negative lavage), CT has documented a superficial cortical laceration, and the patient is clinically stable, observation may be appropriate.

19. Must all renal stab wounds be surgically explored?
The management of renal stab wounds depends on the degree of renal parenchymal damage and the presence of other associated intra-abdominal injuries. Stab wounds occurring anterior to the mid-axillary line which have penetrated the peritoneal cavity are associated with a significant risk of visceral injury and are explored. At the time of laparotomy, the kidney is explored and repaired. Stab wounds occurring posterior to the mid-axillary line are less likely to be associated with visceral injuries. Observation may be appropriate if the peritoneal lavage is negative, there is no evidence of severe blood loss, and CT findings suggest a superficial laceration.

BIBLIOGRAPHY

1. Bright TC, White K, Peters PC: Significance of hematuria after trauma. J Urol 120:455, 1978.
2. Dixon CM, McAninch JW: Traumatic renal injuries: Part I. Patient assessment and management. AUA Update 10(35):273, 1991.
3. Smith EM, Elder JS, Spirnak JP: Major blunt renal trauma in the pediatric population: Is a nonoperative approach indicated? J Urol 149:546, 1993.
4. Spirnak JP, Resnick MI: Revascularization of traumatic thrombosis of the renal artery. Surg Gynecol Obstet 164:22, 1987.
5. Spirnak JP: Blunt renal trauma In Resnick MI, Kursh ED (eds): Current Therapy in Genitourinary Surgery. Toronto, BC Decker, 1987, p 355.
6. Spirnak JP: Penetrating renal trauma. In Resnick MI, Kursh ED (eds): Current Therapy in Genitourinary Surgery. Toronto, BC Decker, 1992, p 403.

70. URETERAL INJURIES

J. Patrick Spirnak, M.D.

1. What percentage of abdominal gunshot wounds involve the ureter?
About 2.5%.

2. What is the blood supply to the ureter?
The ureter derives its primary blood supply from a branch of the renal artery. In most cases, this artery traverses the entire length of the ureter, running in the outer adventitial sheath. Other sources of ureteral blood supply include branches from the aorta, gonadal, hypogastric, and superior and inferior vesical arteries.

3. Are stab wounds to the ureter more common than gunshot wounds?
No. Gunshot wounds account for > 95% of all traumatic ureteral injuries.

4. Is hematuria a reliable finding in patients with suspected ureteral injury?
No. Up to 37% of all traumatic ureteral injuries present with a normal urinalysis.

5. What is the appropriate imaging study to obtain in trauma victims with a suspected ureteral injury?
An intravenous pyelogram (IVP) is obtained in all patients with suspected ureteral injury.

6. What findings on IVP suggest a ureteral injury?
   1. Delayed or nonvisualization of the involved renal unit
   2. Hydronephrosis
   3. Urinary extravasation
   4. Incomplete visualization of the entire ureter.

7. In the presence of a retroperitoneal hematoma and a ureteral contusion, how can one tell if the integrity of the ureter has been compromised?
The intravenous administration of indigo carmine is helpful in identifying urinary extravasation and a devitalized ureter.

8. In the postoperative period, what signs and symptoms are suggestive of a missed ureteral injury?
The findings are nonspecific. The presence of prolonged adynamic ileus, persistent flank or abdominal pain, a palpable abdominal mass, an elevation in blood urea nitrogen, sepsis, prolonged and persistent drainage from operative drain sites, and/or the development of a spontaneous cutaneous fistula all suggest the diagnosis.

9. What types of iatrogenic ureteral injuries commonly occur?
Ureteral injury can occur as a result of either ligating or crushing the ureter with a clamp or ligature. Surgical transection, avulsion, devascularization, or angulation of the ureter may also occur.

10. What is the incidence of iatrogenic ureteral injury?
Due to the silent nature of many surgical ureteral injuries, the exact incidence is unknown. However, an incidence ranging from 0.5%–30% has been reported following gynecologic surgery.

11. What are the common sites of iatrogenic ureteral injury associated with gynecologic surgery?

1. During ligation of the infundibulopelvic ligament
2. While clamping or ligating the uterine artery as it crosses the ureter
3. As it lies in the ovarian fossa
4. During extensive pelvic node dissection accompanying radical hysterectomy
5. While attempting to control pelvic hemorrhage.

12. When ureteral injury is associated with a vascular reconstructive procedure, is repair indicated?

If the urine is sterile, ureteral repair with the use of indwelling stents, drains, and antibiotics is recommended.

13. What are the goals of ureteral reconstructive surgery?

Restoration of normal anatomy and renal preservation while minimizing patient morbidity.

14. What is the recommended treatment of a ligated ureter?

If noted at the time of injury, simple de-ligation seldom leads to postoperative complications. If the injury is noted and repair undertaken more than 24 hours after injury, de-ligation should be accompanied by stent drainage or resection and primary repair. If the injury is noted more than 72 hours from the time of surgery, resection and primary repair are recommended.

15. How is a proximal or midureteral transection commonly repaired?

Proximal and midureteral injuries are best treated by debridement and ureteroureterostomy. The area is also drained.

16. How should distal ureteral injuries be managed?

Distal injuries are best treated by ureteroneocystostomy.

17. List several relative contraindications to transureteroureterostomy.

- Extensive radiation damage to the ureter
- History of recurrent stone disease
- History of transitional cell carcinoma of the upper urinary tract
- Tuberculosis
- Retroperitoneal fibrosis
- Marked discrepancy in the size of the two ureters
- Anomalies of the recipient ureter

18. If extensive loss of ureteral length has occurred, what adjunctive procedures may be performed to gain length and allow a tension-free repair?

Downward mobilization of the kidney with concomitant nephropexy and/or upward mobilization of the bladder with fixation to the psoas tendon (psoas hitch) performed in conjunction, when necessary, with a Boari bladder flap make it possible to surgically replace nearly the entire ureter.

19. What is an ileal ureter?

An ileal ureter refers to the replacement of a damaged ureter with a segment of ileum. It is useful in secondary reconstructive procedures when extensive loss of ureter has occurred.

20. What is the role of cystoscopy with retrograde pyelography and ureteral stent placement in the evaluation and treatment of suspected ureteral injury?

Cystoscopy and retrograde pyelography are indicated when ureteral injury is suspected. It will identify the exact point of obstruction and the length of ureter involved. At the same time, an attempt is made to pass a guidewire beyond the point of obstruction over which a double J tent may be therapeutically placed.

BIBLIOGRAPHY

1. Bright TC: Emergency management of the injured ureter. Urol Clin North Am 9:285, 1982.
2. Gurin JI, Garcia RL, Melman A, Leiter E: The pathologic effect of ureteral ligation with clinical implications. J Urol 128:1404, 1982.
3. Hoch WH, Kursh ED, Persky L: Early aggressive management of intraoperative ureteral injuries. J Urol 114:530, 1975.
4. Kerr WS: Effects of complete ureteral obstruction in dogs in kidney function. Am J Physiol 184:521, 1956.
5. Raney AM: Ureteral trauma: Effects of ureteral ligation with and without deligation-experimental studies and case reports. J Urol 119:326, 1978.
6. Spirnak JP, Resnick MI, Persky LP: The management of civilian ureteral gunshot wounds: A review of 8 patients. J Urol 134:733, 1985.
7. Spirnak JP, Hampel N, Resnick MI: Ureteral injuries complicating vascular reconstructive surgery: Is repair indicated? J Urol 141:13, 1989.

71. BLADDER TRAUMA

J. Patrick Spirnak, M.D.

1. What types of bladder perforation may occur?
Bladder perforation may be intraperitoneal, extraperitoneal, or both.

2. What is the mechanism of intraperitoneal bladder perforation in patients with blunt abdominal trauma?
Intraperitoneal bladder perforation usually occurs during severe, blunt, lower abdominal trauma while the bladder is full or distended with urine. The intravesical pressure becomes acutely elevated, and the bladder perforates at its weakest point, the dome.

3. Explain how extraperitoneal bladder perforation occurs.
There are two accepted theories as to how extraperitoneal trauma occurs.

    1. When associated with pelvic fracture, extraperitoneal tears are thought to occur as a result of an anterior pubic arch fracture with displacement of bony fragments and bladder perforation near the vesical neck.

    2. A second mechanism of injury has been proposed to explain extraperitoneal tears in the absence of pelvic fracture. With the bladder empty, severe lower abdominal trauma may cause a bursting-type injury similar to that which occurs through the dome with the bladder full.

4. What are the indications for bladder evaluation in patients with blunt lower abdominal trauma?
A **cystogram** is performed in all patients with gross hematuria. If the patient is unable to urinate, has blood at the urethral meatus, or has perineal ecchymosis with swelling or a nonpalpable prostate, a **urethrogram** must be performed prior to performing a cystogram.

5. Do patients with pelvic fracture and microscopic hematuria require bladder evaluation?
Studies have shown a low incidence of bladder injury in the absence of gross hematuria, and thus urologic evaluation is not performed in the absence of other signs suggestive of a urologic injury.

6. How is a cystogram performed?
An 18F Foley catheter is placed into the bladder, and contrast material is administered under gravity to fill the bladder (300–500 ml). Once the inflow of contrast material has stopped, an additional 10–15 ml of contrast is injected under slight pressure to ensure complete bladder filling and to avoid a false-negative study. With the catheter clamped, an abdominal radiograph is obtained. A complete bladder study requires oblique and drainage films.

7. What are the cystographic findings suggestive of an extraperitoneal bladder perforation?
Radiographic findings include a teardrop-shaped bladder secondary to compression by a pelvic hematoma associated with extravasation confined to the pelvis. The pattern of extravasation may range from flame-like wisps or linear streaks to a large stellate or sunburst pattern which may be more obvious on drainage film.

8. What cystographic findings suggest intraperitoneal bladder perforation?
Intraperitoneal perforation may produce diffuse extravasation of contrast material through the peritoneal cavity with no filling of the bladder. Contrast material may accumulate in the dependent portion of the pelvis, obscuring the superior aspect of the bladder and resulting in an hourglass configuration. Contrast material may also extend in the paracolic gutters to the diaphragm.

9. What is the appropriate treatment of an intraperitoneal bladder rupture?

All patients with intraperitoneal bladder perforation undergo surgical exploration and watertight bladder closure.

10. How are extraperitoneal bladder perforations treated?

The treatment of extraperitoneal bladder perforation is controversial. If surgical exploration is performed for other associated injuries, the bladder is explored and repaired. If the patient has an isolated extraperitoneal bladder injury, a nonoperative approach consisting of catheter drainage and broad-spectrum antibiotics is recommended. A cystogram is performed prior to catheter removal, usually after 7–14 days. Severe bleeding with clots, sepsis, and persistent urinary extravasation are indications for exploration.

11. How are gunshot wounds to the bladder treated?

Penetrating wounds to the abdomen and bladder are surgically explored. The bladder is repaired and the area drained.

BIBLIOGRAPHY

1. Brosman SA, Fay R: Diagnosis and management of bladder trauma. J Trauma 13:929, 1973.
2. Carroll PR, McAninch JW: Major bladder trauma: Mechanism of injury and a unified method of diagnosis and repair. J Urol 132:254, 1984.
3. Spirnak JP, Resnick MI: Intraoperative consultation for the bladder. Urol Clin North Am 12:439, 1985.
4. Spirnak JP: Lower urinary tract trauma. In Resnick MI, Kursh ED (eds): Urology Problems in Primary Care. Oradell, NJ, Medical Economics Co., 1987, pp 303–306.
5. Spirnak JP: Pelvic fracture and injury to the lower urinary tract. Surg Clin North Am 68:1057, 1988.

72. URETHRAL INJURY

Kenneth W. Angermeier, M.D.

1. Define the components of the anterior and posterior urethra in the male.
The anterior urethra consists of the glanular, pendulous (penile), and bulbous portions of the urethra. It extends from the urethral meatus to the perineal membrane and is surrounded by the corpus spongiosum throughout its course. The posterior urethra consists of the membranous and prostatic portions of the urethra and extends from the perineal membrane to the bladder neck. The membranous urethra is encompassed by the striated urethral sphincter and the prostatic urethra by the prostate gland.

2. What is the most common cause of traumatic injury to the anterior urethra?
Blunt perineal trauma, usually in the form of a straddle injury, is the most common etiology of disruptive anterior urethral injuries. Other causes include penetrating injury as a result of gunshot or stab wound, urethral instrumentation such as catheterization or endoscopy, disruption in association with a penile fracture, and iatrogenic injury during penile surgery.

3. In what setting are injuries to the posterior urethra most commonly encountered?
Virtually all posterior urethral injuries occur in association with traumatic pelvic fracture, as in a motor vehicle accident. Penetrating trauma to the posterior urethra is seen infrequently.

4. When should one suspect a urethral injury?
Patients with a history of perineal or pelvic trauma, particularly in the presence of a pelvic fracture, should be suspected of having a urethral injury. Blood at the urethral meatus is a common finding, and the patient may be unable to void. These signs are not always present, however, and a high level of suspicion is necessary. Severe urethral injuries may be associated with swelling and ecchymosis of the penis and/or perineum.

5. Describe the fasical layers and attachments that may contain extravasated urine or blood from a urethral injury.
The deep penile fascia (Buck's fascia) is the layer immediately surrounding the corpora cavernosa and corpus spongiosum. It is attached distally to the undersurface of the glans penis at the corona. Proximally Buck's fascia encloses each crus of the corpora cavernosa and the bulb of the corpus spongiosum. Injuries to the anterior urethra with extravasation confined to Buck's fascia may result in swelling and ecchymosis of the penis alone. The superficial fascia of the perineum (Colles' fascia) curves around the superficial transverse perinei muscles and attaches laterally to the ischia and inferior rami of the pubis as well as the fascia lata of the thigh. Anteriorly Colles' fascia is continuous with the dartos layer of the scrotum and Scarpa's fascia of the abdominal wall until its superior attachment to the coracoclavicular fascia. Extravasation penetrating through Buck's fascia and confined by Colles' fascia may result in a "butterfly" perineal and scrotal hematoma and potentially may extend along the anterior abdominal wall to the level of the clavicles.

6. What finding on rectal examination is associated with pelvic fracture and a posterior urethral distraction injury?
A superiorly displaced, "high-riding" prostate on rectal examination is helpful in the diagnosis of a posterior urethral distraction injury. Distraction and separation of the membranous urethra in association with pelvic fracture allow the prostate to be displaced superiorly by the pelvic hematoma that fills the surrounding area.

7. How often does a pelvic fracture result in urethral injury?
Approximately 10% of pelvic fractures are associated with injuries to the lower urinary tract. Urethral injuries are present in approximately 3.5–5.0% of cases.

8. What is the evaluation of the patient with possible urethral injury?
Retrograde urethrography is the first step in the diagnosis of urethral injury. It is important to use contrast suitable for intravenous administration, because extravasation into the corpus spongiosum and surrounding tissues may occur. A Foley catheter should not be passed until a retrograde urethrogram has confirmed that the urethra is normal; the catheter may disrupt or worsen an incomplete urethral injury if present.

9. Describe the different types of posterior urethral injury.
The vast majority of posterior urethral injuries occur within the membranous urethra. The developed prostate gland tends to protect the prostatic urethra, and distraction injuries are primarily located distal to the prostatic apex. Injury may involve the proximal, mid, or distal membranous urethra. In the mildest case, the membranous urethra is stretched by surrounding hematoma without disruption, as radiography demonstrates. Partial disruptions of the membranous urethra demonstrate varying degrees of contrast extravasation with visualization of the more proximal prostatic urethra. Complete posterior urethral distraction injuries are the most severe and demonstrate complete extravasation of contrast into the pelvis and/or perineum.

10. How is an injury to the anterior urethra managed?
Blunt injury to the anterior urethra that results either in partial disruption with significant extravasation of contrast or in complete disruption should be managed with placement of a suprapubic catheter to divert the urine. After several weeks the patient is evaluated with urethrography and endoscopy. If a significant urethral structure has developed, the area is allowed to completely heal over several months, and urethral reconstruction is undertaken as described in chapter 45. Penetrating injury to the anterior urethra should be explored, and associated injuries should be repaired. If tissue loss is minimal, primary urethral repair may be accomplished. The urethra is stented, and a suprapubic catheter is placed for urinary diversion. If tissue loss is extensive, a suprapubic catheter is placed, and the injury is debrided, with care to preserve as much viable tissue as possible. Urethral reconstruction is accomplished at a later date.

11. What are the initial steps in the management of the patient with a posterior urethral distraction injury?
At the time of the acute injury, suprapubic cystotomy is performed. The bladder is inspected for evidence of injury, and repair is undertaken if necessary. If the patient is stable, an attempt to place an aligning urethral catheter is reasonable. This procedure is often accomplished with a combination of retrograde and antegrade passage of catheters, with or without endoscopy. If the procedure is successful, the urethral catheter is capped, and a suprapubic catheter is secured into position. If the patient is unstable, a suprapubic catheter alone is placed in the most expeditious manner possible. In general, placement of an aligning urethral catheter does not prevent formation of a urethral stricture but may help to align the prostatic apex with the distal urethra and may facilitate subsequent posterior urethral reconstruction.

12. What is the timing of posterior urethral reconstruction after a posterior urethral distraction injury?
In general, posterior urethral reconstruction is delayed for approximately 4–6 months to allow complete healing of the perineum and resolution of the pelvic hematoma. In most instances, resolution of the hematoma allows the prostate to return near its original location, with a resulting scar defect of approximately 1.5–2 cm between the ends of the urethra.

13. What operative approach is used for posterior urethral reconstruction?
Posterior urethral reconstruction almost always can be performed through a perineal incision with

the patient in the exaggerated lithotomy position. Excision of the scar with a primary urethral anastomosis affords the best chance for success and is technically feasible in most cases.

14. Describe several techniques that may be used to gain length on the anterior urethra to allow a tension-free primary urethral anastomosis.
After excising the scar and preparing the proximal urethral opening, the anterior urethra is mobilized away from the corpora cavernosa to the level of the suspensory ligaments of the penis. Buck's fascia is completely dissected from the corpus spongiosum to allow maxima extension of the urethra. Subsequently, the corporal bodies may be divided proximally in the midline to shorten the distance to the proximal urethral opening. This distance may be further shortened by performing an inferior pubectomy, with or without spuracrural rerouting of the urethra. Using such maneuvers in a progressive fashion allows a tension-free primary urethral anastomosis in the majority of cases.

15. Are there any concerns about subsequent transurethral resection of the prostate (TURP) after posterior urethral reconstruction?
Yes. By their nature, posterior urethral distraction injuries often result in damage to the striated urethral sphincter mechanism. After posterior urethral reconstruction, urinary continence is maintained primarily by the smooth muscle at the level of the bladder neck. TURP results in resection and obliteration of this continence mechanism. Patients undergoing this procedure after posterior urethral reconstruction are at high risk for significant urinary incontinence. Therefore, symptomatic benign prostatic hyperplasia in such patients is best managed with medical therapy or, if necessary, by intermittent self-catheterization.

BIBLIOGRAPHY

1. Angermeier KW, Devine CJ Jr: Anatomy of the penis and male perineum. Part 2. American Urological Association Update Series. Vol. 13, Lesson 3, 1994.
2. Corriere JN Jr: Trauma to the lower urinary tract. In Gillenwater JY, Grayhack JT, Howards SS, Duckett JW (eds): Adult and Pediatric Urology. Chicago, Year Book, 1987, pp 450–463.
3. Devine CJ Jr, Angermeier KW: Anatomy of the penis and male perineum. Part 1 American Urological Association Update Series. Vol. 13, Lesson 2, 1994.
4. Jordan GH: Treatment of urethral stricture disease. In Stein BS (ed): Practice of Urology. New York, Norton, 1993, pp 1–38.
5. Lowe MA, Mason JT, Luna GK, et al: Risk factors for urethral injuries in men with traumatic pelvic fractures. J Urol 140:506, 1988.
6. Peters PC, Sagalowsky AI: Genitourinary trauma. In Walsh PC, Retik AB, Stamey TA, Vaughan ED Jr (eds): Campbell's Urology, 6th ed. Philadelphia, W.B. Saunders, 1992, pp 2583–2589.
7. Pierce JM Jr: Disruptions of the anterior urethra. Urol Clin North Am 16:329, 1989.

73. TESTICULAR TRAUMA

Anthony J. Thomas, Jr., M.D.

1. What types of injury befall the testicles?

Probably every man over the age of 18 years has experienced some form of testicular trauma. Although most instances are not severe enough to require medical attention, at the time of even relatively minor injury many a strong man has been brought to his knees. Blunt trauma is by far the most common cause of testicular injury, followed by penetrating, self-inflicted, and, finally, dislocation injuries. Testicular trauma has been reported to occur during breech delivery, but most instances occur in the adolescent and young adult under 40 years of age. Most are solitary testicular injuries, although some, particularly those caused by a penetrating object, may involve the contralateral testis or penis and urethra.

2. What is the goal of treatment for a serious testicular injury?

With any testicular injury, the primary objective is to preserve as much functional tissue as possible. The spermatogenic portion is the most sensitive to insult compared with the more resilient Leydig cells, fibrous tissue, and blood vessels. Numerous studies indicate that early surgical exploration and repair of a testicular rupture lead to a higher salvage rate and lower morbidity than a more conservative watchful-waiting approach.

3. Can testicular torsion or tumors occur as a result of trauma?

Direct trauma causes neither torsion nor tumor. Torsion may be associated with strenuous physical activity, including contact sports (e.g., football, rugby, martial arts), and the physician must differentiate by taking a careful history to determine whether there was a direct hit to the scrotum. Swelling due to traumatic hematocele is generally greater than that found with torsion. Minor trauma may bring a patient with a testicular neoplasm to the attention of a physician. If the degree of swelling is out of proportion to the type of injury reported, the presence of a testicular neoplasm should be considered, and appropriate evaluation and treatment should be carried out.

4. What action should be taken when a patient has sustained blunt testicular trauma?

If possible, an accurate history should be obtained to determine the cause of the injury and thus to allow a fuller appreciation of the severity of the incident. Blunt trauma causes testicular rupture when a significantly strong blow forces the testis abruptly against the pubic bone. If the testis is still palpable and the swelling is not excessive, gentle examination of the testis, epididymis, and, finally, the cord structures should be undertaken. Any defect that can be palpated in the tunica albuginea is large enough to require surgical repair. Often a thorough examination of the scrotum and its contents is difficult, because the area may be quite swollen and exquisitely sensitive. If scrotal swelling is marked and the testis is not palpable, and if the patient's condition is otherwise stable, an ultrasound examination is helpful in determining the extent of the injury. With a high degree of suspicion that the tunic has been ruptured with or without ultrasound confirmation, surgical intervention should be considered. In the operating room the testis is examined. If a tunica tear is found, the loosely extruded tubules are cut sharply from the healthy tissue, and the albuginea is closed with absorbable sutures. The tunica vaginalis should be closed over the testis, if possible, leaving within the tunica vaginalis a small (1/4-inch diameter) Penrose drain that exits through the inferior portion of the scrotum.

5. How does the evaluation of the testis after penetrating injury differ from evaluation after blunt trauma?

Penetrating injuries within an urban setting are caused most commonly by knives or bullets. Falls onto sharp objects also may damage the testis, but they are a more rare occurrence. Little diagnostic skill is needed to identify the type and severity of the injury caused by a sharp object or projectile. Most, if not all, injuries need to be explored carefully. Large hematomas should be evacuated, the testis debrided, and viable tissues closed with absorbable sutures. With injuries from a bullet, cloth fragments from the victim's clothes often are brought into the wound and imbedded in the tissue. Such fragments should be removed, the wounds cleansed thoroughly, and the scrotum drained, as with blunt injuries. High-velocity projectiles may cause particularly severe injuries that are not initially appreciated. Delayed tissue necrosis may occur at the area of injury. In most instances, if a high-velocity bullet strikes the testis, little is left to be repaired. The cord structures may need to be debrided, the open vessels secured, and the wound adequately drained and closed.

6. Are antibiotics needed for the treatment of blunt or penetrating testicular injury?

Penetrating injuries require broad-spectrum antibiotic coverage. Blunt injuries, particularly those that cause only a contusion and do not require surgery, generally do not require antibiotics unless significant hematocele is associated with the injury. In some reports subsequent infection has been associated with hematocele. If operative intervention is performed for a blunt injury, of course, it is prudent to administer antibiotics before and after the procedure.

7. What is a dislocation injury? How serious is it?

Blunt trauma does not always result in contusion or rupture. Sudden force may push the testicle upward toward or through the inguinal canal. It may then be held in position at the external ring, within the inguinal canal or even in the abdomen. This dislocation injury can be extremely painful. At times, the testis may twist on its cord, compromising circulatory integrity, or the tunica albuginea may rupture. Such injuries appear to be more frequent during motorcycle accidents, perhaps as a result of a sudden impact against the wide gas tank, which the driver straddles. Most serious motorcycle accidents result in multiple organ injury, and the "missing testis" may not be noticed. If the patient is conscious, he may complain of severe inguinal pain. Examination reveals the empty hemiscotum, and often the testis can be palpated in the groin area. If no more serious injuries are present and if the testis is palpably normal, the patient is given intravenous analgesia for sedation and pain relief. With gentle massage an attempt is made to push the testis back into the scrotum. If this approach fails or if the structural integrity of the testis is in question, the patient is taken to the operating room for a formal exploration; the testis is repaired and replaced in the scrotum.

8. If the cord structures are damaged, should an attempt be made to revascularize the testis?

Blunt injury to the cord structures is relatively uncommon. The cord is fairly well protected, and generally the injuries are limited to contusions that do not require surgery unless a large hematoma is present. Gunshot wounds of the cord usually destroy the vasculature and require orchiectomy and ligation of the vessels. Injuries that may require microsurgical expertise either result from accidental avulsion of the scrotum and testes or are self-inflicted by mentally disturbed men. The patient with accidental avulsion usually reports working with a large piece of machinery when his pants get trapped in the gears or teeth and drag parts of him into the machinery before it can be shut down. Certain types of farm equipment are notorious for such mutilating injuries. In most instances, the testis is damaged beyond repair. Self-inflected injuries are often cleaner, and if the testis is brought in with or by the patient, an attempt at reimplantation may be considered, depending on the condition of the patient, the time lapse between injury and presentation, and, of course, the condition of the testis(es).

9. Can testicular trauma affect fertility adversely?

Immediately following any significant traumatic event, sperm production may be altered adversely, at times to an azoospermic state. Most patients resume active spermatogenesis in time, but recovery may take 3–9 months after injury. Some evidence from laboratory experiments suggests that unilateral testicular injury may cause permanent changes in the contralateral testis that lessen fertility. Whether all patients who have sustained significant trauma to a testis should be followed with subsequent semen analysis remains to be seen. Men presenting with infertility problems, however, should be questioned about a past history of testicular trauma.

10. What are the basic principles for treatment of a traumatic testicular injury?

1. Identify the cause of the injury, if possible.

2. Use ultrasound, if available, to look at the testis and help to determine if the tunica albuginea is ruptured.

3. Do not depend totally on ultrasound to give the right answer every time. Use clinical judgment.

4. Surgery may result in less morbidity than watchful waiting if there is any doubt that more than a simple contusion is present.

BIBLIOGRAPHY

1. Altarac S: A case of testicular replanatation. J Urol 150(5 pt 1):1507–1508, 1993.
2. Bhandary P, Abbitt PL, Watson L: Ultrasound diagnosis of testicular rupture. J Clin Ultrasound 20:436–438, 1992.
3. Cass AS, Luxenberg M: Testicular injuries. Urology 37:528–530, 1991.
4. Corrales JG, Corbel L, Cipolla B, et al: Accuracy of ultrasound diagnosis after blunt testicular trauma. J Urol 150:1834–1836, 1993.
5. Gomez RG, Castanheira AC, McAninch JW: Gun shot wounds of the male external genitalia. J Urol 150:1147–1149, 1993.
6. Masui Y, Ueda K, Ootaguro K: Traumatic dislocation of the testis: A case report. Hinyokika Kiyo 35:1417–1420, 1989.
7. Sauvage P, Geiss S, Leculee R, Hideux S: Injuries of the testis in children. Chirurgie Pediatrique 29:136–141, 1988.
8. Singer AJ, Das S, Gavrell GJ: Traumatic dislocation of the testes. Urology 35:310–312, 1990.
9. Tiwary CM: Testicular injury in breech delivery: Possible implications. Urology 34:210–212, 1989.

74. PRIAPISM

Drogo K. Montague, M.D., and Milton M. Lakin, M.D.

1. What is priapism?
Priapism is a prolonged, usually painful erection not associated with sexual desire.

2. Describe the types of priapism.
- Low-flow (ischemic) priapism
- High-flow (nonischemic) priapism

3. What are the causes of priapism?
1. **High-flow priapism** is secondary to penile or perineal trauma and results when injury creates an arterial-sinusoidal shunt within the corpus cavernosum.

2. **Low-flow priapism** may result from sickle cell disease, leukemia, anticoagulants, spinal cord lesions, fat emboli, malignant penile inflammation, autonomic neuropathy, and drugs, and many cases have unknown etiologies. Low-flow priapism, which is painful, is much more common than nonpainful high-flow priapism.

4. How do drugs cause priapism?
- **Psychotropic agents** may have peripheral α-blocking activity and/or central serotonin-like activity. A commonly used antidepressant associated with priapism is trazodone (Desyrel).
- **Intracavernous pharmacotherapy** is a technique used to treat erectile dysfunction (impotence). Drugs commonly injected into the corpora cavernosa for this purpose include papaverine, phentolamine, and prostaglandin E_1. While this technique is very effective in the treatment of erectile dysfunction, it is associated with low-flow priapism in a small percentage of cases.

5. Does priapism have any distinctive features on physical examination?
Yes. A normal erection involves both corpora cavernosa, the corpus spongiosum, and glans penis. With priapism, only the corpora cavernosa are erect. The glans penis is small and flaccid and the ventral surface of the erect penis is flat, since the bulge of erect corpus spongiosum which surrounds the urethra in normal erection is absent.

6. Is priapism an emergency?
Yes. Most cases of priapism are of the low-flow, ischemic variety. When oxygen levels in the blood trapped within the corpora drop, pain occurs and time-dependent damage to cavernosal smooth muscle ensues.

7. What are the consequences of delayed or nontreatment of priapism?
Cavernosal fibrosis results, and subsequent ability to obtain normal erections is lost.

8. How soon should priapism be treated?
Ideally, any erection lasting 4 hours should cause the man to seek prompt urologic attention. In reality, most patients present with an erection of at least 24 hours' duration. Successful reversal of the priapism at this point may still preserve subsequent erectile function, but with increasing duration of priapism, the incidence of erectile dysfunction rises sharply.

9. Describe the initial encounter with the patient who has low-flow ischemic priapism.
The history should document the duration of the priapism and elicit factors which may be responsible. Physical examination confirms the presence of priapism by its characteristic

findings. The patient, and whenever possible the partner or family, are then counseled regarding the possibility of permanent erectile dysfunction (impotence) regardless of success in the treatment of the priapism.

10. What is the first step in the treatment of low-flow, ischemic priapism?

Non-operative treatment should always be tried first. A 19-gauge butterfly needle is inserted into one corpus cavernosum. (The septum between the corpora is incomplete and entry into one side provides access to both corporeal bodies.) Blood is aspirated and sent for blood gas determination to document the degree of ischemia. Blood is then aspirated from the corpora (10–15 ml), discarded, and then replaced with an equal amount of normal saline. This process is repeated until the aspirate is bright red. A solution of phenylephrine is prepared by taking 1 ml containing 10 mg and diluting it to 100 ml with normal saline. Three to 5 ml of this dilute solution are then injected into the corpora, and this process is repeated at 10-minute intervals until the erection subsides. The patient's pulse and blood pressure should be monitored during this procedure.

11. Why is phenylephrine used to reverse priapism?

Any sympathomimetic amine can be used to reverse priapism. However, when the priapism subsides, the sympathomimetic drug which was injected into the corpora is released into the systemic circulation. If epinephrine is used, tachycardia and arrhythmia often result. If metaraminol is used, severe hypertension often results. Phenylephrine has minimal systemic side effects.

12. How does operative treatment play a role in the treatment of low-flow, ischemic priapism?

If nonoperative treatment of priapism fails, prompt operative intervention is indicated. Surgical treatment of priapism involves establishing a shunt between the erect corpora cavernosa and the glans penis, or corpus spongiosum, or saphenous vein system.

13. How is the presence of high-flow, nonischemic priapism established?

A history of penile or perineal trauma is invariably present. Color duplex ultrasonography is useful in revealing the presence of an arterial-sinusoidal shunt.

14. Describe the treatment of high-flow, nonischemic priapism.

Selective internal pudendal arteriography confirms the presence of the arterial-sinusoidal shunt, and then selective embolization of the artery feeding the shunt is performed.

15. What is stuttering priapism?

Stuttering priapism consists of recurrent episodes of priapism, which either subside spontaneously after several hours or are successfully reversed by corporeal aspiration and phenylephrine injection. These episodes occur frequently, often daily.

16. Describe the treatment of stuttering priapism.

Stuttering priapism has been treated by all of the following methods:
- Systemic sympathomimetic amines (phenylpropanolamine, pseudoephedrine, or terbutaline)
- Monthly injections of a luteinizing hormone-releasing hormone agonist, leuprolide acetate (Lupron)
- Self-administered intracorporeal injections of a sympathomimetic amine

BIBLIOGRAPHY

1. Brock G, Breza J, Lue TF, Tanagho EA: High flow priapism: A spectrum of disease. J Urol 150:968–971, 1993.
2. Carson CC, Mino RD: Priapism associated with trazodone therapy. J Urol 139:369–370, 1988.

3. Dittrich A, Albrecht K, Bar-Moshe O, Vandendris M: Treatment of pharmacological priapism with phenylephrine. J Urol 146:323–324, 1991.
4. Fouda A, Hassouna M, Beddoe E, et al: Priapism: An avoidable complication of pharmacologically induced erection. J Urol 142:995–997, 1989.
5. Fowler JE, Koshy M, Strub M, Chinn SK: Priapism associated with the sickle cell hemoglobinopathies: Prevalence, natural history and sequelae. J Urol 145:65–68, 1991.
6. Klein EA, Montague DK, Steiger E: Priapism associated with the use of intravenous fat emulsion: Case reports and postulated pathogenesis. J Urol 133:857–859, 1985.
7. Levine LA, Guss SP: Gondadotropin-releasing hormone analogues in the treatment of sickle cell anemia-associated priapism. J Urol 150:475–477, 1993.
8. Lue TF, Hellstrom WJG, McAninch JW, Tanagho EA: Priapism: A refined approach to diagnosis and treatment. J Urol 136:104–108, 1986.
9. Molina L, Bejany D, Lynne CM, Politano VA: Diluted epinephrine solution for the treatment of priapism. J Urol 141:1127–1128, 1989.
10. Shantha TR, Finnerty DP, Rodriquez AP: Treatment of persistent penile erection and priapism using terbutaline. J Urol 141:1427–1429, 1989.
11. Winter CC, McDowell G: Experience with 105 patients with priapism: Update and review of all aspects. J Urol 140:980–983, 1988.

VI.   Calculus Disease

75. RENAL CALCULI

J. Patrick Spirnak, M.D.

1. What causes renal calculi to form?
Many theories have been proposed to explain the cause of renal stone formation. Unfortunately, no one mechanism fully explains the cause in all stone formers.

In one commonly accepted model of stone formation, a period of abnormal crystalluria is required. For crystals to form and grow, the urine must be supersaturated with the salt of the stone-forming crystal. Urinary substances which act as inhibitors to crystal formation must be reduced or absent from the urine, and certain proteins which act as the framework for crystal depositions must be present in the urine.

2. What risk factors enhance stone formation?
1. Metabolic state (influenced by patient's genetic background)
2. Hormonal imbalances
3. Environmental factors
4. Dietary excesses
5. Anatomic abnormalities leading to chronic infection or stasis

3. Where do renal stones form?
Stones form in the collecting tubules and pass into the calyces, renal pelvis, and ureter.

4. List the four most common types of stones found in North America.
1. Calcium-containing stones (calcium oxalate, calcium phosphate, mixed), 70%
2. Infection stones (struvite, magnesium ammonium phosphate), 15–20%
3. Uric acid stones, 5–10%
4. Cystine, 1–5%.

5. Name the most common stone found in American men.
Calcium.

6. Name the most common stone found in American women. Why?
Infection stones. Women are more prone to urinary tract infections than men.

7. What stone is inherited as an autosomal-recessive trait?
Cystine.

8. How does the typical patient present with a nonobstructing caliceal stone?
Nonobstructing caliceal stones are usually discovered as incidental findings on radiographs obtained for the evaluation of other organ systems or during the evaluation of hematuria.

9. Describe the typical presentation of a patient with an obstructing renal pelvic stone.
Obstruction occurring at the level of the ureteropelvic junction causes sharp, intermittent, colicky

pain typically localized to the flank or costovertebral angle. The pain is not related to activity and may be accompanied by nausea and vomiting.

10. What are the expected urinalysis findings in patients with renal colic?
Microscopic or gross hematuria is common. However, the absence does not exclude renal stone disease. Pyuria may be present without infection. Crystals may be seen.

11. Is urine pH important in determining the type of stone present?
Yes. An acid urine (pH <5.5) is suggestive of a uric acid stone, whereas a pH of 8 suggests an infectious stone.

12. Is a KUB film sufficient to diagnose a renal stone?
No, only 90% of stones are radiopaque. Pure uric acid stones are usually radiolucent and do not appear on a plain film of the abdomen.

13. What x-ray study should be performed?
An excretory urogram (IVP) is obtained in all patients suspected of having a renal stone, unless they are allergic to the contrast.

14. List the indications for surgical stone removal.
• Persistent pain
• Recurrent, gross hematuria
• Obstruction with progressive renal damage
• Recurrent urinary tract infection

15. What type of stone can be dissolved?
Pure uric acid stones can almost always be dissolved by oral alkalinization therapy.

16. Is pyelolithotomy the treatment of choice in managing a 1-cm obstructing calcium pelvic stone?
No. Extracorporeal shock-wave lithotripsy is the treatment of choice and is successful in > 90% of cases.

17. Can all renal stones be treated by extracorporeal shock-wave lithotripsy?
Stones larger than 2.5 cm in diameter are frequently associated with obstruction following this form of treatment. These patients may be best managed by either percutaneous or open surgical stone removal.

BIBLIOGRAPHY

1. Pak CYC: Medical management of nephrolithiasis. J Urol 128:1157, 1982.
2. Resnick MI, Spirnak JP: Calculus disease: General considerations. In Pollack HM (ed): Clinical Urography. Philadelphia, W.B. Saunders, 1990, p 1752.
3. Sarmina I, Spirnak JP, Resnick MI: Urinary lithiasis in the black population: An epidemiologic study and review of the literature. J Urol 138:14, 1987.
4. Spirnak JP, Resnick MI: ESWL. In Pak C, Resnick MI (eds): Urolithiasis. Philadelphia, W.B. Saunders, 1990, pp 321–362.
5. Spirnak JP, Resnick MI: Urinary stones. In Tanagho EA, McAninch JW (eds): Smith's General Urology. Norwalk, CT, Appleton & Lange, 1992, pp 271, 298.

76. STAGHORN CALCULI

Stevan B. Streem, M.D.

1. How did staghorn calculi get their name?
Here is a plain abdominal x-ray in a patient with bilateral staghorn calculi. Now you know.

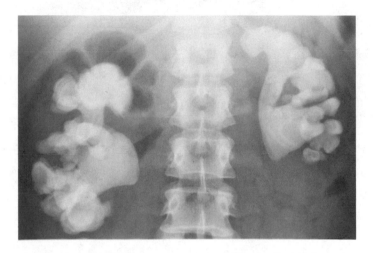

Bilateral staghorn calculi in a woman with recurrent proteus infections of the urinary tract.

2. What causes them?
Most stones of "staghorn" size and shape are infection related and composed of magnesium ammonium phosphate (struvite) along with calcium phosphate. These minerals precipitate on a matrix "cast" of the pyelocalyceal system in a staghorn configuration. The basic abnormality in these patients is a chronically alkaline urine that results from infection with urease-producing urinary pathogens.

3. Are all staghorn stones related to infection?
Most stones of staghorn size and shape are infection related. However, uric acid stones and cystine stones may also develop in a staghorn configuration. Calcium oxalate and calcium phosphate stones, which are the most frequent stones, rarely grow in a staghorn shape or to such a large size.

4. Should staghorn stones be removed even if they are not causing symptoms?
Many studies have shown that the natural history of these stones is progressive obstruction, infection, and loss of kidney function. Therefore, the presence of this stone is itself an indication for intervention, even in the absence of symptoms.

5. How are they removed?
In the past, a "kidney-splitting" operation called anatrophic nephrolithotomy was often performed. Now, various combinations of percutaneous stone removal and extracorporeal shock-wave lithotripsy can be used as an alternative to such surgery.

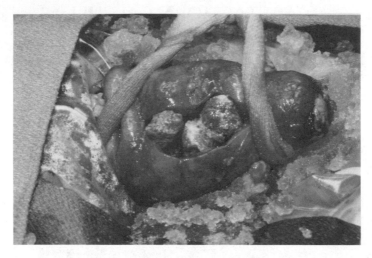

"Anatrophic" nephrolithotomy is performed by incising the kidney in a relatively avascular plane. The renal artery is clamped during this time to allow the surgery to be performed in a bloodless field. Renal ischemia is prevented by intraoperative cooling of the kidney while the artery is clamped. (From Novick AC, Streem SB: Surgery of the kidney. In Walsh PC, et al (eds): Campbell's Urology, 6th ed. Philadelphia, W.B. Saunders, 1992, p 2461; with permission.)

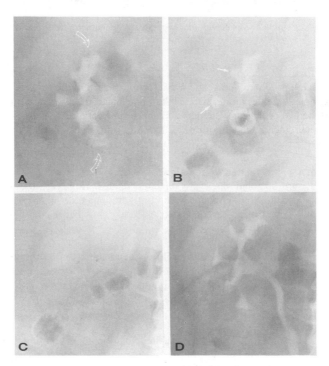

A. Plain abdominal radiograph reveals a "staghorn" calculus. **B.** Most of the stone has been removed by percutaneous ultrasonic nephrostolithotomy. Residual fragments inaccessible to the percutaneous tract (*arrows*) are treated with extracorporeal shock-wave lithotripsy. **C.** Follow-up plain x-ray shows no residual stones. **D.** Follow-up pyelogram reveals an excellent functional and anatomic result.

BIBLIOGRAPHY

1. Blandy JP, Singh M: The case for a more aggressive approach to staghorn stones. J Urol 115:505, 1976.
2. Boyce WH, Elkins IB: Reconstructive renal surgery following anatrophic nephrolithotomy: Followup of 100 consecutive cases. J Urol 111:307, 1974.
3. Gil-Vernet J: New surgical concepts in removing renal calculi. Urol Int 20:255, 1965.
4. Nickel JC, Emtage J, Costerton JW: Ultrastructural microbial etiology of infection induced urinary stones. J Urol 133:622, 1985.
5. Novick AC, Streem SB: Surgery of the kidney. In Walsh PC, Retick AB, Stamey TA, Vaughan ED Jr (eds): Campbell's Urology, 6th ed. Philadelphia, W.B. Saunders, 1992.
6. Kahnoski RJ, Lingeman JE, Coury TA, et al: Combined percutaneous and extracorporeal shock wave lithotripsy for staghorn calculi: An alternative to anatrophic nephrolithotomy. J Urol 135:679, 1986.
7. Smith MJ, Boyce WH: Anatrophic nephrotomy and plastic calyrhaphy. J Urol 99:521, 1968.
8. Streem SB, Lammert G: Long-term efficacy of combination therapy for struvite staghorn calculi. J Urol 5:245, 1987.
9. Vargas AB, Bragin SR, Mendez R: Staghorn calculus: Its clinical presentation, complications and management. J Urol 127:860, 1982.

77. URETERAL CALCULI

Mark A. Wainstein, M.D., and Martin I. Resnick, M.D.

1. Where in the collecting system do ureteral calculi become impacted?

Uroliths create symptoms when they become trapped in a segment of the upper urinary tract. To become impacted, a calculus must have a diameter > 2 mm. Areas where a calculus may become impacted include:

   1. **Ureteropelvic junction.** Here, the large diameter of the renal pelvis decreases to that of the ureter (2–3 mm). Beyond the ureteropelvic junction, the ureter develops a diameter of 10 mm (30F), and small calculi can pass distally to the iliac vessels.

   2. **Ureters cross the pelvic brim.** The ureters, as they arch over the iliac vessels, narrow to approximately 4 mm (12F).

   3. **Ureterovesical junction.** The ureter here narrows to a diameter of 1–5 mm, and it is here where most ureteral stones lodge. Another area, in women, is in the posterior pelvis, where the ureter is crossed anteriorly by the pelvic blood vessels and the broad ligament.

2. What variables affect spontaneous passage of ureteral calculi?

The size and location of the calculus are the two most important variables in planning therapy. Ninety percent of stones in the distal ureter and measuring < 4 mm in diameter will pass spontaneously, compared to only 50% of stones 4–5.9 mm in diameter. Only 20% of stones > 6 mm will pass without surgical intervention. Proximal ureteral stones are less likely to pass than distal ureteral stones.

3. What is Steinstrasse?

Steinstrasse is a term meaning ''stone street'' and describes the fragments of urinary calculus created after extracorporeal shock-wave lithotripsy, which stack up and obstruct the ureter. Some pass spontaneously while others require intervention.

4. How do calculi create symptoms?

Ureteral calculi create symptoms when they become trapped in a segment of the upper collecting system. Ureteral pain (or colic) is characterized as an extremely intense pain, sudden in onset, and stabbing in nature. The pain and associated symptoms are often related to the location of the calculus within the ureter.

5. Describe the symptoms stones produce according to their location.

   Caliceal calculi. Small nonobstructing caliceal calculi are often asymptomatic but are detected when a patient develops gross hematuria or incidentally on a radiograph. These calculi can result in urinary tract infections, persistent hematuria, or flank pain if they become large enough to obstruct an infundibulum.

   Renal pelvic stones. Small renal pelvic calculi are usually asymptomatic. If they become impacted at the ureteropelvic junction pass or the proximal ureter, the resultant obstruction of urine may cause symptoms of localized flank or costovertebral angle tenderness. If urinary infection is associated, the patient can develop pyelonephritis or even florid sepsis.

   Proximal ureteral calculi. Patients experience sharp intermittent flank pain of acute onset associated with hematuria. As the stone passes distally to the pelvic brim, pain may radiate to the lateral flank of the abdominal region.

   Distal ureter. As the stone enters the distal ureter, pain frequently radiates along the inguinal canal into the corresponding groin and genitals. Calculi lodged at the ureterovesical junction create symptoms of vesical irritability, including urinary urgency and frequency.

6. What are the indications for hospitalizing a patient with a ureteral calculus?
1. A stone in a solitary kidney
2. Fever, leukocytosis, or bacteriuria
3. Azotemia
4. Colic and associated nausea and vomiting too severe to be managed on an outpatient basis
5. Uncontrollable pain requiring parenteral analgesics

7. Where do ureteral calculi form?
Ureteral stones originate in the renal pelvis and pass into the ureter, where they frequently become lodged. Calculi that primarily develop in the ureter are rare. Instances in which they can develop in the ureter have been seen in association with ureteroceles, neoplasms, ectopic ureters, ureteral strictures, and foreign body such as a suture in the ureter. Right and left ureteral calculi occur with equal frequency.

8. What is the composition of ureteral calculi?
Since most ureteral calculi originate in the kidney, they possess the same composition as renal calculi. Calcium oxalate stones are the most frequent.

9. How quickly do ureteral calculi need to be treated?
If infection exists behind an obstructed ureter, the obstruction must be relieved as soon as possible. If there is no infection and minimal discomfort, use your clinical judgment. With complete obstruction (in dog studies), renal deterioration begins within 18–24 hours. Within 5 days to 2 weeks, some irreversible changes in function have occurred. After 16 weeks of obstruction, only partial return of function is expected. Partial obstruction, of course, modifies these values. However, studies by Schweitzer found that chronic partial obstruction results in significant renal damage, and therefore early intervention is recommended.

10. What are phleboliths? How are they different from ureteral calculi?
Phleboliths are calcifications within pelvic veins. They differ from ureteral calculi in that they are rounder, cast shadows lateral to the course of the ureter, and have centers that are radiolucent.

11. Describe the expectant strategy for ureteral calculi.
Most calculi < 5mm in diameter will pass spontaneously. Expectant management consisting of hydration, analgesia, and serial abdominal x-rays obtained at 1–2-week intervals to assess stone passage. Patients should be instructed to strain all their urine and save the stone for analysis. The patient should be instructed to watch for signs of fever, urinary tract infection, increasing pain unresponsive to oral medications, or severe nausea or vomiting.

12. What are the indications for surgical intervention?
- Infection unresponsive to antibiotics
- Severe colic unresponsive to oral medications
- Complete urinary obstruction of a solitary kidney
- Impaction

13. Describe the invasive treatment options for ureteral calculi.
Treatment options for ureteral calculi include extracorporeal shock-wave lithotripsy, endourologic stone extraction, and open surgery. No single modality is superior for treating all ureteral calculi. The choice of treatment needs to be individualized to the patient as well as the experience of the surgeon.

   Extracorporeal shock-wave lithotripsy (ESWL). Since its introduction in 1980, ESWL has become the noninvasive treatment-of-choice for upper ureteral and most renal calculi. Response rates are much higher for upper ureteral (98%) compared to iliac (70%) and distal ureteral (85%) calculi. Calculi in the lower ureter are more difficult to localize and thus treated with ESWL. Other factors influencing the success of ESWL include the stone composition, size, and degree of impaction.

Ureteroscopy. Although ESWL is effective in managing most urinary calculi, a significant proportion of patients do not respond to this therapy alone. With the advent of ureteroscopes with significantly reduced diameters (5–11F), endourologic intervention has become an increasingly safe and effective means of therapy for ureteral calculi. Success rates of 97% have been reported with ureteroscopic techniques. Calculi > 6 mm require fragmentation prior to extraction, usually by ultrasound or electrohydraulic and laser lithotripsy.

Ureterolithotomy. Ureterolithotomy is now used in < 2% of patients, when ESWL or endourologic intervention has failed. Other indications for ureterolithotomy include conditions requiring concomitant surgical correction of an anatomic abnormality, such as ureteral stricture, ureterovesical obstruction, and vesicoureteral reflux.

14. When is chemolysis used?

In chemolysis, urinary calculi are dissolved by alterations in the urinary environment. This process can be accomplished systemically by oral or parenteral therapy (systemic chemolysis) or by direct irrigation of the renal pelvis (direct contact chemolysis). Cystine, struvite, uric acid, and apatite calculi are all amenable to this therapy. The success of ESWL and endourologic intervention has limited the role of this therapy. Currently, percutaneous chemolysis is used as adjunctive therapy for residual stones after ESWL, open stone surgery, and endourologic procedures.

BIBLIOGRAPHY

1. Drach GW: Urinary lithiasis: Etiology, diagnosis, and medical management. In Walsh PC, Retik AB, Stamey TA, Vaughn ED Jr (eds): Campbell's Urology, 6th ed. Philadelphia, W.B. Saunders, 1992.
2. Dretler SP: Ureteral stone disease: Options for management. Urol Clin North Am 17(1):217–229, 1990.
3. Kumar S, Menon M: Ureteral calculi. In Resnick MI, Kursh ED (eds): Current Therapy In Genitourinary Surgery, 2nd ed. St. Louis, Mosby-Year Book, 1992.
4. Morse RM, Resnick MI: Ureteral calculi: Natural history and treatment in an era of advanced technology. J Urol 145:263, 1991.
5. Spirnak JP, Resnick MI: Urinary stones. In Tanagho EA, McAninch JW (eds): Smith's General Urology, 13th ed. Norwalk, CT Appleton & Lange, 1992.

78. BLADDER CALCULI

Nehemia Hampel, M.D.

1. Who is most often affected by bladder calculi?

Bladder calculi are most commonly found in adult men with bladder outlet obstruction and in children who live in lesser developed countries.

2. What are primary and secondary bladder calculi?

Primary bladder calculi are endemic and involve only children. Secondary bladder calculi occur primarily in adults and are secondary to urinary stasis with or without associated infection or foreign bodies. Whenever foreign bodies, such as chronic indwelling catheters, are present, bladder calculi should be suspected.

3. Has the incidence of bladder calculi in children changed?

In the past bladder calculi were more common in children than in adults. With industrialization, increase in average income, and dictary and nutritional progress, bladder calculi are disappearing from previously afflicted areas.

4. What is the composition of pediatric bladder calculi?

In endemic areas most calculi are composed of ammonium acid urate, calcium oxalate, or mixtures of both.

5. What is the chemical composition of bladder calculi in adults?

The chemical composition of bladder calculi is similar to the spectrum seen in upper tract calculi. Calcium oxalate is the most common constituent of calculi in the United States. In Europe uric acid and urate stones are more prevalent.

6. What is the sex distribution of bladder calculi?

Bladder calculi are predominantly a disease of males of all ages and all nationalities. The most important factor for male preponderance is associated with urine stasis due to obstruction.

7. What are the symptoms of bladder calculi?

Patients with bladder calculi may be free from specific symptoms, particularly in the pediatric age group. The history, however, may provide a clue to diagnosis. The symptoms in most cases are those of bladder outlet obstruction or urinary infection. Typical symptoms of bladder calculi are intermittent voiding with sudden painful interruptions, perhaps in association with terminal hematuria. The pain may be in the lower abdomen and referred to the tip of the penis, along the course of the second to fourth sacral nerves. Irritating voiding symptoms of frequency, urgency, and dysuria are usually present.

8. What are the specific laboratory findings?

There are no specific laboratory tests to identify bladder calculi. Proteins, erythrocytes, and leukocytes usually are found in the urine, and urine cultures may be positive in the presence of infection. None of these findings is specific to bladder calculi.

9. How do you establish the diagnosis of bladder calculi?

The absence of shadow on the plain roentgenogram does not exclude bladder calculus. About 50% of calculi are missed on plain radiographs. Cystogram may detect radiolucent calculi. The best and surest method for detecting bladder calculi is cystoscopy. No stones should be missed on direct inspection of the bladder.

10. Is there a difference in treatment plans for primary and secondary bladder calculi?
Primary and secondary bladder calculi present different problems and require individual approaches. In primary (endemic) calculi, the stones have to be removed, and the patient should be followed with proper dietary correction. In secondary calculi, eradication of the calculi does not prevent recurrences. The underlying obstructive lesion and infection should be corrected. Foreign bodies should be removed whenever possible.

11. What are treatment options to eliminate bladder calculi?
Standard treatment options include chemodissolution, transurethral extraction, fragmentation with mechanical electrohydralic or ultrasonic instruments and evacuation or open surgical removal (cystolithotomy). Chemodissolution, though attractive, requires long periods of time, and therefore is impractical compared with other options. Most calculi can be removed transurethrally, and open surgery is seldom required. In boys, due to the relatively large stones at presentation, and the narrow urethra, stones are usually removed through open surgery.

12. What is the prognosis for patients with bladder calculi?
Primary bladder calculi are gradually eliminated in developed countries. They are more of a socioeconomical problem than medical. Recurrence of secondary bladder calculi is mostly related to the correction of the underlying obstruction and infection. With proper care and regular urologic follow-up, there should be very few recurrences.

BIBLIOGRAPHY

1. Dalton DC, Hughes J, Glenn JF: Foreign bodies and urinary stones. Urology 6:1, 1975.
2. Gillenwater JY, Grayhack JT, Howards SS, Duckett JW (eds): Adult and Pediatric Urology, 2nd ed. Chicago, Year Book, 1991.
3. Rous SN: Stone Disease: Diagnosis and Management. Orlando, FL, Grune & Stratton, 1987.
4. Walsh PC, Retik AB, Stamey TA, Vaughan ED Jr (eds): Campbell's Urology, 6th ed. Philadelphia, W.B. Saunders, 1992.

79. CALCIUM OXALATE STONES

Stevan B. Streem, M.D.

1. How common are calcium oxalate stones?

In the United States, the incidence of urinary stone disease is estimated to be 0.1–0.3%. Therefore, 240,000–720,000 Americans suffer a metabolic stone event each year, with men more frequently affected than women. The prevalence of stone disease is estimated to be 5–10%, meaning that in the United States alone, 12–24 million people will develop a stone at some time during their life.

Calcium oxalate stones, with or without a calcium phosphate component, account for approximately 75% of all urinary calculi.

2. How do calcium oxalate stones usually present?

Calcium oxalate calculi may first come to medical attention when they cause pain or hematuria. The symptoms usually result from acute obstruction, such as when a stone moves to the ureter. Occasionally, otherwise asymptomatic calcium stones may be found serendipitously at radiographic evaluation for an unrelated abdominal or musculoskeletal disorder. Radiographic evaluation of asymptomatic stones may also be prompted by microhematuria or pyuria found at routine urinalysis.

3. Describe the radiographic characteristics of calcium oxalate stones.

On a plain radiograph, calcium oxalate stones are opaque, with a radiodensity similar to that of iodinated contrast. Therefore, after contrast is administered for a urogram or during a retrograde study, the stone may be obscured. Ultrasound and computed tomography can identify stones, although these studies cannot distinguish calcium oxalate calculi from stones of other composition.

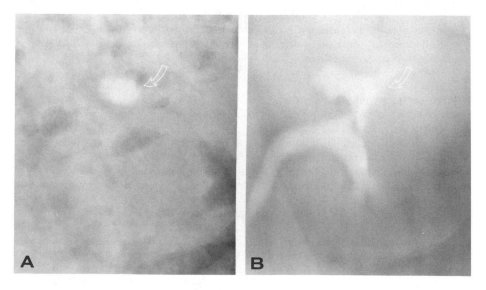

A. A plain x-ray reveals opacity overlying the renal shadow, consistent with a calcium stone. **B.** During intravenous urography, the stone itself is obscured by radiographic contrast media, which has the same radiodensity.

4. What causes calcium oxalate stones?
In simplest terms, they form when the urine is supersaturated with calcium oxalate—i.e., when the concentration of calcium oxalate in the urine exceeds its solubility.

5. What are some of the environmental risk factors?
A low urine volume is clearly associated with an increased risk of stones. Though not well documented, there does appear to be an increased risk for patients in hotter climates or working conditions, at least during an initial acclimatization period.

6. Is it true that people with calcium oxalate stones should avoid dairy products?
Probably not. Although it might seem reasonable that dairy products, with their relatively high calcium content, might predispose to calcium oxalate stones, there is little scientific evidence to support that concept. In fact, in otherwise healthy people, a diet high in calcium may provide protection from these stones. One possible explanation is that the dietary calcium is needed to find oxalate in the intestinal tract, which then prevents absorption of the oxalate.

7. What dietary advice should be given to prevent calcium oxalate stones?
A high fluid intake is most important, as it will increase urinary volume and decrease the concentration of calcium oxalate. A diet low in oxalates is more reasonable than a calcium-restricted diet. Tea, nuts, and some green leafy vegetables are high in oxalates. Studies have also shown a benefit in restriction of salt and fat intake as well as increased dietary fiber. Actually, a healthy diet in general is a stone-prevention diet.

8. When should a patient be evaluated for metabolic risk factors?
There is some difference of opinion here, but certainly any patient with recurrent calcium stones should be offered a metabolic evaluation. Even a single kidney stone event should prompt metabolic evaluation when it occurs in a child.

9. What should the metabolic evaluation include?
- Serum calcium, phosphate, uric acid, electrolytes, and creatinine
- 24-Hour urinary calcium, oxalate, uric acid, citrate, sodium, and, to be sure it is an adequate collection, creatinine
- Fasting urine pH

10. What are these studies looking for?
The most frequent cause of recurrent calcium oxalate stones is **"idiopathic" hypercalciuria.** A reasonable definition for this is a 24-hour urinary calcium excretion exceeding 300 mg in men or 250 mg in women, although others define hypercalciuria as 24-hour urinary excretion of > 4 mg Ca/kg. The uric acid level is also important even for calcium stones, as hyperuricosuria is clearly associated with an increased risk for calcium oxalate stones. The citrate levels are important, as hypocitraturia is a well-known risk factor for recurrent calcium stones and may also be associated with renal tubular acidosis. Sodium excretion is an important marker of sodium intake, and elevated salt intake is associated with increased calcium excretion.

11. Can any treatment prevent stones?
That depends on the result of the metabolic evaluation. Hypercalciuria is usually treated with diuretics that decrease urinary calcium excretion. The most frequently used and perhaps best studied one has been **hydrochlorothiazide,** which is very effective in these cases. Patients with hyperuricosuria may benefit to some degree from a purine-restricted diet, though dietary restriction alone may not be adequate. In those cases, **allopurinol** is used to decrease urinary uric acid excretion and has proven effective in then reducing the recurrence rate of calcium oxalate stones. Patients with hypocitraturia can be treated with **citrate supplements.** Patients with renal tubular acidosis require large doses of **alkalinizing agents.**

12. Is it true that some calcium stones can be dissolved?
No.

13. When is surgical intervention indicated for calcium stones?

Indications for Surgical Intervention for Calcium Oxalate Calculi
Progressive obstruction
Intractable pain
Associated infection
Significant hematuria
Stone growth
Socioeconomic concerns
Stone too large to pass

Basically, stones require intervention whenever they cause progressive obstruction or intractable pain. When stones are associated with infection or significant hematuria they also require intervention, though calcium oxalate stones are only rarely infection-related. Stones that increase in size despite appropriate medical management also require intervention. Some patients have stones that might pass spontaneously, but they require intervention to allow them to get back to work; this would be a socioeconomic indication. Finally, any calcium stone in the ureter judged too large to pass on its own requires intervention. Stones < 4 mm generally pass spontaneously, whereas those 4–7 mm have a 50% chance of doing so. Stones in the ureter > 7 mm are unlikely to pass spontaneously.

14. What forms of intervention are available?
These days, most stones in the kidney and upper ureter are treated with **extracorporeal shock-wave lithotripsy,** as this is an effective, safe treatment that can generally be done on an outpatient basis. Stones in the lower ureter can be managed with extracorporeal shock-wave lithotripsy or with **ureteroscopy,** at which time they can be either removed intact or fragmented using ultrasound, laser, or electrohydraulic lithotripsy. **Open surgical intervention** is only rarely indicated for management of calcium stones (failure of or contraindication to the less-invasive forms of management, or when an associated anatomic abnormality requires open operative reconstruction).

BIBLIOGRAPHY

1. Barcelo P, Wuhl O, Servitge E, et al: Randomized double-blind study of potassium citrate in idiopathic hypocitraturic calcium nephrolithiasis. J Urol 150:1761, 1993.
2. Borghi L, Meschi T, Amato F, et al: Hot occupation and nephrolithiasis. J Urol 150:1757, 1993.
3. Curhan GC, Willett WC, Rimm EB, Stampfer MJ: A prospective study of dietary calcium and other nutrients and the risk of symptomatic kidney stones. N Engl J Med 328:833, 1993.
4. Laminski NA, Meyers AM, Kruger M, et al: Hyperoxaluria in patients with recurrent calcium oxalate calculi: Dietary and other risk factors. Br J Urol 68:454, 1991.
5. National Institutes of Health Consensus Development Conference on Prevention and Treatment of Kidney Stones. J Urol 141:705–808, 1989.
6. Pak CYC, Resnick MI: Urolithiasis: A Medical and Surgical Reference. Philadelphia, W.B. Saunders, 1990.
7. Sakhaee K, Harvey JA, Padalino PK, et al: The potential role of salt abuse on the risk for kidney stone formation. J Urol 150:310, 1993.

80. URIC ACID CALCULI

Mark A. Wainstein, M.D., and Martin I. Resnick, M.D.

1. What percentage of urinary calculi are uric acid stones?
Uric acid stones account for 5–10% of all urinary calculi in the United States. The incidence varies among other countries, with the Middle Eastern countries, such as Israel, having an incidence as high as 25%.

2. In what other mammal does uric acid calculi form?
Dalmatian coach dog is the only mammal, other than humans, that is at risk for formation of uric acid urinary lithiasis. Its risk is roughly equal to that of humans.

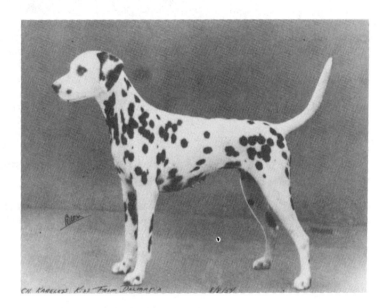

3. Why are humans affected but not other mammals?
Humans do not possess the hepatic enzyme **uricase** found in other mammals, which transforms the water-insoluble uric acid into allantom, which is freely soluble and excreted by the kidney. The consequence of this enzymatic defect is that humans (and Dalmatian dogs) have uric acid levels that are 10 times greater than those of other mammals.

4. What are the four categories of uric acid nephrolithiasis?
1. **Idiopathic uric acid lithiasis.** Patients have normal serum and urinary levels of uric acid, but a chronically low urinary pH. Patients with chronic diarrhea, ileostomies, and those on medications that acidify their urine are included in this category.
2. **Hyperuricemia associated with uric acid calculi.** Approximately 25% of patients with uric acid calculi are hyperuricemic, including those with gout, myeloproliferative disorders, and Lesch-Nyhan syndrome. Approximately 25% of patients with symptomatic gout form uric acid calculi, and 25% of patients who form uric acid calculi will prove to have gout. Patients with myeloproliferative diseases, including lymphoma, develop elevated serium levels of uric acid presumably from increased cell turnover. In addition, patients receiving chemotherapy for neoplastic disease may also develop increased serum and urinary levels of uric acid. Lesch-Nyhan

syndrome, an X-linked genetic deficiency of the enzyme hypoxanthine-guanine-phosphoribosyltransferase (HGPRT), is characterized by choreoathetosis, striking growth, mental retardation, spasticity, and compulsion for self-mutilation. Patients with this syndrome develop both uric acid calculi and gouty arthritis.

3. **Uric acid calculi associated with chronic dehydration.** Patients have concentrated and acidic urine as a result of chronic diarrhea, ileostomies, inflammatory bowel disease, or excessive perspiration.

4. **Uric acid calculi associated hyperuricosuria without hyperuricosemia.** Patients in this group include those who ingest uricosuric medications (salicylates, thiazides, sulfinpyrazone, probenecid) or have a dietary excess of purine-rich foods (organ meats and sardines).

5. Describe the etiology of uric acid calculi formation.

Uric acid is the end product of purine metabolism, and the supersaturation of urine with the undissociated uric acid is needed for the development of uric acid crystals. Normal 24-hour urinary excretion of uric acid is 800 mg in males and 750 mg in women.

Uric acid exists in the urine in two forms: uric acid and urate salt. The salt form compounds with sodium and is 20 times more soluble than free uric acid. Uric acid is a weak acid with a pKa of 5.75. At this pH, half of the molecules exists in the insoluble acid form, and the other half in the soluble salt form. As the urine becomes more acidic, more ions dissociate into the insoluble form. Patients with uric acid calculi have persistently acidic urine with urine pH < 6 and often at 5.0. Some investigators postulate that the mechanism for this disturbance is a deficiency in renal production of ammonium which is available for urinary buffering.

6. What factors are responsible for the formation of uric acid calculi?
1. Urinary pH
2. Low urine volume
3. Uric acid concentration

Probably the most important factor, and most commonly encountered problem related to uric acid formation, is a persistently acid urine. The interaction of all three of these variables, however, influences uric acid crystallization and subsequent stone formation.

7. What is the differential diagnosis of a stone or obstruction seen on intravenous urography?

Filling Defect of the Renal Pelvis	Radiolucent Stone
Urothelial tumor	Uric acid calculi
Blood clot	Sodium urate stones
Sloughed renal papilla	Ammonium urate stones
Fungal ball	Xanthine stones
	2,8-Dihydroxyadenine stones (rare)

8. What diagnostic tests are typically used for evaluating possible uric acid calculi?

Urinalysis will show a urine pH of < 5.5 and uric acid crystals which appear as needles under ordinary light microscopy. Under polarized light, these crystals appear as strongly negatively birefringent.

Intravenous urogram demonstrates a radiolucent filling defect.

Ultrasound is a noninvasive study that can detect calculi as small as 0.5–1.0 cm. With this technique, the uric acid calculus produces a negative shadow that is not seen with blood clots or tumor.

Computed tomography, done without intravenous contrast, is simple and can detect calculi as small as 0.5 cm. It can clearly differentiate uric acid calculi from nonopaque masses (the density of a uric acid calculus is 350–400 Hounsfield units on a ± 1000 scale). It also provides greater density discrimination than conventional radiography as well as a means to follow stone dissolution therapy.

Other more **invasive measures** include retrograde pyelography and retrograde brushing in association with urinary cytology. Ureteroscopy may be required to visualize a defect and to obtain a biopsy.

Biochemical values measured include serum levels of uric acid and a 24-hour uric acid. The upper limit of normal for serum uric acid is 7 mg/dl in males and 5.5 mg/dl in females. Most patients with uric acid calculi have normal levels of uric acid excretion and normal serum levels. Patients with evidence of hyperuricemia should undergo a brief evaluation to rule out the possibility of myeloproliferative or neoplastic disease.

9. How are patients with uric acid calculi managed?

Uric acid calculi are unique in that of all calculi of the urinary tract, they are the most easily dissolved with appropriate diet and therapy. Goals of management including raising urinary pH and lowering the urinary uric acid concentration by decreasing excretion and increasing urinary volume.

Hydration. Patients must increase their oral fluid intake to ensure their urine output is > 1500–2000 ml/day. Higher urinary outputs also result in some increase in urinary pH secondary to the diuretic effects of the water.

Diet. Instruct patients on how to maintain a diet low in purine, limiting the dietary protein to 90 g/day. Patients should reduce their intake of red meat, beef, chicken, and peanuts.

Alkalinization. Uric acid stone formers typically have low urinary pH of 5.0–5.5. Various agents can be used to alkalinize the urine, and the choice depends on the clinical situation. Nitrazine paper can be used to monitor and maintain urinary pH between 6.5 and 7.0. Excessive alkalinization can be detrimental because patients begin to form stones that precipitate in alkaline solution, including calcium oxalate.

10. What agents are used to achieve urinary alkalinization?

1. **Oral agents.** Sodium bicarbonate (650 mg or more every 6–8 hours) or potassium citrate (15 mEq 3–4 times a day). In patients with malabsorption problems or chronic diarrhea, a liquid preparation of potassium citrate or sodium-potassium citrate is of particular value. The liquid preparation allows for better absorption in patients with rapid intestinal transit time.

2. **Intravenous agents.** If the patient requires hospitalization because of nausea, vomiting, and pain, intravenous infusion of 1/6 molar lactate provides rapid alkalinization. A disadvantage of this treatment is that because of the increased sodium load, patients must be monitored for signs of congestive heart failure.

11. Is invasive therapy ever warranted?

Chemolysis of uric acid stones can be accomplished with direct irrigation of the renal pelvis with sodium bicarbonate solution via a transureteral or percutaneous catheter. Though rarely used today, it has application in debilitated patients who are poor candidates for operative procedures.

12. What is the role of allopurinol?

If the patient is hyperuricosuric, efforts should be made to reduce uric acid excretion. Aside from dietary measures already described, medications such as allopurinol (300–600 mg/day) can be given. Allopurinol decreases uric acid synthesis by inhibiting the enzyme xanthine oxidase, which catalyzes the conversion of hypoxanthine to uric acid.

BIBLIOGRAPHY

1. Drach GW: Urinary lithiasis: Etiology, diagnosis, and medical management. In Walsh PC, Retik AB, Stamey TA, Vaughan ED Jr (eds): Campbell's Urlogy, 6th ed. Philadelphia, W.B. Saunders, 1992.
2. Kursh ED, Resnick MI: Dissolution of uric acid calculi with systemic alkalization. J Urol 132:286–287. 1984.
3. Resnick MI: Uric acid stones. In Resnick MI, Kursh ED (eds): Current Therapy in Genitourinary Surgery, 2nd ed. St. Louis, Mosby, 1992.
4. Resnick MI, Kursh ED, Cohen AM: Use of computerized tomography in the delineation of uric acid calculi. J Urol 131:9–10, 1984.
5. Seftel A, Resnick MI: Metabolic evaluation of urolithiasis. Urol Clin North Am 17(1), 1990.

81. STRUVITE STONES

J. Patrick Spirnak, M.D.

1. What is a struvite stone?
A struvite stone is an infectious stone.

2. What does a struvite stone consist of?
A mixture of magnesium ammonium phosphate and carbonate apatite.

3. What percentage of all stones are struvite?
Approximately 15–20%

4. Are struvite stones more common in men or women?
Women, by an approximate ratio of 2:1. Women have a higher incidence of urinary tract infections, which predispose them to stone formation.

5. How does infection cause struvite stone formation?
The association between struvite stone formation and urinary tract infection has long been recognized, but it is still unclear whether the stone or the infection is the initiating factor.

The presence of a struvite stone is evidence for either a past or current infection with urea-splitting bacteria. The enzymatic breakdown of urea by urease increases the bicarbonate and ammonia concentrations with a resultant increase in urinary pH above 7.0. When alkaline, the urine becomes supersaturated with magnesium, ammonium, phosphate, and carbonate apatite, leading to stone formation.

6. Can struvite stones form in the absence of an alkaline urine?
No. A pH >7.0 is necessary for stone formation to occur.

7. Name three common bacteria which are known to produce urease.
Proteus, Pseudomonas, and *Klebsiella.*

8. List three conditions predisposing to struvite stone formation.
1. Congenital anomalies such as ureteropelvic junction obstruction, duplication anomalies, or vesicoureteral reflux are associated with a higher incidence of urinary tract infection and struvite stone formation.
2. Neurogenic bladder or an enlarged prostate may prevent patients from emptying the bladder completely, making them prone to infection and struvite stone formation.
3. Urinary diversion or chronic catheter drainage also make patients prone to struvite stone formation.

9. What is a staghorn stone?
It is a large branched stone which may grow to fill the entire renal collecting system. About 60–90% of staghorn stones are struvite. [*See also* Chapter 76.]

10. Do asymptomatic struvite stones in a healthy individual require treatment?
Large struvite stones should be surgically removed in order to avoid the potential infectious complication of perinephric abscess and sepsis. Loss of renal function and patient mortality are also increased if the stone is not removed.

11. What role do antibiotics play in the treatment of struvite stones?
Antibiotics are important in controlling the acute infection. They are also used to sterilize the

urine in the perioperative period. Antibiotics may also be used prophylactically once the stone has been removed if an anatomic abnormality is present that may predispose to future infection and stone formation.

12. Why are patients with struvite stones susceptible to recurrent infections?
Bacteria exist in the stone itself and persist even after the patient completes a course of culture-specific antibiotics. It is possible to sterilize the urine temporarily, but once the antibiotic is stopped, the bacteria reemerge from the stone to reinfect the urine.

13. What surgical interventions are used to treat struvite stones?
Open surgical procedures, such as **anatrophic nephrolithotomy,** have long been the primary means to eradicate struvite stones. More recently, a combined approach using percutaneous lithotripsy and extracorporeal shock-wave **lithotripsy** have proven successful in eradicating struvite stones.

14. Are fragments left after treatment significant?
If a large (> 1 cm) struvite stone fragment is left after treatment, the most likely outcome will be recurrent urinary tract infection and stone formation.

15. Is it possible to dissolve struvite calculi?
Yes. The use of 10% hemiacidrin irrigation has been used to dissolve struvite calculi. When combined with percutaneous and extracorporeal shock-wave lithotripsy techniques, hemiacidrin use may enhance stone-free rates.

16. Does hemiacidrin use have any contraindications?
The presence of an uncontrolled urinary tract infection is an absolute contraindication. In the presence of an infection, sepsis may occur.

17. What are urease inhibitors?
Urease inhibitors (acetohydroxamic acid) inhibit the bacterial enzyme urease, thereby reducing the alkalinity of the urine and the subsequent precipitation of struvite.

18. When is the use of urease inhibitors indicated?
The primary indications are patients who have residual stone fragments after incomplete surgical removal and patients with intractable urinary tract infections that cannot be eradicated (e.g., cutaneous urinary diversion).

BIBLIOGRAPHY

1. Blandy JP, Singh M: The case for a more aggressive approach to staghorn stones. J Urol 115:505, 1976.
2. Griffith DP: Struvite stones. Kidney Int 13:372, 1978.
3. Resnick MI: Evaluation and management of infection stones. Urol Clin North Am 8:265, 1981.
4. Spirnak JP, Resnick MI: Urinary stones. Prim Care 12:735–104, 1985.
5. Spirnak JP, DeBaz BP, Green HY, Resnick MI: Complex struvite calculi treated by primary extracorporeal shock wave lithotripsy and chemolysis with hemiacidrin irrigation. J Urol 140:1356, 1988.

82. CYSTINE STONES

Stevan B. Streem, M.D.

1. About how many patients does a busy family practitioner see each year with cystine stones?
None.

2. How common are cystine stones?
Cystine stones are rare. Only 1–2% of all stone patients have cystine stones.

3. What causes them?
Cystine stones result from an inherited defect of renal tubular reabsorption of cystine. Actually, the tubular defect affects the reabsorption of the four dibasic amino acids.

4. How can I remember which four?
With the mnemonic **COLA:**

    C = Cystine
    O = Ornithine
    L = Lysine
    A = Arginine

5. Is there a specific radiographic appearance suggestive of cystine stones?
Cystine stones are opaque, though not as opaque as most calcium stones. They may have a homogeneous "ground-glass" appearance. Because they are less opaque than radiographic contrast, they may appear to be lucent during intravenous or retrograde pyelography.

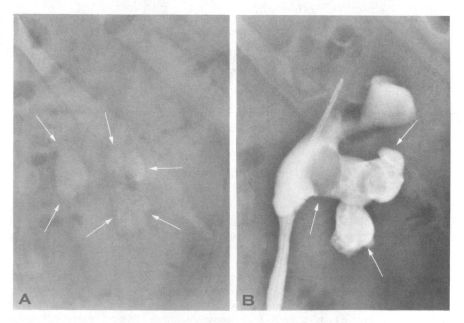

A. A plain abdominal radiograph reveals multiple, lightly opaque, homogeneous calculi (*arrows*) suggestive of cystine stones. **B.** After retrograde injection of contrast, the stones are visualized as filling defects. Though cystine stones are opaque, they are relatively lucent compared to contrast material.

6. Why aren't there ornithine, lysine, or arginine stones?

Those three amino acids are very soluble. Only cystine is relatively insoluble and will precipitate in urine to form stones.

7. How is the propensity for cystine stones inherited?

In an autosomal recessive fashion. If both parents are carriers or a sibling has cystine stones, you have a 25% chance of being affected.

8. How do I know if a stone patient has cystine stones?

Often, the urinalysis will reveal classic hexagonal crystals, and this finding alone is diagnostic of cystinuria. A 24-hour urine study for cystine excretion should always be done in these patients. Normal individuals excrete < 100 mg of cystine/day. Heterozygotes excrete 150–300 mg/day but do not get cystine stones. Homozygous cystinurics excrete > 400 mg/day.

9. Although cystine stones are a genetic problem, can they be prevented?

For many affected patients, cystine stones can be prevented or even dissolved with medical management.

10. What is the best treatment?

Three to 4 quarts of oral fluids per day should be ingested to decrease the urinary concentration of cystine. Also, the urine should be alkalinized because cystine is more soluble in an alkaline urine. When cystine stones form or increase in size with fluid and alkalinization therapy, drugs that bind cystine to form the more soluble cysteine should be prescribed. These include D-penicillamine and α-mercaptopropionylglycine (MPG).

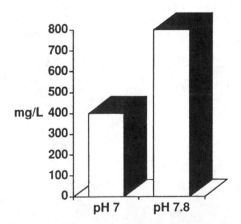

Relative solubility of cystine in urine at pH 7 versus pH 7.8.

11. Why aren't those drugs used for all patients as preventive therapy?

Unfortunately, they are associated with a 30–50% incidence of significant side effects.

12. What is the best way to remove cystine stones?

Of all stone types, cystine stones are the least amenable to extracorporeal shock-wave lithotripsy. However, they do fragment well with ultrasound. Therefore, patients are now treated preferentially with percutaneous or ureteroscopic ultrasonic lithotripsy. "Open" surgery should be avoided whenever possible because of the high rates of recurrence that necessitate repeated intervention.

BIBLIOGRAPHY

1. Crawhall JC, Scowen EF, Watts RWE: Effect of penicillamine on cystinuria. BMJ 1:585, 1963.
2. Crawhall JC, Watts RWE: Cystinuria. Am J Med 45:736, 1968.
3. Dent CE, Rose GA: Amino acid metabolism in cystinuria. Q J Med 20:205, 1951.
4. Dent CE, Senior B: Studies on the treatment of cystinuria. Br J Urol 27:317, 1955.
5. Evans WP, Resnick MI, Boyce WH: Homozygous cystinuria—Evaluation of 35 patients. J Urol 127:707, 1982.
6. Giugliani R, Ferrari I, Greene LJ: Heterozygous cystinuria and urinary lithiasis. Am J Med Genet 22:703, 1985.
7. Harris H, Mittwoch U, Robson EB, et al: Phenotypes and genotypes in cystinuria. Ann Hum Genet 20:57–91, 1955.
8. Kachel TA, Vijan SR, Dretler SP: Endourological experience with cystine calculi and a treatment algorithm. J Urol 145:25, 1991.
9. Knoll LD, Segura JW, Patterson DE, et al: Long-term followup in patients with cystine urinary calculi treated with percutaneous ultrasonic lithotripsy. J Urol 140:246, 1988.
10. Pak CYC, Fuller C, Sakhaee K, et al: Management of cystine nephrolithiasis with alpha-mercaptopropionylglycine. J Urol 136:1003, 1986.
11. Sakhaee K, Poindexter JR, Pak CYC: The spectrum of metabolic abnormalities in patients with cystine nephrolithiasis. J Urol 141:819, 1989.
12. Streem SB: Medical and surgical management of cystine stones. In Preminger G (ed): Evaluation and Treatment of Calculi Disease of the Urinary Tract. Philadelphia, J.B. Lippincott, 1994.

INDEX

Page numbers in **boldface** type indicate complete chapter.